Psychosocial Occupational Therapy

NANCY CARSON, PhD, OTR/L, FAOTA

Associate Professor
Division of Occupational Therapy
Medical University of South Carolina
Charleston, South Carolina

ELSEVIER

Elsevier
1600 John F. Kennedy Blvd.
Ste 1800
Philadelphia, PA 19103-2899

PSYCHOSOCIAL OCCUPATIONAL THERAPY, FIRST EDITION   ISBN: 978-0-323-08982-1

Notice

Practitioners and researchers must always rely on their own experience and knowledge in evaluating and using any information, methods, compounds or experiments described herein. Because of rapid advances in the medical sciences, in particular, independent verification of diagnoses and drug dosages should be made. To the fullest extent of the law, no responsibility is assumed by Elsevier, authors, editors or contributors for any injury and/or damage to persons or property as a matter of products liability, negligence or otherwise, or from any use or operation of any methods, products, instructions, or ideas contained in the material herein.

ISBN: 9780323089821

Content Strategist: Lauren Willis
Content Development Specialist: Angie Breckon
Publishing Services Manager: Shereen Jameel
Project Manager: Nadhiya Sekar
Design Direction: Brian Salisbury

Printed in United States of America

Last digit is the print number: 9   8   7   6   5   4   3   2   1

This textbook is dedicated to the legacy of Dr. Maralynne D. Mitcham, an exceptional mentor to me and many other educators. Maralynne always made you feel like you were one of the most important people in her life. She was a wonderful and compassionate mentor; the most influential one I have had in my career. She encouraged me to see the big picture and stretch my boundaries professionally. I miss her tremendously and I am very grateful for the many lessons I learned from her.

LIST OF CONTRIBUTORS

Nancy Carson, PhD, OTR/L, FAOTA
Associate Professor
Division of Occupational Therapy
Medical University of South Carolina
Charleston, South Carolina

Tina Champagne, OT, OTD, FAOTA
Chief Executive Officer
Cutchins Programs for Children and Families, Inc.
International Consultant
Champagne Conferences & Consultation
Northampton, Massachusetts
Adjunct Professor
Occupational Therapy
American International College
Springfield, Massachusetts

Joy Crawford, OTD, OTR/L
OTA Program Coordinator
Trident Technical College
Charleston, South Carolina

Gail Fisher, PhD, OTR/L, FAOTA
Clinical Professor
Department of Occupational Therapy
University of Illinois at Chicago
Chicago, Illinois

Michael Iwama, PhD, MSc, BSc, BScOT
Dean & Professor
School of Health and Rehabilitation Sciences
MGH Institute of Health Professions
Boston, Massachusetts

Monica Keen, MS, OTR/L
Adjunct Instructor
Occupational Therapy
Medical University of South Carolina
Charleston, South Carolina

Carol Lambdin-Pattavina, OTD, OTR/L
Assistant Professor
Department of Occupational Therapy
University of New England
Portland, Maine

Nicole Maxham, MS, OTR/L
Occupational Therapist
BAYADA Home Health Care
White River Junction, Vermont

Jane O'Brien, PhD, OTR/L, FAOTA
Professor
Department of Occupational Therapy
University of New England
Portland, Maine

Ashley Stoffel, OTD, OTR/L, FAOTA
Clinical Associate Professor
Department of Occupational Therapy
University of Illinois at Chicago
Chicago, Illinois

Heather Thomas, PhD, OTR/L
OTA Program Director
American Career College
Los Angeles, California

This textbook provides an overview of psychosocial practice in occupational therapy, as it is impossible to write a text that includes everything that an occupational therapy practitioner needs to know about mental health and occupational therapy practice. Recognizing that most occupational therapy practitioners do not work in behavioral health care settings or in settings where mental illness is the primary diagnosis for which the individual is receiving care, this text is intended to provide an overview of therapeutic skills and an understanding of basic mental health diagnoses, including assessment and practice considerations. Regardless of the practice setting, the mental health and well-being of the client should always be addressed. Occupational therapy practitioners should understand the implications of mental illness on occupational performance and be prepared to incorporate appropriate strategies into treatment to address mental health and well-being.

The first part of this text is an introduction and includes an overview of historical and current perspectives related to the practice of occupational therapy in mental health. A brief overview of the history of occupational therapy and mental health is included with a focus on the Recovery Model for mental health. An overview of therapeutic interpersonal skills, group processes and the *Occupational Therapy Practice Framework* is also included in part one. The second part is focused on theoretical approaches and occupational therapy assessment with a focus on occupation-centered practice models, psychosocial theories, cognitive approaches, and sensory modulation. The third part is focused on mental disorders and occupational therapy practice. The primary mental disorders from the DSM-5 are presented with a review of symptomology and implications for occupational therapy practice. The fourth part includes practice considerations. The emotional impact of physical illness or injury and trauma-informed care are two topics that are discussed. A chapter on issues related to pediatric mental health is included. The final chapter is focused on mental health wellness, prevention, and advocacy. This book includes case studies throughout each chapter that are consistent with the *Occupational Therapy Practice Framework*. The use of case studies promotes clinical reasoning and understanding. Suggested learning activities and reflection questions are included in each chapter to promote further learning.

CONTENTS

1

Occupational Therapy in Mental Health: Historical and Current Perspectives

Nancy Carson

LEARNING OBJECTIVES

1. Describe the influence of mental health treatment and culture during the emergence of the occupational therapy profession.
2. Understand the context for occupational therapy workforce practice trends in mental health.
3. Consider the prevalence of mental health disorders in the general population.

4. Understand the concepts and application of the Recovery Model in mental health.
5. Discuss the role of occupational therapy in the recovery process for people with mental illness.

HISTORICAL PERSPECTIVE

The roots of occupational therapy are strongly grounded in the mental health domain. The profession developed during the moral reform and mental hygiene movements of the 1800s and early 1900s.[1-3] Before this time the treatment of the mentally ill was often inhumane. The causes of mental illness were not understood and were often considered the result of evil spirits. Practices such as trepanation occurred, in which holes were drilled into the skulls of individuals exhibiting mental illness to let the evil spirits out.[4] As the population increased and the number of mentally ill individuals grew, asylums were built to house the mentally ill. The conditions and the care provided at these asylums were often deplorable and inhumane.[4]

The first of four reform movements in mental health services in the United States, the moral reform movement, occurred from 1800 to 1850.[5] It was toward the end of this time that Dorothea Dix (1802–1887) became a prominent

force in the movement that suggested that people with mental problems could be helped and possibly even cured. She was supportive of moral treatment and actively criticized the cruel and inhumane treatment of many individuals institutionalized with mental disorders. In the 1830s, Dix spent time in Europe and met a prison reformer by the name of Elizabeth Fry; she also met Samuel Tuke, found of the York Retreat for the mentally ill. These encounters, along with her understanding of the work of French psychiatrist Philippe Pinel, led to her embracing and advocating for a model of compassionate care for those with mental illness.[6]

Another reformer of the time, Horace Mann (1796–1859), also supported the idea of humane treatment for individuals with mental illness. Along with Dix, he supported asylums that provided a combination of somatic and psychosocial treatments that were controlled and designed to improve the individual's mental functioning; this was far different from earlier treatments of the mentally ill and thus represented an era of moral treatment.

The second reform movement was called the mental hygiene movement and occurred during the years of 1890–1920. It consisted of elements of the public health concept becoming prominent at this time and included emphasis on scientific medicine and social progressivism.[5] It was during this time, on March 15, 1917 in Clifton Springs, New York, that the National Society for the Promotion of Occupational Therapy was founded. The name was officially changed to the American Occupational Therapy Association in 1923.[7] There were six people in attendance at this first meeting: Thomas Kidner, George Barton, William Dunton, Eleanor Clarke Slagle, Isabel Newton, and Susan Johnson.[8]

Occupational therapy developed as part of the reform movements in mental health services and the changes occurring in mental health treatment. Many of the humane approaches that provided improvement in the mental well-being of institutionalized individuals formed the basis for the occupational therapy profession. Contributions to the formation of the profession were presented by many different individuals, each bringing forth a view of principles supporting the use of occupation to improve the health and well-being of the individual. Although mental well-being was the primary focus for some of the earlier proponents of occupation, the benefits to overall health were also addressed. Contributions and beliefs of some of the founders of the profession were shared to provide an understanding of the mental health roots in the development of the profession as well as the importance of occupation to the emotional well-being of the individual.

Eleanor Clarke Slagle, a founding member of the profession, was a social worker who was born in 1871. Her work with mental patients and her perspective on habit training and occupational engagement to restore health is a foundational concept of the profession. In 1911, while a social work student, she became interested in "invalid occupations" and the therapeutic usefulness of both occupations and recreation for patients in a state mental hospital. Her observations were that these individuals were experiencing negative effects from idleness, and occupational engagement provided a positive alternative.[9] In 1912 she worked with Adolf Meyer at the Phipps Psychiatric Clinic at Johns Hopkins Hospital, and developed and administered a habit-training program designed for individuals with severe schizophrenia. While at Johns Hopkins, she taught 3-week courses on occupation to nurses in training.[7] In 1915 she started the Henry P. Favill School of Occupations in Chicago to provide an educational program focused on habit training and purposeful activity.[9] From 1921 to 1942 she was the Director of Occupational Therapy at the New York State Department of Mental Hygiene, managing up to 255 staff. She oversaw occupational therapy service provision in a network of hospitals in which occupational therapy was an essential component

of the treatment programs for patients with psychiatric conditions.[9] Slagle was unique for her time. She was a pioneer who was innovative in her development of programs for providing services to patients. She was independent, with professional ambitions, and she strived to educate herself and promote the profession.[7,10] The Eleanor Clarke Slagle Lectureship was created in 1953 and serves to recognize her significant contributions to the profession. Each year the lectureship is awarded to an outstanding occupational therapist (OT) who has also made significant contributions to the profession.[7]

William Rush Dunton, Jr., a founding member of the profession, was a physician who treated psychiatric patients in an institutional setting. He is referred to as the "father of occupational therapy" because of his role in the development of the profession.[11] His treatment method of choice was occupation therapy, a term he used to describe activities or occupations designed to improve the individual's health. He believed in the value of therapeutic occupation and he had a lifelong interest in arts and crafts.[7] He served as President of the National Society for the Promotion of Occupational Therapy and he published over 120 books and articles about occupational therapy.[1] At the second annual meeting of the National Society for the Promotion of Occupational Therapy, Dunton presented nine principles for the use of activity in the practice of occupational therapy, which resonate with the current view of occupation. These principles focused on work that should be curative, interesting, have a useful end, occur with others, and preferably increase knowledge. Additionally, the principles included observation of the patient's level of fatigue and encouragement to the patient, and the principle that "work resulting in a poor or useless product is better that idleness."[12]

Dunton's view of occupation is further illustrated in his Credo to his text in which he states "That occupation is as necessary to life as food and drink. That every human being should have both physical and mental occupation . . . . That sick minds, sick bodies, sick souls, may be healed thru occupation."[13] The focus on the healing power of occupation, particularly for the mind and soul, is evident in Dunton's philosophy. You cannot separate the two when treating the individual. Occupation is a necessity to life because of its healing power to the individual as a whole, and because of the sense of purpose it evokes.

George Barton, a founding member of the profession, was an architect who contracted tuberculosis and dealt with other health issues preventing his return to his former work. He became despondent and sought counsel, after which he embarked on opening Consolation House. This was a place for individuals to recover that was different from the institutional environment of hospitals. Consolation House provided an environment conducive to physical, emotional, and spiritual healing through the use of occupations such as carpentry, gardening, and craft activities.[7,14] Barton coined the term *occupational therapy* and organized the first meeting of the National Society for the Promotion of Occupational Therapy in 1917.[1,7]

Susan Cox Johnson was a teacher of arts and crafts who was recruited by Barton. She believed that occupations have the power to improve the mental and physical well-being of patients and that occupational engagement is morally uplifting. She believed that the use of crafts was extremely beneficial to the mental well-being of the individual and could redirect thoughts and build confidence.[10]

Adolf Meyer, a professor of psychiatry, also had a significant impact on the founding beliefs of the profession and contributed to the initial philosophy of occupational therapy. His view of occupational therapy as a connection between an individual's activities and mental health was apparent in his approach to clinical psychiatry. He emphasized occupation as essential in the treatment of individuals with mental illness.[1] He also focused on the balance of work, play, rest, and sleep in his paper, *The philosophy of occupational therapy*. He viewed activity as an opportunity that should be provided to the individual, indicating that opportunities should at times be provided in place of prescriptions, as activities allow the individual to do and create, which promotes healing.[15]

As can be seen, the founding of the profession was in response to the mental health culture of the time and the belief by many of the founders in the role of occupation in treating the mentally ill. As knowledge of psychiatry and changes in psychiatric treatment advanced, so has the practice of occupational therapy.

WORKFORCE PRACTICE TRENDS

As the profession evolved over the years, the emphasis on the use of occupation to improve the physical and mental well-being of an individual has never faltered, and continues to be an essential element of the practice of occupational therapy today. However, despite the strong beginnings of the profession in mental health, the number of OTs working in mental health settings has decreased over time. In the first half of the history of the profession, more than 50% of OTs were working in mental health settings.[11] The number of OT practitioners working in settings that primarily provide services to individuals with mental illness started declining rapidly as the 20th century came to a close. The decline from 1980 to 2017 is reported in practice setting trends data[3,16-20] in Table 1.1. For some years the data is reflected separately as the percentage of OTs practicing in mental health and the percentage of occupational therapy assistants (OTAs) practicing in mental health; for some years this data was combined when reported. The

TABLE 1.1 Workforce Practice Trends for Occupational Therapy Practitioners in Mental Health Settings.

Year	OT	OTA	OT & OTA
1982	10%	13%	
1990	9%	12%	
1998	4%	4%	
2000	5%	5%	
2006			3.6%
2010			2.9%
2015	2.4%	1.4%	
2017			2%

OT, Occupational therapist; *OTA*, occupational therapy assistant.

most recent data[19] reflect only 2% of OT practitioners (OT and OTAs combined) working in mental health settings.

As OT became more focused on physical rehabilitation, more opportunities arose for OTs to specialize and work in a variety of health care settings. Additionally, Congress passed the Community Mental Health Act in 1963 that led to widespread deinstitutionalization of psychiatric facilities. The transition of occupational therapy practitioners from inpatient to community-based service provision was not widespread, with many OT positions being absorbed by other professions. The reasons for the decline of occupational therapy in mental health practice incudes (1) lack of advocacy on the part of occupational therapy practitioners, (2) lack of research documenting the effectiveness of OT services in mental health practice, (3) insufficient documentation of the role of OT in mental health treatment, and (4) less reimbursement for mental health in general, which translates to lower salaries for occupational therapy practitioners[21,22] With increasing costs for higher education, many graduates are seeking higher salaries to pay off student loan debt.[22]

Despite the decrease in mental health practitioners working primarily in mental health settings, the need to understand mental health and well-being and its impact on the individual remains strong. Every client treated by an occupational therapy practitioner has psychosocial needs. Mental well-being impacts the outcome of services provided regardless of the reason for service provision, therefore it is essential to understand and address the psychosocial needs of every client. Ultimately, you cannot provide occupational therapy without addressing the psychosocial aspect of the individual. Diseases and injuries can have a significant emotional impact on the individual, and that affects therapy and occupational functioning. Consider the individual who may have psychological distress following a burn injury[23] or amputation,[24] and how that can be addressed in occupational therapy. Many diseases affect mental health and are well documented in the literature, such as depression and anxiety following stroke and spinal cord injury.[25,26]

MENTAL HEALTH STATISTICS

It is also significant to consider the prevalence of mental illness in the general population. Conceptually, there are two categories of mental illness: any mental illness (AMI), defined as a mental, behavioral, or emotional disorder excluding developmental and substance use disorders; and serious mental illness (SMI), defined as a mental behavioral or emotional disorder resulting in significant limitations or impairment in functional abilities.[27] In a given year, about 1 in 5 adults (18.5%) in America experiences a mental illness or AMI, and 1 in 25 adults (4.0%) experiences SMI,[28] which is a subset of AMI. Overall, mental illness affects approximately 44 million adults in the United States each year. Mental illness also affects children and adolescents: approximately 21.4% of youths aged 13–18 and 13% of youths aged 8–15 experiences a severe mental disorder at some point during their life.[28] Considering these statistics, it is unavoidable that the therapist who is treating clients primarily for physical illness or injury will at times have clients who also have a mental illness. Although the primary referral may not be for mental illness treatment, behavioral or emotional needs often present in the course of treatment, and an understanding of mental illness by the therapist provides for optimal therapeutic intervention. Likewise, an understanding of the connection of mind, body, and spirit for all individuals necessitates a holistic approach to treatment at all times.

The Occupational Therapy Practice Framework (OTPF)[29] directs occupational therapy practitioners to evaluate client factors and their effect on occupational performance. Body functions include specific and global mental functions as part of client factors. Examples of specific mental functions include higher-level cognitive skills, attention, memory, perception, thought, and regulation and range of emotions. Examples of global mental functions include consciousness, orientation, temperament, personality, and energy and drive. Furthermore, performance skills are evaluated, which includes process and social interactions skills that are components of mental and behavioral functioning. As stipulated in the OTPF, occupational performance is reliant on physical, mental, emotional, and social skills; each domain must be evaluated to provide effective intervention. "Analyzing occupational performance requires an understanding of the complex and dynamic interaction among client factors, performance skills, performance patterns, and contexts and environments, along with the activity demands of the occupation being performed."[29]

Two AOTA official documents published as AOTA Statements focus specifically on the role of occupational therapy in mental health. These documents are useful for occupational therapy practitioners as well as various external audiences. *Mental health promotion, prevention, and intervention in occupational therapy practice*[30] provides a description of the knowledge and skills occupational therapy practitioners share with other core mental health professionals as well as the knowledge and skills specific to occupational therapy practitioners. Some areas of knowledge for OTs that are required by the Accreditation Council for Occupational Therapy education (ACOTE) standards[31] that are listed in this document include knowledge of:

- the development of mental illness, including neurophysiological changes and environmental factors
- the effect of mental illness on human development and behavior
- perspectives on mental health treatment such as the recovery approach and trauma-informed care
- current clinical diagnostic criteria and prognosis for mental disorders
- comorbidities with mental illness
- effects of psychiatric medications
- therapeutic use of self.

Additionally, knowledge of legal and ethical issues, reimbursement issues, and standards for service delivery and documentation in mental health are also required for OTs.[31]

Occupational therapy services in the promotion of mental health and well-being[32] "describes the role of occupational therapy practitioners in addressing the psychological and social aspects of human performance as they influence health, well-being, and participation in occupations."[32] Examples of occupational therapy interventions with a focus on mental health are provided. Case examples include individuals referred to occupational therapy services for various reasons, including orthopedic injury, neurological disorders, and disease processes as well as mental disorders. For each case example, challenges to occupational performance and occupational therapy interventions that focus on mental health are highlighted. These two documents, along with the OTPF, clearly outline the role of occupational therapy in the evaluation and treatment of mental health.

RECOVERY MODEL

The idea that one could recover from mental illness, especial SMI, was not considered by health care providers prior to the 1970s. It was widely believed that individuals with SMI would never get better, that they would be institutionalized frequently, and they would not be able to function in society.[33] These ideas were challenged when individuals with mental illness began believing that they could recover,[34] and several long-term studies supported the concept of recovery.[35] Researchers found that individuals who had been previously institutionalized were able to achieve long-term remission, reintegrate into the community, and lead satisfying, productive lives.[36] These findings and the empowerment of individuals with mental illness led to the development of the recovery movement. At first, the recovery movement was primarily advanced by people with mental illness, as most mental health practitioners were not trained in the concept of recovery and viewed SMI as a chronic debilitating process. Traditional mental health treatment, focused on medication and psychotherapy, remained the focus until the 1990s. Although traditional treatment is essential for many individuals, it does not promote recovery in the sense of the individual moving toward remission, independence, and personal satisfaction.

The Stress Vulnerability Model[37] was introduced in 1977 to offer a general theory for the cause and course of psychiatric disorders. It also serves as a guide for recovery. The model identifies three components responsible for mental illness and its progression for the individual: biological vulnerability, stress, and protective factors. Biological vulnerability is determined by many factors, including genetics, prenatal health and delivery, and adverse childhood experiences. Genetics can a play a role in some disease processes, but they do not explain the majority of biological factors. Environmental factors ranging from prenatal health to experiencing abuse or growing up without adequate societal or familial support can increase vulnerability for mental illness. When an individual experiences stressful events or situations, positive or negative, it has the capacity to worsen symptoms. Everyone experiences stress, but it can vary greatly in the degree of challenge it presents to the individual and the degree of adaptation or change it requires to deal with it effectively. Stress can be considered mild, such as in waking up late or missing an appointment, to severe, such as in losing a loved one. Positive events or occurrences are not typically thought of as stressful; however, they can be. Consider, for example, the birth of a child or starting a new job, both considered very positive situations but also very stressful. It can also be stressful for people who do not have meaningful occupations in their life. If illness has resulted in job loss or the inability to maintain roles, routines, and daily occupations, this lack of engagement in daily life creates enormous stress for the individual. Protective factors include anything that assists the individual in dealing with both the biological vulnerability and the stress. This can include medications, traditional therapy, lifestyle changes, coping mechanisms, environmental adaptations, and anything else that is meaningful to the individual and supports recovery. This model ignited the

move toward understanding recovery as a possibility for individuals with mental illness.

Another significant impetus for the Recovery Movement was the publication of the report from the US President's New Freedom Commission on Mental Health entitled *Achieving the Promise: Transforming Mental Health Care in America*.[38] This report paved the way for many mental health organizations and systems to develop recovery oriented approaches for individuals with SMI. A central theme is that consumers and family members are closely involved with health care providers in determining the services needed for the individual and those services are focused on a recovery approach. Despite the support of the recovery model for mental health, many providers are still not adequately trained in evidence-based practice and lack the skills for implementation.[39]

Before 2010 there were varying definitions of recovery being used by different agencies and organizations. There were also different definitions in use by the Substance Abuse and Mental Health Services Administration (SAMHSA)[40] for recovery from mental disorders and substance use disorders. The lack of a common definition made it difficult to develop recovery programs to be used widely, and made it difficult to engage in conversations regarding reimbursement and policy. In 2010 behavioral health leaders, along with individuals in recovery from mental health and substance use problems, met to begin developing a common definition of recovery from mental disorders and/or substance use disorders.

The resulting working definition of recovery provided by SAMHSA[40] defines recovery as "a process of change through which individuals improve their health and wellness, live a self-directed life, and strive to reach their full potential."[40] Along with this definition, four key components that support recovery include (1) healthy choices that support positive physical and emotional well-being; (2) a stable home environment; (3) purpose in daily life, including independence and social participation; and (4) a community with supportive relationships. The occupational therapy profession is closely aligned with the concept of recovery. The OTPF defines occupational therapy as "the therapeutic use of everyday life activities (occupations) with individuals or groups for the purpose of enhancing or enabling participation in roles, habits, and routines in home, school, workplace, community, and other settings."[29]

The 10 guiding principles of recovery identified by SAMHSA[40] are listed below and an overview of how they align with occupational therapy is provided.

1. **Recovery emerges from hope**

   Hope is necessary for the individual to initiate the recovery process. Hope is the belief that one can get better. OT is client-centered and fosters hope by engaging the individual in goal setting. OT works with the individual to identify and overcome obstacles and recognize existing abilities.

2. **Recovery is person-driven**

   In using a client-centered approach, OT collaborates with the individual to design treatment activities that are defined by the client. The client is provided choices and has the power to choose services and resources that support recovery. The client is empowered to develop a path to recovery and quality of life as defined by personal standards.

3. **Recovery occurs via many pathways**

   Each person is a unique being with specific preferences, abilities, and life experiences. Recovery pathways are based on all aspects of the individual and therefore are highly personalized. No two paths to recovery will look the same. Through the occupational profile, occupational therapy practitioners are skilled at identifying the individual's strengths and abilities and can assist the individual in identifying potential pathways to recovery. The occupational therapy practitioner is also skilled at evaluating the environment and adapting activity to enable recovery. Recovery is a nonlinear process that may involve periodic setbacks and require continual adaption, which occupational therapy can support.

4. **Recovery is holistic**

   Recovery requires a focus on every component of the individual's life. Mind, body, and spirit are interwoven, therefore isolated abilities, preferences, and resources do not provide an accurate portrayal of the individual. An understanding of the individual as a whole person is necessary for moving forward in recovery. Occupational therapy practitioners are trained in holistic evaluation and treatment intervention.

5. **Recovery is supported by peers and allies**

   Peer support plays a vital role in recovery. Peers with similar challenges can provide a wealth of knowledge and the insight of real-life experience to support the individual with mental illness. Peers can provide a sense of belonging and a level of support that is different than that provided by family members or professionals. Occupational therapy practitioners can foster peer support by connecting individuals with appropriate peer support resources and facilitating participation and interaction to learn from others.

6. **Recovery is supported through relationship and social networks**

   Encouraging healthy relationships and social activities supports the recovery process. Occupational therapy practitioners can enable the individual with the skills to build positive relationships and identify satisfying roles as well as develop a greater sense of belonging and community participation.

7. **Recovery is culturally based and influenced**

   Through the occupational profile the therapist identifies values, traditions and beliefs inherent to the individual, which directs the individualized pathway to recovery for that person. OTs are trained to provide services that consider the cultural context of the individual in relation to service provision.

8. **Recovery is supported by addressing trauma**

   For those individuals experiencing the effects of trauma, occupational therapy practitioners evaluate functional performance, identifying areas adversely affected by trauma, and design appropriate treatment approaches. Approaches such as sensory modulation, mindfulness, stress management, and a focus on health habits and routines may be used in treatment.

9. **Recovery involves individual, family, and community strengths and responsibility**

   Occupational therapy practitioners work with individuals to identify personal strengths and empower them toward personal responsibility in the journey of recovery. They engage families and communities in supporting the recovery process through education and provision of resources.

10. **Recovery is based on respect**

   Through advocacy, occupational therapy practitioners work with communities and organizations to ensure societal acceptance and respect for people with mental health disorders. Decreasing and ultimately eliminating the negative effects of stigma and the occurrence of discrimination is crucial in supporting the recovery process for all individuals with mental health disorders.

Occupational therapy and the recovery model both promote collaboration, personal growth, client participation, and empowerment. Occupational therapy practitioners working with individuals in recovery can assist the individual by teaching the active use of coping strategies, supporting the implementation of healthy habits and routines, supporting the use of a wellness recovery plan, educating the individual on community resources, empowering self-awareness and monitoring for personal physical and mental well-being, and supporting the individual in identifying personal recovery goals and a plan for long-term wellness.[41] There are numerous strategies and approaches for occupational therapy practitioners to employ in support of the recovery process. Any occupation that is meaningful to the individual supports recovery.

SUPPORTING RECOVERY

There are a variety of structured tools and resources available to support recovery. Examples of tools available include the Wellness Recovery Action Plan[42,43] or WRAP, the Living Skills Recovery Workbook,[44] the Recovery Curriculum for People with Serious Mental Illnesses and Behavioral Health Disorders,[33] and the Illness Management and Recovery evidence-based practices curriculum.

Wellness Recovery Action Plan

WRAP is an individualized, self-designed self-help system that is used by individuals with mental illness to promote self-recovery.[42,43] It was developed in 1997 by a group of people that included people who experience psychiatric symptoms. Mary Ellen Copeland, PhD, worked with this group. It provides a plan for individuals to overcome mental health issues and move toward recovery and a fulfilling life. It is now used by people with all kinds of health conditions to improve both physical and mental well-being. It is a structured system for identifying and monitoring distressing symptoms, with a personally designed plan for reducing, modifying, or eliminating those symptoms. It also includes a plan for others to be involved when a person's symptoms have made it too difficult for decision-making and self-care. Individuals report feeling empowered by focusing on personal strengths and self-directed plans for moving toward and maintaining recovery. WRAP is listed in the National Registry of Evidence-Based Programs and Practices.[42,43]

The development of a personal plan includes the following sections.

Wellness Toolbox

The toolbox is a listing of strategies and resources that are the "tools" for developing your personal WRAP. It can include things you have done previously that have worked well for you or things you could do to feel better. Examples include things like talking with friends or family, peer support, relaxation and stress management techniques, journaling, exercise, and listening to music.

Daily Maintenance Plan

In this section, the individual describes how it feels to feel well personally and makes a list of daily activities that should be done to maintain wellness.

Triggers

In this section, the individual identifies events or circumstances that can lead to negative feelings. If the person is unable to cope with these external events, they can make the person feel worse.

Early Warning Signs

These are subtle signs that indicate to the person that things are not going well. The challenge is to identify what those signs are so that they can be addressed and therefore prevent a downward progression in mental status. Examples might include mild restlessness or inattention, difficulty sleeping, or irritability. Over time the person works toward developing self-awareness to allow for early identification of warning signs.

When Things Are Breaking Down

These are more pronounced signs that indicate a definite decline in mental functioning. Examples might include profound feelings of sadness, hearing voices, and sleeping much more than normal. The individual should have a definitive plan to engage in activities that can potentially prevent further worsening and allow for improvement. The personal Wellness Toolbox provides the resources for identifying and following through on wellness activities.

Crisis Plan

The purpose of the crisis plan is to alert others to the behaviors that let them know they need to assist the individual and make decisions for care if necessary. The plan should identify these individuals and types of support and services that are desired. Being proactive provides a sense of control even though the individual may not feel in control with the moment-to-moment occurrences during a crisis.

Post-Crisis Plan

This plan can be developed after going through a crisis by recording those activities, resources, and people that are most helpful during the recovery process.

In developing a personal WRAP, there are five definitive recovery concepts that provide the foundation and support for progress. They are hope, personal responsibility, education, self-advocacy, and support. Through this process the individual becomes empowered to continue to move forward with the goal of long-term recovery.

Living Skills Recovery Workbook

This workbook was developed by an OT to support individuals with dual diagnoses in the recovery process.[44] It was published in 2015 and provides the occupational therapy practitioner with tools for addressing functional living skills in relation to recovery and relapse prevention. It includes activities and worksheets for the client to complete to increase self-awareness. Topics such as stress management, social skills, and basic living skills are addressed. It is client-centered, allowing for individualization to the client's lifestyle and personal challenges. A focus on improving quality of life and progressing to the highest level of recovery is emphasized.

Recovery Curriculum for People With Serious Mental Illnesses and Behavioral Health Disorders

This curriculum was designed by the American Psychological Association in 2014, and its purpose is to train mental health professionals in recovery-oriented principles and practices to implement with individuals with serious mental illnesses.[33] The curriculum consists of 15 modules, each with learning objectives, required readings, and a sample activity related to the content of the module. The modules are evidence-based and provide knowledge of the concept of recovery from severe mental illness, rehabilitation assessments, and psychosocial rehabilitation (PSR) interventions to assist individuals with severe mental illnesses to achieve their highest level of function. Other module topics include person-centered planning, health disparities, issues in forensic settings, peer support services, and systems transformation. This curriculum is an excellent resource for occupational therapy practitioners working with individuals in recovery.

Illness Management and Recovery

This is an evidence-based practices curriculum developed by the Center for Mental Health Services in the SAMHSA of the U.S. Department of Health and Human Services.[45] The overall goals of illness management and recovery (IMR) are to learn about mental illnesses and treatment strategies, decrease symptoms, reduce relapses, and progress toward recovery. IMR can be offered over a course of 3 to 10 months, with weekly or biweekly sessions either individually or in group sessions.

The Recovery Model and Occupational Therapy

As noted in the history of occupational therapy, the principles of occupational therapy align closely with the recovery model. The power of occupation in improving the lives of individuals with mental illness was a significant factor in the development of the profession, and continues to be a powerful force for clients as they move through the recovery process. Research supports meaningful occupation-based interventions in reducing symptoms of mental illness and fostering recovery.[46] Occupational therapy practitioners use the key principles of the recovery model when performing function-based assessments and designing and implementing client-centered interventions.[47,48] Clients participating in recovery-based occupational therapy report favorable outcomes.[49] These first-person narratives are the most compelling evidence of the influence of occupation on recovery.[50]

SUGGESTED LEARNING ACTIVITIES

1. Watch the classic movie *One Flew Over the Cuckoo's Nest* and reflect on the negative effects of institutionalization on occupational performance and the human spirit.
2. Contact your local mental health department and interview a peer counselor about their path to recovery.
3. Develop your own personal Wellness Recovery Action Plan. Share your plan with your peers and discuss strategies that work well for you.
4. Download the Illness Management and Recovery curriculum developed by the SAMHSA at https://store.samhsa.gov/shin/content/SMA09-4463/PractitionerGuidesandHandouts.pdf and download the Recovery Curriculum for People with Serious Mental Illnesses and Behavioral Health Disorders developed by the American Psychological Association at https://www.apa.org/pi/mfp/psychology/recovery-to-practice/all-curriculums.pdf.

   Read through the curriculums and explore some of the learning activities provided.

REFLECTION QUESTIONS

1. The founders of the profession believed in the power of occupation for improving the lives of individuals with mental illness. Crafts and work tasks were the primary occupations prescribed for therapy. Choose two specific occupations typical of this time period and reflect on the benefits of these occupations for individuals with mental illness. Would these be appropriate occupations for clients today? Why or why not?
2. Most occupational therapy practitioners today do not work in settings focused primarily on mental health treatment. For occupational therapy practitioners in other settings, what do you think are the primary mental health concerns that are observed? How can the practitioner address these concerns?
3. What do you consider to be the most important aspect of the Recovery Model?

REFERENCES

1. Bing RK. Occupational therapy revisited: a paraphrastic journey. *Am J Occup Ther*. 1981;35:499-518. Available at: https://search.ebscohost.com/login.aspx?direct=true&db=ccm&AN=107994949&site=ehost-live.

2. Engelhardt HTJ. Defining occupational therapy: the meaning of therapy and the virtues of occupation. *Am J Occup Ther*. 1977;31:661-672.

3. Peloquin SM. Moral treatment: contexts considered. *Am J Occup Ther*. 1989;43:537-544.

4. Baumeister AA, Hawkins MF, Lee Pow J, Cohen AS. Prevalence and incidence of severe mental illness in the United States: an historical overview. *Harv Rev Psychiatry*. 2012;20:247-258.

5. U.S. Department of Health and Human Services. *Mental Health: A Report of the Surgeon General*. Rockville, MD: U.S. Department of Health and Human Services, Substance Abuse and Mental Health Services Administration, Center for Mental Health Services, National Institutes of Health, National Institute of Mental Health; 1999. Available at: https://profiles.nlm.nih.gov/ps/access/NNBBHS.pdf.

6. Parry MS. Dorethea Dix (1802-1887). *Am J Public Health*. 2006;96:624-625.

7. Schwartz KB. Reclaiming our heritage: connecting the founding vision to the centennial vision. *Am J Occup Ther*. 2009;63:681-690.

8. Peloquin SM. Occupational therapy service: individual and collective understandings of the founders, part 1. *Am J Occup Ther*. 1991;45:352-360.

9. Cromwell FS. Eleanor Clarke Slagle, the leader, the woman. *Am J Occup Ther*. 1977;31:645-648.

10. Peloquin SM. Occupational therapy service: individual and collective understandings of the founders, part 2. *Am J Occup Ther*. 1991;45:733-744.

11. Quiroga VAM. *Occupational Therapy: The First 30 Years, 1900 to 1930*. Bethesda, MD: The American Occupational Therapy Association, Inc; 1995.

12. Dunton WR. *Occupation Therapy A Manual for Nurses*. Philadelphia and London: WB Saunders Company; 1918.

13. Dunton WR. *Reconstruction Therapy*. Philadelphia and London: WB Saunders Company; 1919.

14. Licht S, Features Submission HC. The early history of occupational therapy. *Occup Ther Ment Health*. 1983;3:67-88.

15. Meyer A. The philosophy of occupation therapy. *Arch Occup Ther*. 1922;1:1-10.

16. American Occupational Therapy Association. *Workforce Trends in Occupational Therapy*. 2006. Available at: https://www.aota.org/~/media/Corporate/Files/EducationCareers/StuRecruit/Working/Workforce%20Trends%20in%20OT.pdf.

17. American Occupational Therapy Association. *Workforce Trends in Occupational Therapy*. 2010. Available at: https://www.aota.org/~/media/Corporate/Files/EducationCareers/Prospective/Workforce-trends-in-OT.PDF.

18. American Occupational Therapy Association. Surveying the profession: the 2015 AOTA salary & workforce survey. *OT Pract*. 2015;20:7-11.

19. AOTA State Affairs Group. *Occupational Therapy Fact Sheet*. 2017. Available at: https://www.aota.org/~/media/Corporate/Files/Advocacy/Federal/Tips-and-Tools/OT-Fact-Sheet-2017.pdf.

20. Fisher G, Cooksey J. The occupational therapy workforce, part I: context and trends. *Adm Manag Spec Interest Sect Q*. 2002;18:1-4.

21. Fisher G, Cooksey J. The occupational therapy workforce, part two: impact and action. *Adm Manag Spec Interest Sect Q*. 2002;18:1-3.

22. Gutman SA. Special issue: effectiveness of occupational therapy services in mental health practice. *Am J Occup Ther*. 2011;65:235-237.

23. Fauerbach JA, McKibben JF, Bienvenu OJ, et al. Psychological distress after major burn injury. *Psychosom Med*. 2007;69:473-482.

24. Pedras S, Carvalho R, Pereira MG. A predictive model of anxiety and depression symptoms after a lower limb amputation. *Disabil Health J*. 2018;11:79-85.

25. Fang Y, Mpofu E, Athanasou J. Reducing depressive or anxiety symptoms in post-stroke patients: pilot trial of a constructive integrative psychosocial intervention. *Int J Health Sci*. 2017;11:53-58.

26. Le JF, Dorstyn D. Anxiety prevalence following spinal cord injury: a meta-analysis. *Spinal Cord*. 2016;54:570-578.

27. National Institute of Mental Health. *Mental Illness*. November, 2017. Available at: https://www.nimh.nih.gov/health/statistics/mental-illness.shtml.

28. National Alliance on Mental Illness. *Mental Health Facts in America*. n.d. Available at: https://www.nami.org/NAMI/media/NAMI-Media/Infographics/General MHFacts.pdf.

29. American Occupational Therapy Association. Occupational therapy practice framework: domain & process. 3rd edition. *Am J Occup* Ther. 2014;68(suppl 1):S1-S51.

30. American Occupational Therapy Association. Mental health promotion, prevention, and intervention in occupational therapy practice. *Am J Occup Ther*. 2017;71(suppl 2):S1-S19.

31. Accreditation Council for Occupational Therapy Education. 2011 Accreditation council for occupational therapy education (ACOTE) Standards. *Am J Occup Ther*. 2012;66:S6-S74.

32. American Occupational Therapy Association. Occupational therapy services in the promotion of mental health and well-being. *Am J Occup Ther*. 2016;70(suppl 2):S1-S15.

33. American Psychological Association, Jansen MA. Introduction to recovery based psychological practice. *Reframing Psychology for the Emerging Health Care Environment: Recovery Curriculum for People with Serious Mental Illnesses and Behavioral Health Disorders*. Washington, DC: American Psychological Association; 2014.

34. Deegan PE. Recovery as a self-directed process of healing and transformation. *Occup Ther Ment Health*. 2002;17:5-21.

35. Warner R. Does the scientific evidence support the recovery model? *Psychiatrist*. 2010;34:3-5.

36. Zipursky RB, Reilly TJ, Murray RM. The myth of schizophrenia as a progressive brain disease. *Schizophr Bull*. 2012;39:1363-1372.

37. Zubin J, Spring B. Vulnerability; a new view of schizophrenia. *J Abnorm Psychol*. 1977;86:103-126.

38. President's New Freedom Commission on Mental Health. *Achieving the Promise: Transforming Mental Health Care in America. Final Report*. DHHS Pub. No. SMA-03-3832. Rockville, MD: Author; 2003.

39. Mueser KT. Evidence-based practices and recovery-oriented services: is there a relationship? Should there be one? *Psychiatr Rehabil J*. 2012;35:287-288.

40. Substance Abuse and Mental Health Services Administration. *SAMHSA's Working Definition of Recovery*. 2012. Available at: https://store.samhsa.gov/shin/content/PEP12-RECDEF/PEP12-RECDEF.pdf.

41. American Occupational Therapy Association. *Occupational Therapy's Role in Mental Health Recovery*. Fact Sheet. 2016. Available at: https://www.aota.org/~/media/Corporate/Files/AboutOT/Professionals/WhatIsOT/MH/Facts/Mental%20Health%20Recovery.pdf.

42. Advocates for Human Potential, Inc. *WRAP Is . . .* n.d. Available at: http://mentalhealthrecovery.com/wrap-is/.

43. Copeland ME. Wellness recovery action plan. *Occup Ther Ment Health*. 2002;17:127-150.

44. Precin P. *Living Skills Recovery Workbook*. Brattleboro, VT: Echo Point Books & Media; 2015.

45. Substance Abuse and Mental Health Services Administration. *Illness Management and Recovery: Practitioner Guides and Handouts*. HHS Pub. No. SMA-09-4462, Rockville, MD: Center for Mental Health Services, Substance Abuse and Mental Health Services Administration, U.S. Department of Health and Human Services; 2009.

46. Anderson Clarke LM, Warner B. Exploring recovery perspectives in individuals diagnosed with mental illness. *Occup Ther Ment Health*. 2016;32:400-418.

47. Clay P. Shared principles: the recovery model and occupational therapy. *Mental Health Spec Interest Sect Q*. December, 2013;36:1-3.

48. Getty SM. Implementing a mental health program using the recovery model. *OT Pract*. February, 2015;20:CE-1-CE-8.

49. Synovec CE. Implementing recovery model principles as part of occupational therapy in inpatient psychiatric settings. *Occup Ther Ment Health*. 2015;31:50-61.

50. Pitts DB. Understanding the experience of recovery for persons labeled with psychiatric disabilities. *OT Pract*. March, 2004;9:CE-1-CE-6.

Therapeutic Interpersonal Skills

Nancy Carson

LEARNING OBJECTIVES

1. Define therapeutic use of self.
2. Describe the Intentional Relationship Model and relevance to occupational therapy practice.
3. Recognize therapeutic and nontherapeutic interaction skills for use in practice.

4. Define motivational interviewing and understand purpose and techniques for implementation.

THERAPEUTIC USE OF SELF

How do you define therapeutic use of self and what does that really mean? Many words are associated with the concept of therapeutic use of self, i.e., empathy, caring, concern, effective communication, trust, and understanding. Reflecting on personal experiences, consider times when you felt comfortable with your health care provider and times when you did not feel comfortable. What was it that made the difference? A health care provider may be selected based on experience, perceived knowledge, and critical thinking skills, which are all very important, but there may still be a lack of trust and ability to communicate with this person. Without trust and good communication, health care outcomes may not be as effective; patients may be less likely to ask questions and less likely to understand important information related to their illness or injury.

In the occupational therapy literature, Punwar and Peloquin[1] define therapeutic use of self as "A practitioner's planned use of his or her personality, insights, perceptions and judgements, as part of the therapeutic process."[1] Cole and McLean[2] constructed a definition of the therapeutic relationship by comparing common words used by therapists to define therapeutic relationships in the literature. Themes identified through qualitative analysis of what these words mean to therapists were also compared. The resulting definition of the therapeutic relationship is "a *trusting* connection & *rapport* established between therapist & client through *collaboration*, *communication*, therapist *empathy* & mutual *understanding* and *respect*."[2] Solman and Clouston[3] discuss the importance of therapeutic use of self, yet see it as a vague aspect of practice lacking in clarity, theory, and evidence.

A national study of 568 randomly selected practicing occupational therapists revealed that more than 80% of the respondents considered therapeutic use of self to be the most important determinant in therapy outcomes.[4] Interestingly, less than half of these respondents felt that they were trained adequately regarding therapeutic use of self in their educational curriculum, with only 4.3% reporting that they took a course that primarily emphasized "therapeutic use of self" skills. Support for the Intentional Relationship Model is suggested as a way to conceptualize, understand, and practice therapeutic use of self.

INTENTIONAL RELATIONSHIP MODEL

The Intentional Relationship Model (IRM) is a conceptual practice model based on research with occupational therapists regarding their use of self.[5] The IRM defines the relationship of therapeutic use of self with occupational engagement and includes methods for the development of interpersonal skills and their use in the therapist–client relationship. The IRM consists of four components that compose this relationship: (1) the client, (2) the interpersonal events that occur during therapy, (3) the therapist, and (4) the occupation.[5] The model is illustrated in Fig. 2.1.

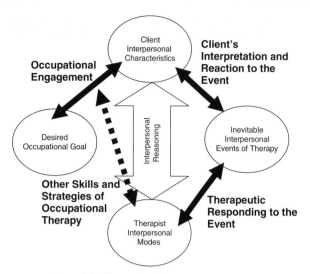

Fig. 2.1 A model of intentional relationship in occupational therapy. (From Taylor RR and VanPuymbrouck L. Therapeutic use of self: applying the Intentional Relationship Model in group therapy. In: JC O'Brien and JW Solomon (Eds). *Occupational Analysis and Group Process*. Elsevier; 2013.)

To understand the client, an awareness of their interpersonal characteristics is essential. These are a client's emotional responses and behaviors that are observed during treatment. They can be categorized as enduring or situational characteristics. Enduring interpersonal characteristics include lifelong behavioral patterns reflecting the client's temperament, personality, and cultural background. Situational characteristics are situation-specific and may differ from the individual's usual or predicted behavioral response. The IRM model identifies 12 dimensions of characteristics that have variable behaviors associated with them and that can be observed in clients and used to understand their unique interpersonal characteristics. These 12 dimensions include:

- communication style
- capacity for trust
- need for control
- capacity to assert needs
- response to change and challenge
- affect
- predisposition to giving feedback
- capacity to receive feedback
- response to human diversity
- orientation toward relating
- preference for touch
- capacity for reciprocity[5]

Challenges to the client–therapist relationship are described in the interpersonal events of therapy. The IRM describes 11 categories of interpersonal events that may occur and need to be addressed during a therapy session. These events are emotionally charged and if not responded to appropriately, they have the capacity to negatively influence the therapeutic relationship and the client's occupational engagement. Examples include boundary testing, power dilemmas, expressions of strong emotion, and intimate self-disclosure.[5]

The interpersonal skills that the therapist possesses also influences the therapeutic relationship. These may be skills that are natural to the therapist's interaction style or they may be skills that the therapist has mindfully practiced and developed. Examples include being friendly, attentive, flexible, motivating, humorous, caring, direct, gentle, and empathetic. In the IRM, six therapeutic modes or interpersonal styles are also identified, each describing a specific manner of client interaction: advocating, collaborating, empathizing, encouraging, instructing, and problem-solving. A brief description of each mode is provided in Table 2.1. The

TABLE 2.1	The six therapeutic modes
Mode	**Definition**
Advocating	Therapist: • Assists client in obtaining resources for optimal occupational performance • Supports client in managing physical, social, and environmental barriers to promote access • Addresses legal and civil rights issues that impede occupational performance • Functions as a facilitator or consultant
Collaborating	Therapist: • Involves client in decision making • Encourages participation and feedback from client • Empowers client to problem-solve • Functions as a partner in the therapeutic process

TABLE 2.1 The six therapeutic modes—cont'd	
Mode	**Definition**
Empathizing	Therapist: • Authentically validates client emotions • Actively listens to client and strives for deeper understanding of client needs • Responds to client changes in behavior and affect • Functions as a supporter through astute awareness of client's emotional state
Encouraging	Therapist: • Promotes a sense of hope for the future • Provides consistent reinforcement in a variety of ways • Adapts activities to respond to client values and preferences • Functions as a cheerleader or motivator for occupational engagement
Instructing	Therapist: • Shares technical and educational information as needed for skill development • Structures the therapeutic sessions for optimal learning • Provides directive feedback and focused discussion for goal attainment • Functions as a teacher or coach for skill attainment in occupational performance
Problem solving	Therapist: • Possesses focused technical abilities • Promotes use of complex assistive devices • Employs creativity in adapting activities to promote occupational performance • Functions as a skilled technician in the therapeutic process

Modified from Taylor RR. *The Intentional Relationship: Occupational Therapy and Use of Self.* Philadelphia PA: FA Davis Company; 2008:87-95.

therapist also needs to possess the capacity for interpersonal reasoning, which is a process of evaluating and responding appropriately to the interpersonal events that occur in therapy.[5]

The remaining component is the occupation, which is the activity of choice for the therapy session. The IRM is intended to support occupational engagement by positively facilitating the therapeutic relationship, thus enabling occupational participation that is meaningful and therapeutic for the client. For effective implementation, the IRM assumes principles such as in-depth self-awareness, a desire to strengthen interpersonal skills, a client-centered focus, and cultural competence.[5]

INTERPERSONAL TECHNIQUES

When considering how to apply therapeutic use of self and what it means in daily interactions, it is helpful to review specific therapeutic and nontherapeutic techniques. Awareness of personal skills that are used in daily client-therapist interactions is helpful to achieve therapeutic use of self. It is also important for the therapist to avoid using medical jargon and avoid overloading the client with too much information. Assessing the client's ability to understand, communicating at an appropriate level, and focusing on one issue at a time can enable effective communication and understanding. Other factors to consider include the individual's ability to hear and the individual's native language. If needed, a translator should be provided. Therapeutic and nontherapeutic techniques can be categorized as follows, and definitions and examples are provided to foster understanding and personal reflection of skill use.

Therapeutic Techniques
General Skills

Active listening. Active listening is the simplest and arguably the most important skill to use when interacting with a client. If you listen to the client, they will tell you what is wrong. Additionally, it is human nature to want to be heard. Even if you cannot offer a solution or answer a question, active listening can build trust and make the individual feel better by talking about concerns and feelings. To actively listen, the therapist should sit with the client at a comfortable distance, maintain eye contact, and avoid looking past the client or looking at an electronic device or their watch while the client is talking. The therapist should demonstrate a relaxed and attentive posture that demonstrates interest in the client. The therapist should focus on what the client is saying and should avoid thinking ahead to formulate responses and avoid thinking of issues not related to the client. People know when someone is actively listening to them, and when this occurs it builds trust in the therapeutic relationship.

Use silence. At times, using silence can provide an opportunity for the client to reflect on what has been said and allow organization of thoughts and feelings for further discussion. Just as important as active listening is the active physical support provided by sitting quietly with a client. Maintaining an attentive, expectant silence lets the client know that silence is acceptable and therapeutic. For distressed clients, periods of silence can be essential for maintaining emotions and synthesizing verbal dialogue. For clients in severe distress, offering to sit with them without any conversation can be very therapeutic as the presence of another human being can be comforting and decrease feelings of isolation and loneliness. It is important for the therapist to observe the client's nonverbal behavior to assess when to break the silence and either encourage discussion or leave the client alone.

Demonstrate empathy. Understanding another person's perceived feelings and experience is an important skill for the therapist in building the therapeutic relationship. It is important for the therapist to routinely assess how empathy is demonstrated and communicated to others. Statements such as "It must be difficult to want to go back to work but not be able to right now" can effectively communicate empathy to a client. Awareness of tone of voice and body language can also demonstrate empathy.

Instill hope. Providing encouragement and communicating a sense of self-empowerment to an individual can foster hope for the future. Encouragement should be provided appropriately within the context of the individual's current circumstances. It is important to avoid the perception of instilling false hope or appearing to lack understanding and empathy. Statements such as "I believe you have the strength to deal with this setback; you have faced challenges in the past and have been successful in facing them" can foster hope within a client. Actively listening to a client can help determine when to provide encouragement and hope.

Use of humor. In some situations, humor can be used effectively to build a common ground in awkward or uncomfortable settings and create a sense of togetherness. Laughter can be very effective in diffusing uncomfortable situations and/or emotions. Humor may allow people to laugh at a situation or themselves, thus creating a sense of closeness with others who have had similar experiences and can share in the laughter. As with many therapeutic skills, the therapist needs to be acutely aware of when to use humor appropriately. In times of profound loss or feelings of despair, humor is discouraged. "Laughter is the best medicine" is a cliché but one that does have some evidence to support it.[6,7]

Use of touch. Human touch is a profound form of nonverbal communication. The presence and closeness provided by holding someone's hand, placing a hand on someone's shoulder, or providing a hug, can be extremely powerful in communicating a sense of closeness and support when words do not seem appropriate or when one is at a loss for words. Some individuals may be resistant to touch, therefore if unsure, it is important to be aware of the client's response to touch and to ask if it is acceptable to touch or hug the person. The evidence for touch when working with distressed clients is supported in the literature.[8,9]

Directing the Conversation

Offer broad openings. At times the individual needs encouragement to start talking. The use of a broad opening question such as "Is there anything you would like to talk about?" provides the client with an opportunity to identify a topic or express a concern or feeling. The client can then choose and direct the conversation if desired. The conversation is focused on the client, and a sense of concern and interest in the client is communicated by the therapist. Other broad opening questions can be used as appropriate such as "Is there something you are concerned about?" or "What is most important to you at this time?" As the conversation progresses, the therapist follows the client's lead and may use additional broad questions to facilitate further discussion.

Encourage dialogue. At times it may be necessary to provide general leads to encourage the client to continue the dialogue. Some clients are hesitant to speak more despite having a desire or need to talk. They may not feel comfortable with the therapist or may not be able to tell if the therapist is truly interested in what they are saying. Using general leads conveys interest in the conversation and prompts the client to continue the narrative. It is important to let the client talk so that concerns, feelings, and thoughts can be expressed as desired. The therapist can gather valuable information about the client during these conversations. By offering general leads, the therapist avoids speaking for the client or leading the client into responding to the therapist's perceived concerns of the client. If after offering several general leads, the client declines to continue talking, the therapist should abstain from further conversation and assess the need to offer other forms of support for the client. General leads are simple statements such as "Tell me more," "Yes, I hear you," and "I would like to hear more about this." Nonverbal leads such as acknowledgment of the conversation through nodding in agreement or use of varying facial expressions are also effective.

Request orienting information. During conversation, it can be helpful to request logistical information from the client to understand the context of the narrative. If a client is telling a story or describing a situation without providing clarity, it can be helpful to ask questions such as "When/where did this happen?", "Who was present at this time?" and "What happened first, second, third…?" It is important to not assume facts of a story or conversation that the client relates, as these details may change your understanding of the client's concerns.

Encourage descriptive perceptions. If appropriate, it can also be helpful to facilitate conversation regarding how the client was feeling when discussing a situation or telling a story. If a client relates general feelings during conversation, you can ask questions such as "You stated you were upset, can you describe how you felt?" This prompts the client to discuss feelings more in detail and may reveal specific triggers or circumstances that were not apparent thus far in the conversation. This also prevents the therapist from making assumptions regarding the client's feelings.

Seek clarification. There will be times when the therapist will need to clarify what the person is saying. The person may be distressed and relating information that is vague and confusing or the person may be rambling. The person may also use phrases or words that are culturally relevant, personally relevant, or have more than one meaning. Asking relevant questions, focusing, exploring, and encouraging comparison are techniques that can be used to clarify the information being provided by the client. One example of a relevant question to clarify the meaning of a client's words is "I want to be sure I understand what you mean by 'I feel bad today.' How is today different from a usual day for you?" The therapist may also want to obtain more specific information by asking questions that focus the client such as "Do you have any difficulty bathing and dressing independently at home or does someone assist you?" It may be necessary to break the question down into separate activities to assess independence or to ask questions related to the ability to complete activities of daily living (ADLs) when home alone to assess for safety. The person may present self as more or less independent based on personal perception.

The therapist may also need to ask focused questions to clarify the meaning of a specific word or phrase if it is unclear to the therapist or to obtain specific information. An example of a question with a very specific focus is "On a scale of 0 to 10 with 0 being no pain and 10 being unbearable pain, how would you rate the level of pain in your back right now?" Exploring is another technique that can be used to obtain more information. Questions such as "Would you describe what happened to you when you went grocery shopping?" or "Can you tell me more about your sister's visit?" can provide more detailed information about topics that the client has shared and the therapist feels is relevant to provision of care. It the client does not want to provide more detailed information, the therapist should respect the client's wishes and use other therapeutic techniques to move the conversation forward or end the session as needed. Topics should not be explored out of curiosity or to meet personal needs of the therapist.

If there is difficulty in understanding the meaning of the client's words, another technique is to encourage comparison. For example, the therapist can ask "Is this situation similar to what happened to you last week?" If the person is struggling to explain something, the therapist may also choose to provide examples for the client to use in comparison; however, it is important to be careful that therapist-provided examples do not falsely represent the meaning of the client's words.

Asking questions demonstrates interest in what the client is saying and a desire to fully understand the client. Every effort to ensure a clear understanding of the client's meaning is important. For those individuals who may have disorganized thought processes or confusion related to their illness, it is important to consider what is factual versus nonfactual information. It is important not to dismiss what a client is saying because of their diagnosis or the therapist's perception of the ability to communicate effectively.

Confront. There may be times when it is therapeutic to confront the client. Confronting a client, or voicing doubt, should only be used when trust has been established between the therapist and the client. The goal is to help the client develop awareness of inconsistencies in what is being expressed and inconsistencies with observed or stated behaviors or feelings. An example of gently confronting a client is "You say you don't have time to practice stress management techniques; however, you report that you are bored most of the time." The therapist should avoid statements such as "That's hard to believe that you don't have time." Such statements do not provide the reason for the therapist's perception and therefore do not encourage the client to reflect on the apparent discrepancy in words and/or behaviors.

Feedback on Verbal Dialogue

Reflect. Reflection can be used to foster the individual to think more in depth either about what they want to do or how they feel about an issue. For example, if the individual states "I don't like my job anymore, it is too hard for me now, I think I should quit," the therapist could respond, "In what way is it too hard that you think you should quit?" The goal is to encourage the individual to develop more insight into a situation and how it should be addressed. If a client discusses an option and asks the therapist what he should do, the therapist should avoid advising the client as the therapist may be imparting personal values and beliefs onto the client. In this situation the therapist may simply state, "Do you think you should…?"

Summarizing. When responding to an individual, it can be helpful to summarize the key aspects of the conversation by restating or paraphrasing the narrative. This demonstrates to the client that the therapist is listening and understands what has been said. This allows the therapist to verify the content of what has been said and it allows for further reflection and discussion with the individual. The individual can correct the message if needed, and verification also ensures accuracy for documentation. Verifying the information is important for therapist documentation too.

Orient to reality. There are many reasons why an individual may not be oriented to reality. Individuals may be confused from medication side effects or interactions, anxiety, psychosis, dementia, substance abuse, or generally confused due to environmental changes and changes in their regular roles and routines. It is common for many inpatients to be somewhat disoriented when dealing with illness or injury, and interacting with many different health professionals can be confusing. Providing basic orientation information regularly can be very reassuring to the person. This can include consistently stating your name, why you are seeing the person, and may include other basic information as appropriate such as day of the week and name of the facility. Providing this type of information can help the person who may be slightly disoriented to feel more secure and engage. For those individuals who are delusional or are experiencing hallucinations, it is important to present reality in a calm and reassuring manner without arguing or belittling the individual. The intent is to assist the individual in determining what is real and provide reassurance through orientation. For example, the therapist might say, "I am not your sister, I am your therapist and I will be helping you get dressed this morning," or "I don't hear anyone else talking, I am the only person in the room with you right now."

Provide information. Research has shown that patient anxiety can be caused by a lack of information about the individual's condition and treatment; likewise, the constantly changing and evolving hospital routine and staff can also provoke anxiety.[10,11] Providing relevant and necessary information is important for creating trust and enabling understanding and security when facing health issues.[12,13] Information should be relayed in a manner that is appropriate for the individual, with opportunities provided for asking questions. When the therapist is unable to answer questions or provide information, the individual should be referred to someone who can. When facing uncertainties, the therapist should support the individual through use of other relevant therapeutic techniques.

Feedback on Behavior and Feelings

Give recognition. Providing recognition of an individual's behavior gives support for progress made toward therapeutic or personal goals. Examples of recognition include "You expressed your frustrations about the changes in your schedule in an assertive manner today," and "I see that you were able to prepare your meal by yourself today." Acknowledging these types of behaviors provides support to the individual by recognizing success. Positive feedback and recognition supports a therapeutic relationship.

Make observations. At times it can be beneficial to share observations of an individual's behavior to create awareness of how they are perceived and to determine if perceptions of observed behavior are accurate. For example, an individual who is engaging in behaviors such as pacing, wringing hands, fidgeting, or frowning may be doing so for a variety of reasons and may not be aware of these behaviors. The assumption is that the person is distressed or frustrated. By sharing these observations, the individual is encouraged to respond and the meaning of the behaviors may be revealed. At times the person may not be aware of the behaviors, therefore sharing these observations may encourage the person to consider potential sources of stress that have been suppressed. It is best to share objective observations such as "I notice you have been pacing back and forth for the past hour and looking at your phone every few seconds, is everything OK?" Being objective brings attention to the behaviors. Asking questions such as "Why are you anxious?" may not resonate with the individual as they may be angry, frustrated, or possibly excited. If possible, it is best to have the individual describe their emotions rather than the therapist sharing perceptions that the individual may agree to when it is not an accurate representation of their emotional state. When the therapist attempts to label the individual's emotions, it can also result in an immediate denial, even if accurate, if the individual is uncomfortable with discussing their feelings.

Validate client's feelings. When an individual expresses feelings or emotions, it is therapeutic to acknowledge those feelings and allow further expression if desired. The therapist should avoid approving or disapproving of the feelings expressed, thereby avoiding a judgmental reaction to the individual. When the feelings are negative or upsetting, it can be difficult for the individual to express them, therefore the therapist should be sensitive and demonstrate compassion, saying for example, "It must be frustrating to feel that you are not making any progress on your goals."

Verbalize client's implied thoughts/feelings. If the therapist feels that the individual is not comfortable or willing to verbalize a thought or feeling but the implication is strong, the therapist can verbalize the implied thought and allow the individual the opportunity to verify it. For example, if the individual states, "Everyone avoids me when I go to school," the therapist could reply, "Do you think they don't like you?" When the implication is strong, it is likely that the individual is willing to acknowledge and discuss the feeling, but is too vulnerable to address it directly. If the feeling is denied, the therapist should not pursue the topic at that time as it is possible that the perceived feeling is inaccurate or the person is too uncomfortable to discuss it at the present time.

Therapist Communication

Sharing feelings. It can be therapeutic for the therapist to share personal feelings with the client if done in an intentional manner. In doing so the therapist can model appropriate reactions and expressions of varying emotions. For example, relaying disappointment, expressing regret, or verbalizing frustration when experiencing difficulties demonstrates that everyone experiences challenges. It is crucial to avoid trivializing the client's feelings or emotions by insinuating that all challenges are of the same magnitude and therefore the individual should be able to manage feelings and emotions in the same manner as the therapist.

Self-disclosure. There are times when the therapist can share a past personal experience with the intent of illustrating a similarity that is helpful to the individual in considering options. Self-disclosure can also serve to build empathy and develop a strong therapeutic relationship. The emphasis is always on the client and care is taken to only disclose that which is relevant to the client. The therapist might say, "I had a similar experience and I struggled with choosing an appropriate way to deal with the situation; it was really hard to know what was best; writing down pros and cons for different ways really helped me to move forward."

Suggest collaboration. When an individual is having a difficult time deciding what to do, the therapist may suggest collaborating to brainstorm different options. The therapist can offer different ideas in a collaborative manner and can offer to work together with the individual to identify different solutions. For example, the therapist may offer to brainstorm with the client to identify potential sources of anxiety when the client is struggling to do so. The intent is to help move the client forward in personal awareness and understanding; not to make decisions for the person or tell the person why they feel a certain way. It is important for the therapist to remain nonjudgmental and avoid influencing the individual to agree with concepts or ideas that are not reflective of personal self-discovery and awareness.

Nontherapeutic Techniques
Lack of Compassion

Ignoring, changing the subject. As mentioned earlier, active listening is an essential skill for therapeutic interaction; ignoring the individual or changing the subject demonstrates a lack of empathy and lack of interest in the individual. It is important to allow the client to talk and take the lead in conversation. What may seem insignificant to the therapist can be very meaningful to the individual and it can be very therapeutic to allow the individual to talk without interruption or redirection. There may be times that redirection is appropriate or time constraints are unavoidable; however, the therapist may also consciously or unconsciously change the subject if they are uncomfortable with the topic. Good self-awareness and insight is necessary to assess the flow of the conversation and maintain therapeutic conversation.

Giving literal responses. At times, the individual may say things that do not make sense to the therapist. This may occur when the individual is confused or anxious and has difficulty expressing feelings and emotions. They may state things in a way that does not make sense to the therapist, therefore care should be taken to avoid literal interpretations or responses and the reply should be "Tell me more about how you are feeling or what you mean." Individuals who are delusional or hallucinating may make bizarre statements and the therapist should not respond as if the statements are true. The therapist should gently orient the individual to reality as previously discussed.

Challenging. Asking questions or making statements that are challenging or argumentative will most likely alienate the individual. Asking questions such as "What do you have to be depressed about?" or making statements such as "You should not feel lonely when you have such a nice home and people who care about you" are counterproductive and insinuate that the person's perceptions are wrong. Challenging individuals with statements such as "You can't say you don't have any friends, you have had lots of visitors this week!" implies that the person is lying about his situation and being deceitful. The therapist must avoid making assumptions about the individual and must respect that the individual's perceptions can be very different from the therapist's perceptions.

Asking personal questions. It is not appropriate to ask questions or request information that is irrelevant to the conversation or situation. The individual should feel comfortable answering questions and have an understanding that information shared is for therapeutic purposes. It may be necessary for the therapist to provide rationales for why some questions are posed. Questions should never be asked out of curiosity because the therapist just wants to know.

Sympathy. Sympathy is different from empathy in that sympathy is about the therapist's feelings as opposed to the individual's feelings. Sympathy is a subjective perspective of the individual that interferes with understanding how the individual feels. "I'm so sorry you lost your job because of your illness, I would be so upset not being able to work" focuses on how the therapist feels. Saying "Losing your job is significant, how will this change your daily routine and your self-concept?" is a more empathetic response that puts the focus on the individual.

Belittling feeling expressed. Saying "Everybody gets depressed at times" or "I know how you feel" implies that the individual does not have a legitimate reason for the feelings being experienced, and the person's emotions are devalued and not important. Instead, the therapist should acknowledge the individual's feelings and in doing so communicate understanding, respect, and trust; for example, "This situation must be very upsetting for you, is there anything I can do to help?"

Lack of Understanding

Reassurance, false reassurance. When an individual is facing a difficult situation, or is ill or distressed, the therapist should not provide false reassurance. Statements such as "Don't worry," "You will be fine," or "Everything will be OK" do not offer sincere or genuine encouragement. Instead, they may indicate a lack of compassion and understanding and may discourage the individual from expressing concerns and seeking emotional support. Instead, the therapist could offer assistance by saying, "I see how concerned you are, can I do anything for you?"

Patronizing. Patronizing is another type of response that indicates a lack of understanding and compassion on behalf of the therapist. An example is stating "I know exactly how you feel."

Stereotyped responses. Automatic or stereotypical responses do not encourage meaningful conversation. Statements such as "Tomorrow will be a better day" or "The grass is always greener on the other side of the fence" are superficial and do not demonstrate awareness for the individual's personal concerns. Stereotyped comments such as "Older people are set in their ways" or "Women are more

emotional than men" are also counterproductive. Use of stereotyped responses can indicate stereotypical attitudes and beliefs by the therapist. By using superficial or stereotypical responses, the therapist does not encourage expression of personal feelings and meaningful conversation.

Therapist Focused

Giving approval. Statements such as "That's the best way to deal with this issue" or "I think you are making the right decision, that's what I would do" can sound supportive; however, care should be taken to make sure that the therapist is not implying that certain actions and behaviors are the only acceptable behaviors. The therapist should be careful that personal values and beliefs are not setting a standard for judging the client. The client may not feel comfortable discussing different actions and behaviors if the therapist has strongly endorsed one approach over another. It is important to avoid value judgments, as the client may consciously or unconsciously try to adhere to the standard set by the therapist. For example, if the therapist "approves" a certain type of behavior that consequentially makes the individual uncomfortable, it could result in increased distress to the individual if there is a desire to change the behavior yet approval by the therapist is important. It is essential that therapists do not impose personal values, beliefs, attitudes, or moral standards on the therapeutic relationship. It can be hard to remain impartial when one has strong feelings about controversial topics such as abortion, assisted suicide, religion, etc. The therapist needs to have good self-awareness and be mindful of how personal feelings are dealt with when sensitive topics are being discussed. The therapist should strive to remain neutral and encourage clients to explore their own beliefs without concerns of being judged. Asking the client to talk about why they are making a decision, or why they feel a certain way, can facilitate greater awareness for the client of personal beliefs and feelings.

Disapproving. Likewise, the therapist should avoid disapproval of the individual's actions and behaviors. Stating "I don't think you should do that" or "You should stop getting so upset over what your friend says" are negative value statements that can be upsetting and confusing to the individual. Disapproval implies that certain actions and behaviors are unacceptable and the individual may, once again, consciously or unconsciously try to adhere to the standard set by the therapist. Disapproval can also anger or intimidate the individual, thereby preventing therapeutic communication.

Disagreeing with the patient. Similar to disapproval, contradictory statements such as "You are wrong" or "That is not true" can block therapeutic communication by making the individual feel defensive, threatened, upset, or angry. The therapist does not need to agree or disagree with the individual to foster positive communication. Simply stating "I hear what you are saying" and asking the individual to talk more about the situation or issue and/or more about feelings and emotions experienced can make the individual feel accepted and understood.

Advising, giving advice. Advising or telling the patient what to do is similar to giving approval, except that the therapist is very explicit in directing behavior or emotions. The therapist should avoid telling the patient what to do or how to feel. An example of advising is stating, "I think you should quit your job because it is too stressful for you." This is a decision that the individual should make; the therapist's role is to facilitate the individual to explore personal choices and feelings related to work and stress. This can enable the individual to develop more understanding and self-awareness, leading to increased personal decision-making. Even when a client asks the therapist what to do, the therapist should refrain from obliging the individual, as this implies that the individual is not capable of making decisions. The therapist can provide resources and information that are helpful and can guide the individual in a process to identify potential solutions. There are times when an individual may be incapable of making a decision due to cognitive deficits or emotional stress, and it may be necessary to redirect the individual and encourage decision-making to whatever extent is appropriate. It is important to remember that the individual's problem or concern belongs to the individual, not the therapist, therefore the decisions also belong to the individual. Instead of advising the individual, it is best to state, "Let's talk about what options you have for addressing this situation."

Interpreting. The therapist should also avoid interpreting the individual's words. Telling the person "What you really mean is you are happy with things the way they are and you don't want to make any changes" may or may not be a true representation of the individual's feelings. Interpreting the person's words can demonstrate that the therapist is not listening, and therefore makes therapeutic communication difficult.

Defensive responses, defending. It can be easy for the therapist to become defensive when criticism is expressed. Instead, the therapist should acknowledge the patient's feelings without agreeing or disagreeing. The therapist should listen to what is being said with an open mind. This can serve to defuse expressed anger and can help identify concerns. When the therapist defends self or others when criticized, the patient feels rejected and the criticism becomes reinforced.

Requesting an explanation. It can be difficult for the client to provide an explanation for why they feel or behave a certain way. "Why" questions can be interpreted as accusatory and can make the person feel insecure. For example, "Why are you so upset?" or "Why did you yell at your mom?" can be difficult for the person to explain because they require the person to analyze feelings or behavior on the spot. It is more therapeutic to ask questions that are less intensive such as "Can you tell me how you are feeling today?"

MOTIVATIONAL INTERVIEWING

Motivational interviewing (MI) is a specific therapeutic interaction style that occupational therapists can use to elicit behavioral change in clients. The use of MI promotes greater awareness of healthy behaviors that clients want to adopt. MI was first introduced as an approach to therapeutic interactions with individuals with alcohol addiction.[14]

MI has evolved over time and is established as an evidence-based treatment for individuals with substance use disorders and has been expanded to a variety of other populations and settings.[15] MI consists of four elements that capture the spirit of MI: partnership, acceptance, compassion, and evocation.[15] Partnership embodies respect for each other. Acceptance is valuing strengths, potential, and autonomy while providing empathy. Compassion is awareness and support of personal needs. Evocation is eliciting the person's own knowledge, wisdom, strengths, and motivation.

There are four processes that direct the interactions in MI. They are engaging, focusing, evoking, and planning.[15] Engaging is the establishment of a therapeutic relationship that is mutually respectful and trusting. Focusing is the clarification of a goal or desired behavioral change. Evoking is the implementation of the element of evocation for a specific change. Planning is developing a plan that the person is motivated to follow.

The techniques that are used in MI include: open questions, affirmations, reflective listening, and summaries.[15] Open questions are used throughout the four processes of MI and encourage the individual to choose what is personally important to discuss. In doing so, self-reflection is encouraged, and a better understanding of the person's internal frame of reference emerges. Examples include "What would you like to change about this situation?" and "How did you feel when you went out alone today?"

Affirmations are statements that acknowledge a person's strengths and skills while providing support and encouragement. Affirmations build confidence by focusing on specific positive attributes that are apparent in the individual's behavior or response to a situation. Examples include "You showed a lot of patience today when the situation became intense" and "You really helped your group members today when they were struggling to get the job done, that was nice of you to take the time to help others."

Reflective listening is active, mindful listening followed by carefully selected reflective statements that reiterate the person's thought and feelings that were expressed, and add potential meaning beyond what was expressed. This allows the person to consider those thoughts and feelings further and confirm or further explain them. Reflective statements must be carefully selected to be effective. Practice and skill is needed in choosing what aspects of the conversation most warrant reflective statements, and care must be taken to use these statements to facilitate productive conversation. Reflective statements are not questions; they are statements. An example is "You don't think you need to quit smoking," as opposed to "You don't think you need to quit smoking?" The goal is to have the person confirm or deny the reflection with further self-disclosure; posing a question prompts a defensive stance and blocks self-exploration.

Summaries consists of reflective statements based on what the individual has expressed. Summaries help to guide the conversation and can be used throughout the four processes of MI. They serve to demonstrate attention and interest to the individual speaking, and allow for clarification and additional information to be added as well. Overall, summaries serve many purposes, most significantly they are used to emphasize the individual's *change talk*, which is conversation focused on motivation to change. When used, summaries should be focused and concise.

The purpose of eliciting change talk is to have the individual talk themselves into changing. There should not be an attempt to convince the person to change, as this leads to defensiveness and becomes a barrier to change. Allowing the person to explore change and carefully guiding the person in change talk leads to a higher potential of change occurring.[15] Examples of change talk include statements such as:

- I would like to
- I can
- I am able to
- Something has to change
- I wrote down some ideas for
- I practiced some relaxation strategies yesterday

Examples of questions for the practitioner to evoke change talk include:

- How might you go about it, in order to succeed with making this change?
- On a scale of 0 to 10, how important is it for you to make this change?
- What concerns you absolutely most about…?
- How would you like things to be different a year from now?
- What's most important to you in life?
- How does this fit with your life goals?

MI is a person-centered approach; however, information and suggestions can be offered to the individual for consideration and discussion. It is important to limit offering suggestions to occasions that warrant it. The individual may need information to make informed choices, or it may be apparent that providing expert knowledge would be helpful to the person. There will be times when the person asks for more information as well. The therapist should be mindful that information is provided not to direct the person to a specific conclusion. It is offered to allow the person to make a conclusion with information that is valuable to the situation. The therapist should always acknowledge that it is the individual's decision to make, therefore emphasizing personal choice and control.

Motivational interviewing is more than just motivating clients. Although some therapists may feel they are already engaging in MI with their clients because they provide motivating messages during therapy sessions, they are most likely not providing MI as a therapeutic skill they have honed with practice. A review of these skills and their application to practice is useful to reap the full benefits of MI.

Examples in practice emphasize the psychosocial nature of MI in empowering the client and enabling a holistic approach to regaining occupational functioning, such as in pain management.[16] Additional examples are found in the literature in treating clients with hand injuries[17] and disabling musculoskeletal disorders.[18]

The use of MI in everyday practice can enable a therapist to have greater success with clients who present with difficulty in focusing on therapeutic goals and for some clients who are difficult to engage during therapy sessions. Like any skill, careful reflection of the components needed and practice of these skills are needed to maintain a high level of effectiveness. The focus on client-centered care supports the use of MI in everyday practice.

SUGGESTED LEARNING ACTIVITIES

1. Watch the classic movie *The Doctor* and reflect on the experience of the doctor as the patient. How did his experience change his perspective as a doctor?

2. Consider several potential therapist–client interactions that could be difficult for you to navigate. Role-play with your peers and discuss optimal approaches to each scenario.

3. Practice motivational interviewing (MI) skills by role-playing as the therapist with a peer who role-plays as the client. Choose one of the following situations to role-play:
   a. Incorporating a healthy behavior or habit into one's daily routine
   b. Consistent use of a stress management technique
   c. Regular use of a sensory diet or sensory approaches
   d. Expressing feelings on a consistent basis or speaking up for self consistently
   e. Engaging in a different routine or starting a new hobby/activity
4. Video record your interaction and after viewing your session, identify the MI methods you successfully implemented, and reflect on ways to improve your skills.

REFLECTION QUESTIONS

1. What are the biggest challenges in the therapist–client relationship?
2. Therapeutic use of self is considered an essential skill for effective practice. Why do you think it is so important?
3. Reflect on your personal skills for therapeutic use of self. What are your strengths?
4. Which personal skills would benefit from more practice?
5. How can you improve your skills?

REFERENCES

1. Punwar AJ, Peloquin SM. *Occupational Therapy: Principles and Practice*. 3rd ed. Philadelphia, PA: Lippincott, Williams and Wilkins; 2000.
2. Cole MB, McLean V. Therapeutic relationships re-defined. *Occup Ther Ment Health*. 2003;19:33-56.
3. Solman B, Clouston T. Occupational therapy and the therapeutic use of self. *Br J Occup Ther*. 2016;79:514-516.
4. Taylor RR, Lee SW, Kielhofner G, Ketkar M. Therapeutic use of self: a nationwide survey of practitioners' attitudes and experiences. *Am J Occup Ther*. 2009;63:198-207.
5. Taylor RR. *The Intentional Relationship: Occupational Therapy and Use of Self*. Philadelphia, PA: FA Davis Company; 2008:87-95.
6. Elliot ML. Finding the fun in daily occupation: an investigation of humor. *Occup Ther Ment Health*. 2013;29:201-214.
7. Southam M. Therapeutic humor: attitudes and actions by occupational therapists in adult physical disabilities settings. *Occup Ther Health Care*. 2003;17:23-41.
8. Morris D, Henegar J, Khanin S, Oberle G, Thacker S. Analysis of touch used by occupational therapy practitioners in skilled nursing facilities. *Occup Ther Int*. 2014;21:133-142.
9. Shaltout HA, Tooze JA, Rosenberger E, Kemper KJ. Time, touch, and compassion: effects on autonomic nervous system and well-being. *Explore*. 2012;8:177-184.
10. Bailey L. Strategies for decreasing patient anxiety in the perioperative setting. *AORN J*. 2010;92:445-460.
11. Refai M, Andolfi M, Gentili P, Pelusi G, Manzotti F, Sabbatini A. Enhanced recovery after thoracic surgery: patient information and care-plans. *J Thorac Dis*. 2018; 10(suppl 4):S512-S516.
12. Bellani ML. Psychological aspects in day-case surgery. *Int J Surg*. 2008;6:S44-S46.
13. Tang PC, Newcomb C. Informing patients: a guide for providing patient health information. *J Am Med Inform Assoc*. 1998;5:563-570.
14. Miller WR. Motivational interviewing with problem drinkers. *Behav Psychotherapy*. 1983;11:147-172.
15. Miller WR, Rollnick S. *Motivational Interviewing: Helping People Change*. 3rd ed. New York, NY: Guilford Press; 2013.
16. Ansara A. Psychosocial aspects of pain management: a mind-body-hand treatment approach. *Phys Disabil Spec Interest Section Quarterly*. December, 2013;36(4):1-4.
17. Flinn S, Jones C. The use of motivational interviewing to manage behavioral changes in hand injured clients. *J Hand Ther*. 2011;24:140-146.
18. Park J, Esmail S, Rayani F, Norris CM, Gross DP. Motivational interviewing for workers with disabling musculoskeletal disorders: results of a cluster randomized control trial. *J Occup Rehabil*. 2018;28:252-264.

Group Processes

Nancy Carson

DEFINITION OF A GROUP

A group can be defined as individuals who share a common purpose that can be attained only by group members interacting and working together.[1] All occupational therapy groups can be described as consisting of content and process. The *content* of a group includes the occupational activity that the group completes during the group time and includes what is said, written, or produced during the course of the group. The *process* of a group refers to the manner in which the occupational activity is conducted and the emotional tone of the verbal and nonverbal content that occurs during the group. Although the occupational activity content of a group may remain constant for a series of groups, the process may vary greatly depending on the interpersonal communication that occurs and the facilitation skills of the group leader during the group process.

GROUP STRUCTURE

There are many elements that describe the structure of a group. The organization and procedures of the group may be well developed and formal or may be loosely developed with no specific format. The *setting* of the group refers to the environment in which the group is conducted. The type of facility and the type of room can influence the group process in many ways. Elements of the environment include esthetic properties such as color scheme and use of art and decoration in the meeting space; comfort of the environment such as type of seating provided and temperature; and ability to attend well by minimizing auditory and visual distractions. Attention to the environment can have a significant impact on the ability of the group to attend to the activity and engage in interpersonal communication.

Logistical factors can also impact the group. Factors include time of day, length of group, frequency of group meetings, and number of participants per group. Whether or not the group is an open or closed group can significantly impact participation. If group membership remains the same over time for groups that meet regularly then the group is considered a *closed* group. *Open* groups allow for new participants to join the group so the membership changes over time. With closed groups there is more opportunity to establish interpersonal relationships with other group members and greater rapport with the group leader as opposed to open groups.

Group participation may also be *voluntary* or *involuntary*. If members are attending based solely on their personal desire to attend the group, they will be more invested in engaging in the group process. Some group members may be participating at the advisement of their physician or attending due to pressure from family and friends. Group participation may even be court ordered or required for obtaining other services. In these cases, the participant may not be as invested in the group process.

Group *size* can influence the amount of interpersonal interactions that occur during the process of the group; the larger the number of participants, the less opportunity there will be for interactions. Up to 10 members will allow for members to participate and interact as desired or as facilitated by the group leader. Greater than 10 members can impede the opportunity for participation of all members. The frequency of group meetings can increase the comfort level of participants and increase participation as well, particularly for groups that have more consistent membership and attendance.

Time of day and *length* of group sessions can also impact participation. Some members may have more difficulty concentrating and participating later in the day. Planning groups with awareness of the participants' schedules can facilitate greater attentiveness and involvement. The length of the group session should be appropriate for the type of group that is planned. Groups that are enjoyable and relaxing can be implemented for longer periods of time whereas groups that are more cognitively intense or physically or emotionally stressful may need to be limited to what the clients are able to tolerate.

CLINICAL CONTEXT

When planning for a stress management group designed to increase the group members' ability to relax, the setting should be conducive to enabling relaxation. Elements to consider include comfortable seating, use of soft colors and calming visual stimuli, the elimination of outside or distracting noises, background music or sounds that are pleasing to the group members, and other elements such as room temperature and tone of voice of group leader.

GROUP MODELS

Occupational therapy practitioners have the opportunity to engage clients in a variety of different groups based on purpose, group goals, and setting. The theoretical basis for group design and the purpose of the group dictates how the group is structured and implemented. Occupational therapy groups may be classified into different categories: activity groups, psychoanalytic or intrapsychic, social systems, and growth groups.[2]

Activity Groups

"Activity groups are small, primary groups in which members are engaged in a common activity or task that is directed toward learning and maintaining occupational performance."[2] Activity groups can be further classified into six different types of groups as described by Mosey.[1,3]

These include evaluation, task-oriented, developmental, thematic, topical, and instrumental groups. *Evaluation groups* allow for assessment of both interpersonal and activity skills. *Task-oriented groups* allow for the focus to be on both self-awareness and interactions with other group members through the activity process. *Developmental groups* focus on teaching group interaction skills that are considered developmentally stage specific. There are five stages, beginning with parallel groups where clients work on individual projects in shared space, to mature groups where the group needs take priority over the individuals' needs. *Thematic groups* focus on the clients learning the knowledge, skills, and activities for a specific activity. *Topical groups* are similar to thematic groups, with the difference being the focus of implementing the group activity in the community. *Instrumental groups* focus on clients maintaining their current level of function and meeting health needs.[3]

Psychoanalytic Groups

Psychoanalytic or intrapsychic groups are focused on increasing insight into the self and increasing understanding of personal behavior. These groups can be thought of as traditional group therapy sessions led by a trained psychiatric professional where the primary means of accomplishing the goal is through talking about personal issues and sharing these with the group. Occupational therapy groups may have the same outcome but are structured with the focus on occupation to achieve insight into the self and to increase understanding of personal behavior. Projective occupational therapy groups and groups that use therapeutic media as a means to understanding behavior are examples of psychoanalytic groups. Therapeutic media may include any form of art, such as painting or working with clay, other forms of media such as wood or leather, or creative media such as music or dance.

Social Systems Groups

Social systems groups focus on the group and learning about group dynamics; an example would be team-building groups. Occupational therapy practitioners working in long-term settings may lead these types of groups. An example may be a residential setting for adolescents with emotional and behavioral problems where the occupational therapy practitioner designs occupational therapy groups to focus on team building and group dynamics. Team building can be a lengthy process and require many sessions, ideally with a closed group membership. The purpose of a team-building group is for the group members to learn how to work together productively to achieve a group goal. Learning to trust others and to communicate effectively are the primary goals of the group process.

Examples include activities where members have to depend on others to achieve the outcome of the group: for example, being blindfolded while completing an activity and relying on other group members for guidance.

Growth Groups

Growth groups focus on increasing self-awareness and sensitivity to others; an example would be self-help groups. Most self-help groups are organized and led by clients who share the diagnosis or behavior that is the focus of the group. An example is Alcoholics Anonymous or a support group for a particular diagnosis. Occupational therapy practitioners may be invited to participate in self-help groups to share knowledge or insight related to the behavior but would not be leading or organizing the group.

Functional Group Model

The functional group model was initially developed by Howe and Schwartzberg[4] and subsequently refined "to incorporate the use of purposeful activity and meaningful occupation into the process and dynamics of group work."[2] The frame of reference for this model is based on research in group dynamics, effectance, needs hierarchy, purposeful activity, and adaptation. Based on a literature review of the research, a variety of assumptions related to people, health, occupation, therapy, social systems, change, function, and action were formed. Some of these assumptions related to people include people as action-oriented and social beings who exist in groups that are models of the social behavior patterns of society. Health assumptions include the support of purposeful activity for the health of the mind and the body, whereas occupation assumptions stress use of purposeful activity and active doing for skill development in self-care, work, and leisure. Therapy assumptions include elicitation of adaptive responses in groups, and change assumptions assert that functional groups provide a supportive environment for practicing the skills of living.[5]

The assumptions provide the foundation for this model and for the structure of the group. "The ultimate goal of the functional group is to promote health or adaptation through purposeful, self-initiated, spontaneous, and group-centered action. A functional group can have multiple goals, incorporating the specific needs and goals of individual members as well as more general goals and needs shared by all members."[2] A wide variety of groups may be designed using the functional group model, as this model provides a method of designing occupational therapy groups that are theory-based in the use of occupation and purposeful activity to support goal achievement.

STAGES OF GROUP DEVELOPMENT

As groups engage in the group process, they typically progress through stages of development. The most well-known explanation of group development is provided by Tuckman and Jenson.[6] Tuckman, an educational psychologist, first described four stages of group development in 1965: forming, storming, norming, and performing.[7] In 1977, the final stage, adjourning, was added to the model of group development.

The first stage, *forming*, may also be referred to as the orientation stage. Group members are focused on understanding the nature of the group task and bonding with group members. They may be eager and have positive feelings about the group process and group members or they may have some anxiety about what they are expected to accomplish in the group and how they are expected to interact with other members. Establishing relationships with others during this stage is important for facilitating positive growth through the rest of the stages. It is important that the group's purpose be clarified as well.

The second stage, *storming*, may also be referred to as the conflict or dissatisfaction stage. Group members may experience differences in their expectations of how to proceed with the group task and become aware of differences in opinions, personalities, and values. Interpersonal communication may be difficult to establish and members may feel frustration and possibly even anger with other members as well as the group leader. For some groups this will be a short stage if the group members are homogeneous and similarly focused on the group task and process. For other groups, they may not proceed past this stage in the initial group meeting and require a subsequent group to deal with the conflict appropriately.

The third stage, *norming*, may also be referred to as the resolution or structure stage. Issues are resolved and positive interpersonal communication increases. The group becomes more unified and focused on establishing group procedures and preparing for the group task. Group members are more trusting and respectful of each other as they begin to work together.

The fourth stage, *performing*, may also be referred to as the task performance or production stage. The focus of the group shifts to the performance of the task and effective occupational outcomes and goal attainment. There is positive interpersonal communication and a positive attitude for handling problems and disagreements. Not all groups may reach this stage completely, as some groups will struggle with the interpersonal interactions even while engaging in task performance. Some groups may engage well with others but have difficultly completing the task. There are varying degrees of effectiveness that may occur in this stage.

The fifth stage, *adjourning*, may also be referred to as the dissolution or termination stage. The group is over and no longer needs to meet. A group's entry into the dissolution stage can be either planned or spontaneous, but even planned dissolution can create problems for members as they reduce their dependence on the group. Group members may feel upset to be ending the group or may feel relieved that they group is over. It is helpful to spend time discussing the group's accomplishments and how best to end the group.

COMMUNICATION

The interpersonal relationship and the communication between the occupational therapy practitioner and clients are important factors for satisfactory group intervention outcomes. Knowing how to treat a client requires more than knowledge of the clients' medical diagnosis and treatment protocols; an understanding of personal psychosocial, environmental, cultural, socioeconomic, and occupational factors affecting the clients' level of function is also required. The practitioner must be able to communicate effectively to gather this information, and a positive interpersonal relationship facilitates the therapeutic process within the group setting. Good communication is a key factor in leading and facilitating effective groups.

Components of verbal communication include written and spoken words. In both instances, the practitioner considers the characteristics of the audience. For written communication, the reading and comprehension levels of the group members should be assessed. This can be a challenge when there are varying levels of ability. Plain-language literature suggests that verbal communication be written at a sixth-grade comprehension level. Some clients may be embarrassed at their inability to read and may not wish to disclose this to the practitioner or group members. Careful observation of the clients' skills is necessary to ensure that any written information provided to the clients is appropriate. Practitioners should consider the use of simple explanations of health information versus medical jargon to ensure understanding in both written and verbal communication. They must be aware of the clients' environment and influence of culture, spiritual beliefs, and socioeconomic status. These influences may affect the ways health information and treatment are perceived by the clients.

Verbal communication includes formality and complexity of language used, content of the message, tone and volume of voice, and speed and length of presentation. It is generally respectful to initially refer to an adult by his or her last name or professional title unless otherwise instructed by the client. Following the lead of the client as to how he or she prefers to be addressed is best in most situations. Assumptions should not be made regarding the level of complexity in verbal communication. When communicating, the language should be simple and direct. Observing the clients in the group setting to assess level of understanding and asking if the client needs clarification is essential. Care should be taken to avoid talking down to the clients or making the clients feel uncomfortable. Content should be concise and clearly express the message that the practitioner is conveying. Providing the clients with large amounts of information at one time can be overwhelming. Providing information in short and direct messages increases the likelihood that the clients will understand and retain the information. Tone of voice should match the content of the message and be appropriate to the group members. Talking to older adults in a childlike voice is never appropriate. Likewise, talking in a loud voice when not required for the clients to hear you can be over stimulating and distressing to clients. Most times, individuals who are hard of hearing do better with a moderate tone of voice and the opportunity to look directly at the practitioner to read lips and nonverbal cues to understand what is being said; this can be more challenging in the group setting. The speed of the verbal message is also important. Care should be taken to speak at an average rate.

Components of nonverbal communication include eye contact, facial expression, and body language such as positioning of self and use of gestures. Looking the client in the eye conveys interest and attention to the conversation. Consistently looking away from the client and demonstrating behaviors such as frequently checking the time indicate a lack of interest and caring. Facial expression should be consistent with the verbal message being provided. Smiling when talking about a serious topic is not appropriate and it does not portray compassion. Body language should be appropriate to the situation as well.

Active listening is another essential component of effective communication in groups. It is through listening to the clients that the practitioner becomes aware of the clients' concerns. Critical information for effective intervention may be missed if the practitioner fails to engage in active listening. The practitioner must convey to the clients a willingness to listen to what the clients say and allow the clients adequate time to express their needs and concerns.

When therapy is provided in the context of a group format, the occupational therapy practitioner must be aware of the interpersonal relationships with all group members individually and collectively, and be aware of the interpersonal relationships that exist among group members. An understanding of the interpersonal communication that is needed within the context of the group dynamics is necessary for a therapeutic group process to occur. People are instinctively social beings. They naturally form relationships with other people and are part of groups through these relationships or as part of their work, family, or leisure pursuits.

ESTABLISHING RAPPORT

For a group to be successful, the group leader needs to establish rapport with the group members; they should feel a sense of unity with each other. The group provides support and reassurance to the individual members. Members should feel comfortable sharing experiences and providing feedback to others. There are many *therapeutic factors* related to establishing rapport that can be facilitated in the group process.[8,9] These factors include:

- instilling hope
- universality
- cohesiveness
- imparting information
- altruism
- corrective recapitulation of the primary family experience
- development of socializing techniques
- imitative behavior
- catharsis
- interpersonal learning
- self-understanding
- existential factors

Instilling hope occurs in a group when a member is encouraged by another member who has dealt with a similar problem or issue. The occupational therapy practitioner as the leader can facilitate this process by asking group members to verbalize problems or issues that they are currently dealing with to see if other members have similar past experiences and are willing to share examples of how they dealt with the situation. This sharing of others' experiences can increase the hope that the individual has for dealing with the issue of concern. This relates to *universality* or the realization that other members have similar concerns and feelings and may have very similar experiences. The idea that one is not alone can be instrumental in improving one's emotional outlook. In realizing that a personal concern or feeling is a common human concern, the individual feels less isolated and more validated in their own experience. As members feel less isolated, a sense of *cohesiveness* develops. Members feel a sense of belonging, validation, and acceptance that enhances the group experience.

Imparting information is often a key element of occupational therapy groups. The group leader generally facilitates this process by sharing information prepared for the group; however, the leader may also ask group members to share factual information that they may have learned based on their personal experiences. This information may be related to accessing services, obtaining products, or learning new skills. This relates to *altruism* through the experience of being able to help another person. The group process can encourage members to be supportive and give unselfishly to another group member through being supportive and sharing experiences and knowledge for the sole purpose of helping a fellow group member.

Members of a group may unconsciously relate to the group leader and group members as if they were their own family members. If there are negative interactive patterns that occurred in the past with significant others, these patterns may be present in current relationships and be expressed during the group process. A skilled group leader can assist the group member in identifying these patterns and in developing healthy interaction skills resulting in *corrective recapitulation of the primary family experience*. The group setting can provide a safe and supportive environment for developing these healthy interaction skills or socializing techniques. The *development of socialization skills* is often a primary focus of occupational therapy groups through working with the other group members during the activity process and group discussion. The individual can improve and develop appropriate social skills through the process of modeling or *imitative behavior*. This is achieved by observing the group leader and other group members interacting in an appropriate socially acceptable manner. Behaviors such as showing empathy, using appropriate language, being polite and respectful, and sharing personal feelings appropriately are examples of behaviors that can be modeled and imitated.

For some individuals, the opportunity to tell their story to a group that is supportive and nonjudgmental is liberating. If the individual is able to talk freely and is able to express emotions in an uninhibited manner, then *catharsis*, the experience of relief from emotional distress, can occur. This can provide relief from chronic feelings of insecurity, shame, guilt, or fear. For many individuals, just the knowledge that others are listening to them and they are being heard is instrumental in their recovery.

An important aspect of occupational therapy groups is the learning that occurs through the group process. *Interpersonal learning* occurs when group members become more aware of their behavior and their interaction skills and how their behavior affects other people. It is closely related to *self-understanding,* the insight one has into one's problems and the understanding of how one's behavior positively or negatively influences the problems one is dealing with in life. A high level of self-understanding includes the understanding of unconscious motivations that affect one's behavior as well. In addition to interpersonal learning and self-understanding, the awareness of the *existential factors* of life such as the meaning of life, acceptance of mortality, and recognition of personal responsibility in one's life can be addressed in the group process. Difficulty coming to terms with these factors is a source of anxiety for many individuals and may not be accomplished by the majority of group members.

When facilitating groups, it is not feasible or necessary to include each of the therapeutic factors into each group. The therapeutic factors that emerge during the group process will be dependent on the purpose of the group, the functional level of the members, the ability of the members to interact with each other, and the group leader's skill at guiding the group process so that the appropriate therapeutic factors are embraced by the group members.

CLINICAL CONTEXT

An outpatient energy conservation group for individuals with chronic obstructive pulmonary disease (COPD) may be primarily designed for imparting information in the form of skills for conserving energy effectively; however, equally important elements may be instilling hope by increasing awareness of what one is able to do, recognizing the universality of concerns of others with COPD, and feeling less isolated as cohesiveness with other group members is established.

PLANNING THE GROUP

Effectively planning and leading groups requires a multitude of skills as well as experience in implementation. Occupational therapy practitioners lead groups in a variety of different settings. Many mental health programs use the group format to effectively provide treatment to individuals with similar diagnoses or skill deficits. Examples of other settings in which the group format works well include work simplification and energy conservation groups for clients in outpatient settings with diagnoses such as arthritis or COPD. Occupational therapy practitioners in pediatric settings may use groups for improving gross and fine motor skills through interactive play. Groups focused on increasing strength and endurance for clients in skilled nursing facilities can also provide increased socialization opportunities for these clients. There are many other examples of settings appropriate for group interventions, and the need for more cost-effective treatment may increase the demand for provision of services through this format in the future.

The importance of careful planning cannot be overestimated in leading groups. In planning the group activity, an activity analysis of the group activity is essential so that an appropriate activity is chosen. The physical, psychosocial, sensory, cognitive, and developmental skill levels of the participants must be considered and matched so that interest is sustained through appropriate task challenges. Tasks that are too easy or too difficult will not sustain interest and can lead to frustration. The ability to adapt activities or tasks should be considered ahead of time so that adaptations can be implemented without disrupting the group process. An example of a *group protocol* for planning a group is provided in Box 3.1.

LEADING THE GROUP

Cole[10] presents a model for learning how to lead groups that can be adapted to meet the goals of a variety of different groups. This model can be used in conjunction with a group protocol to identify the leadership skills for the group activity. Seven steps are outlined in Box 3.2.

Using a format such as the one provided by Cole ensures that the occupational therapy practitioner addresses the key elements for successful group implementation. The group leader is responsible for setting the mood and facilitating the progress of the group. The group leader's interpersonal skills and therapeutic use of self is extremely important in doing this. An awareness of one's leadership style is also beneficial. Group leaders that lean more toward an *authoritarian style* are leaders who employ a high level of control in the decision-making of the group. These leaders are more likely to control the progress of the group by dictating how the group activity progresses and what is discussed, without allowing group members to have input or by not recognizing nonverbal cues of dissatisfaction provided by members. This can lead to frustration and lack of progress in achieving group goals.

Leadership styles can be considered on a continuum from a high level of control to a low level of control. On the other end of the continuum is the *laissez-faire style* in which the leader allows the group to control all decision-making and problem-solving. This is generally not a productive form of leadership for occupational therapy groups, as group members need some guidance for achieving the purpose of the group. Leadership styles that fall in the middle of the continuum include the *paternalistic style*, the *participative style*, and the democratic style (see Box 3.3). A group leader using the paternalistic style closely regulates the behavior of group members to assist in achieving individual and group goals. The participative style of leadership is a more flexible approach where the

BOX 3.1   Group Protocol

Topic: Teen Group: Finding Your Voice!

Purpose: Teens will be able to communicate to others verbally in a positive manner.

Members: Six adolescent girls.

Setting: Acute psychiatric hospital (adolescent unit)

Rationale: This group of teens will meet daily to develop positive coping strategies and communication skills. The teens will benefit from learning how to communicate effectively. During this group they will practice how to communicate to get their needs met to use as a positive coping skill.

Goals

Long term: Develop positive coping strategies to address life events.

Short term:

Communicate with others verbally in a positive manner.

Demonstrate positive communication with peers and adults.

State one's point of view in an effective manner.

Outcome Measures

Express their needs in a positive and effective manner.

Identify resources that support them.

Listen to others' points of view.

Make their points to adults and peers verbally and in writing.

Meeting schedule: 1 hour daily

Materials (for collage group):

List all materials needed—type, number, etc.

Assorted magazines and pictures, paper, scissors, glue, markers.

Include cost of each item: magazines ($5–$8), paper—available in bulk on unit, assorted scissors ($5–$10), glue ($3-$5), markers ($5–$10).

Include method of acquiring each item: Available at local department stores.

Session Plan

1. Introduction (10 minutes): This is the first session, so the practitioner will take more time for the introduction.
   - Introduce leaders and set the tone: Welcome to the teen group. We meet each day at this time. The goal of the group is to help you cope with the difficulties you face. Could you write down some things you find difficult? What are some things you find easy to do?
   - Introduce members (icebreaker): Please introduce yourself and tell the group a bit about yourself.
   - Review purpose and expectations: The purpose of the group is to help everyone develop positive strategies for life. The focus will be on communication and

helping everyone find their voice. Please do not discuss the group outside of group time. You are expected to participate in the activities and let me know if you cannot attend the group. After today's session, the group will decide on the activities. It is meant to be fun and creative.
   - Outline of the session: Today, because we are getting to know each other, we will complete collages. Once completed, you will briefly discuss your collage with others so that everyone can get to know each other.

2. Activity
   - Describe the activity step by step in detail: Use these magazines, pictures, and markers to describe yourself to the group members. Include at least three healthy things you like to do.
   - Identify the physical, cognitive, and psychosocial skills needed for participation:
   - Physical: Sitting endurance 30 minutes; bilateral hand use to reach and manipulate paper; fine motor skills to write on, tear, or cut paper; hand strength is minimal but required to press glue on paper.
   - Cognitive: Ability to follow simple two-step directions (find picture and glue to paper); processing to describe one's self in pictures; writing ability if plan on writing on collage; creativity for design of collage; spatial perception to place pictures; choosing and selecting pictures.
   - Psychosocial: Sharing supplies; asking for materials; identifying appropriate pictures to describe one's self; socially acceptable description; being able to limit information that is not acceptable; knowing when to speak up; using body language and mannerisms acceptably; supporting others; engaging in the process.
   - Describe how the activity can be adapted if needed: The pictures could be precut (requiring that the teens select from limited pictures); more materials such as glitter, stickers, yarn, could increase the demands. Less materials could change the emphasis. The instructions could be more emotionally demanding: "Show a collage of yourself currently and then show your future goals." Teens may be asked to share about their collage verbally or in writing. Sharing with a few teens or only one changes the activity.
   - State the therapeutic goals:
     - Teens will identify healthy activities that promote a positive self-image.
     - Teens will communicate verbally with others in a positive manner.
     - Teens will identify three healthy activities in which they engage.

BOX 3.1 Group Protocol—cont'd

- Teens will listen to others as they describe their collages.

3. Closure
  - Review application to daily life: You did a nice job describing who you were and some activities that promote health. Did you learn about any activities that you would like to do that were not on your collage? What things did you like about the ways your peers presented? What did you learn that may help you in your daily life?
  - Assess goal achievement: How did this group accomplish the goals:

- Did you present yourself in a positive manner?
- Did everyone listen to each other?
- Did you learn anything about yourself?
- What went well? What would you do differently?

4. End Group
  - Based on this discussion, it seems you all really enjoy art. Would you like to do an art project tomorrow? Or we could . . . .
  - See you tomorrow at the same time.

Additional information: Note: This group all picked art projects in their collages. Look into a trip to the art museum as the week progresses.
From Carson N. Interpersonal relationships and communications. In: O'Brien JC, Solomon JW, eds. *Occupational Analysis and Group Process.* Elsevier; 2013.)

BOX 3.2 Model for Group Leadership

1. Introduction
  - Warm-up and setting the mood: This includes lighting, room arrangement, materials, and position of the leader. Is the group formal or informal?
  - Expectations of the group, explaining the purpose clearly: Describe the behavioral expectations and purpose of the group. For example, members are expected to remain in the group and participate. Everyone should support each other. If anyone is having difficulty remaining in the group or following the expectations, let the leader know.
  - Brief outline of the session: Give an overview and show a completed project if applicable. Be sure to include time for cleanup and remind group members to help.

2. Activity
  - Timing and therapeutic goals: Carefully review the therapeutic goals and time each part of the activity. Being aware of time is essential.
  - Physical and mental capacities of the members: Understanding the physical and mental capacities of members helps practitioners design group activities. Monitor the members' capacities as they work to be sure they can complete the activities. Guide members or adapt activities as needed so all can participate.
  - Knowledge and skill of the leader: Be knowledgeable about the activity and skill level required prior to leading the group. Complete the activity and note the areas that may be difficult. Allow extra time for those areas and preplan how to adapt the activity if the group needs it.
  - Adaptation of an activity: Examine each step and determine what changes can be made to the activity

if needed. Have additional materials that are already adapted available. For example, have directions in large print or precut materials.

3. Sharing
  - Clients share experiences: Provide opportunities for each client to share his or her experience in the activity. Relate this experience to others.
  - Leader acknowledges each member: Leaders should acknowledge each member positively, using the person's name and emphasizing improvement.

4. Processing
  - Members express feelings about experience and others: Allow members to express their feelings about the experience and how the group performed. The leader must ask questions and be open to the feedback.

5. Generalizing
  - Address cognitive learning aspects of the group: Reflect on the cognitive aspects of the group and determine how the group went.

6. Application
  - How does this apply to everyday life: Ask members how they might use skills from the group in other settings and in their daily lives. Discuss different scenarios with the group.

7. Summary
  - Review goals, content, process: Emphasize to members how the group addressed their goals. Did they feel challenged? Would they be able to use skills learned in other settings? Are there any areas on which they need to continue to work? What did they like or dislike about the process or content?

From Carson N. Interpersonal Relationships and Communications. In: O'Brien JC, Solomon JW, eds. *Occupational Analysis and Group Process.* Elsevier; 2013.)

BOX 3.3   **Leadership Styles**

Style	Level of Control
Authoritarian	High
Paternalistic	Medium-high
Participative	Medium
Democratic	Medium-low
Laissez-faire	Low

BOX 3.4   **Group Member Roles**[11]

Group Task Roles	Group Building and Maintenance Roles	Individual Roles
Initiator-contributor	Encourager	Aggressor
Information seeker	Compromiser	Dominator/monopolist
Opinion seeker	Harmonizer	Blocker
Coordinator	Gatekeeper	Self-confessor
Information giver	Standard setter	Recognition seeker
Opinion giver	Group observer/commentator	Playboy
Elaborator	Follower	Help seeker
Orienter		Special interest pleader
Energizer		
Evaluator-critic		
Procedural technician		
Recorder		

leader adapts the amount of direction and feedback to the specific needs and abilities of the group members. The democratic style allows for a higher level of involvement from group members in achieving the outcomes of the group; the group leader will delegate responsibility for group tasks to group members as appropriate.

The most appropriate leadership style is dependent on the cognitive and psychosocial abilities of the group members. The three styles in the middle of the continuum are generally more effective when leading most groups. Allowing group members to have some control over the direction of the group results in greater group cohesiveness and increased satisfaction. The group leader provides the level of group guidance that is deemed most appropriate for the clients and the activity planned. This may vary greatly and requires the skill of the practitioner to determine what level will result in the best outcomes.

The sharing, processing, generalizing, and applying steps can be the hardest for the group leader to facilitate. These steps should be carefully planned for by determining the types of questions to ask and the best methods for encouraging the clients to participate. Again, this can vary greatly depending on the types of client present in the group. Being aware of the roles that participants engage in during the group process is important too. Group leaders need to have excellent communication skills to positively facilitate the group process.

FACILITATING THE GROUP

Group members can fulfill various roles that can be productive or nonproductive to the group process. Three main categories of roles have been identified in the literature: group task roles, group building and maintenance roles, and individual roles.[11] The roles for each category are listed in Box 3.4. The two categories of group roles function to help the group achieve its goal by focusing on the group task or purpose and by supporting the group members in the process of the group activity. The individual roles function primarily to satisfy the needs of the individual member and do not consider the group task or the process of achieving the

group goals. This can prove to be disruptive to the group's focus and process.[11,12]

The task roles and the group building and maintenance roles represent different contributions of the members that may be needed to complete the group's goal or purpose. A single member can fill more than one role, and there may be times when there are some group task roles that are not needed or are not assumed by any group members. The lack of group members fulfilling certain roles can negatively affect the outcome of the group.[12] For example, not having a member serve as the initiator-contributor, whose role is to present new ideas or ways to approach the task or discussion, can result in the group stalling and members losing interest. The group leader will need to facilitate members to contribute. The lack of opinion and information seekers as well as opinion and information givers can also negatively affect the group's process. Likewise, it is important that some members assume roles such as encourager, compromiser, harmonizer, and gatekeeper, as these roles move the group forward in a positive manner. A lack of group members filling these important roles can present a challenge to the group leader. The group leader should have an awareness of these roles and should assess which roles are necessary for optimal group functioning. In the absence of these roles, the group leader should be prepared to facilitate members to engage in the needed roles.

The individual roles do not support the group task or process. Individual roles meet the needs of the individual member and may be an attempt to garner attention to self or to promote self as superior to other group members. Individual roles may also be used to deal with feelings of insecurity, anxiety, or poor self-esteem. The individual may try to shift the attention to another member to avoid discussing personal problems. The group leader should have an awareness of these roles and how they can negatively impact the group process. The leader should be prepared to redirect members who are engaging in individual roles that are negatively affecting the group.

The aggressor uses intimidation to control the group process. By criticizing other group members or attacking their contributions, the aggressor creates fear and prevents the group from making progress. The aggressor controls the group either due to a sense of superiority or to prevent the group from discussing issues the aggressor finds uncomfortable or uninteresting. The monopolist dominates the conversation by excessive talking, preventing other group members from moving the discussion forward. The blocker uses resistance by disagreeing with other group members' contributions. The blocker takes a negative stance on issues preventing progress. The self-confessor uses the group as an audience to share personal concerns and keeps the conversation focused on those personal issues. The self-confessor dramatizes personal revelations at times, using the element of shock to captivate the group's attention. The recognition seeker works to bring attention to self, thus stalling the group process. The playboy displays a lack of involvement in the group and distracts the group with frivolous conversation and revelation. This causes the group to get off track and remain superficial. The help seeker uses self-deprecation and expressions of insecurity to get sympathy for personal issues not relevant to the group discussion. The special interest pleader brings up other issues and redirects the discussion from the group issue or task to these other issues. Behaviors that may interfere with the group process include monopolizing the activity or discussion, criticizing others, or refusal to participate.

As a group leader, it is important to be prepared to deal with these problems should they arise. No group goes smoothly all of the time, so it is beneficial to consider potential solutions. The group leader needs to be ready to interject as needed to redirect members who are off topic, encourage group members who are having difficulty speaking up, and facilitate the discussion to stay on topic or to stay focused on the task. Prepared statements can be helpful; a few examples of potential responses are provided in Box 3.5.

Another challenge that group members may face includes varied group membership. The composition of the group may have variations in age, culture, diagnosis, cognitive ability, emotional stability, and physical ability. Group composition affects the group process in many ways and cannot always be controlled. In some settings, the practitioner may not know the group participants ahead of time, particularly in acute care settings where there are short lengths of stay. Every attempt should be made to know who the group participants are ahead of time. If not, an icebreaker activity at the beginning of the group can be beneficial in assessing members' abilities. Having tasks and topics that can be adapted to meet varying needs is essential. It is also hard to predict the level of participation the leader can expect when there are new group members. Some participants will be quiet and hesitant to participate. While these members are not disruptive to the group process, it is important to offer opportunities for engagement.

BOX 3.5 Potential Responses to Group Members

Individual Role	Potential Response
Monopolist	"Thank you, Bob, it is good to hear your thoughts, now let's see who else would like to comment or add to the conversation."
Playboy	"We seem to have gotten off topic, let's review the goal for today's group and refocus our conversation."
Aggressor Blocker	"Let's remember to respect each other's opinions and to be respectful in our conversation."
Special interest pleader	"I agree that what you are discussing is an important topic; however, the focus of this group is time management. We will see if there is another group or time to discuss this."
Help seeker Self-confessor	"Pam, let's talk more after the group about your personal concerns, the focus of this group is share ways that everyone can try to manage anxiety."
Recognition seeker	"Thank you for your contributions, it is very helpful to hear of how you have been successful. Let's hear from someone else and how they have been successful in addressing this issue."

SUMMARY

Understanding interpersonal relationships and developing effective communication skills are essential for leading therapeutic groups. The development of group leadership skills requires experience over time. Learning what works best and understanding personal strengths and weaknesses evolves through the process of doing. Practitioners need to invest time into planning groups that will meet the occupational needs of the members. Practitioners also need to invest time into practicing effective leadership skills. Role-playing with other practitioners is extremely helpful, as is evaluating groups afterwards to identify areas for improvement. Groups offer clients a rewarding and satisfying treatment approach through the opportunity to learn from other clients and to experience a sense of camaraderie and support.

SUGGESTED LEARNING ACTIVITIES

1. Observe a group in action; it can be a therapeutic, social, student, or work group. Identify the group roles that different members fulfilled and how they supported the group's task or purpose.
2. Identify if there are any group roles that were not evident and if you think this negatively affected the group process.
3. Identify if there were any individual roles observed in the group process that negatively impacted the group process.
4. Observe experienced practitioners leading therapeutic groups and identify the strategies for leadership that were used effectively.
5. Role-play with others to practice effective leadership strategies for managing group members engaging in individual roles that distract from the group's purpose.

REFLECTION QUESTIONS

1. What do you consider to be the most significant benefits of working with clients in groups?
2. What are the most important components for you to consider in working with clients in a group setting?
3. What are the biggest challenges to effective group leadership?
4. How comfortable are you leading groups and how can you improve your group leadership skills?

REFERENCES

1. Mosey AC. *Activities Therapy*. New York: Raven Press; 1973.
2. Schwartzberg SL, Howe MC, Barnes MA. *Groups: Applying the Functional Group Model*. Philadelphia, PA: FA Davis; 2008.
3. Mosey AC. *Occupational Therapy: Configuration of a Profession*. New York: Raven Press; 1981.
4. Howe MC, Schwartzberg SL. *A Functional Approach to Group Work in Occupational Therapy*. 1st ed. Philadelphia, PA: Lippincott Williams & Wilkins; 1986.
5. Howe MC, Schwartzberg SL. *A Functional Approach to Group Work in Occupational Therapy*. 3rd ed. Philadelphia, PA: Lippincott Williams & Wilkins; 2001.
6. Tuckman B, Jensen M. Stages of small-group development revisited. *Group Organ Manage*. 1977;2:419-427.
7. Tuckman BW. Developmental sequence in small groups. *Psychol Bull*. 1965;63:384-399.
8. Yalom I. *The Theory and Practice of Group Psychotherapy*. 4th ed. New York, NY: Basic Books; 1995.
9. Yalom I, Leszcz M. *The Theory and Practice of Group Psychotherapy*. 5th ed. New York, NY: Basic Books; 2005.
10. Cole MB. *Group Dynamics in Occupational Therapy*. 4th ed. Thorofare, NJ: Slack Inc; 2012.
11. Benne KD, Sheats P. Functional roles of group members. In: Bradford LP, ed. *Group Development*. 2nd ed. La Jolla, CA: University Associates; 1978:52-61.
12. Mahaffey L. Managing difficult groups. In: O'Brien J, Solomon J, eds. *Occupational Analysis and Group Process*. St. Louis, MO: Elsevier; 2013:155-168.

4

Using the Occupational Therapy Practice Framework

Heather Thomas

INTRODUCTION

The Occupational Therapy Practice Framework (OTPF), also referred to as "the Framework," is a document created by the American Occupational Therapy Association (AOTA) to define the current domain and process of occupational therapy.[1] It was designed to guide practitioners, educate others as to our scope of practice, and help organize our philosophical view of practice. It is not, however, a model of practice or theory. The Framework is to be used to guide our everyday practice and to facilitate growth in our profession. The first edition of the Framework[2] was published in 2002, as a result of attempting to revise the Uniform Terminology for Occupational Therapy,[3] which did not fully describe the domain and process of occupational therapy.[1] Now in the third edition, the Framework has evolved and reflects the exciting changes occurring within our profession.

The Framework details two interrelated aspects of practice: the domain of occupational therapy, and the process of occupational therapy. The *domain* provides a rich and comprehensive description of occupational therapy's area of expertise. It includes the aspects of human engagement that concern occupational therapy practitioners. This includes what aspects of the client we would evaluate when determining barriers and supports to occupational engagement, such as the body functions, performance skills, and contexts. The *process* describes the actions that are taken during the evaluation, reevaluation, and intervention processes. This includes the possible outcomes of intervention, intervention types, and approaches to intervention. Although each section outlines specifics to our profession, the domain and process are interrelated and intersect in practice. Interwoven throughout both the domain and process are the concepts of activity analysis, clinical reasoning, and therapeutic use of self.

Central to the Framework is the principle that engagement in occupations is the core of our profession, and that health and wellness are linked to engagement in meaningful occupations. The Framework defines "clients" as not only being individual persons but also groups of people, or populations. For example, an occupational therapy practitioner could provide services to a group of individuals, such as a group of students in a community college, or at a population level, such as those living a certain city or rural area.

CASE STUDY 4.1

Jessica is a 22-year-old college student who lives at home with her mother, younger brother, and two dogs. Her boyfriend of 2 years lives in the same city. Six months after starting college, Jessica has found it harder and harder to get up every day. She cries herself to sleep and has only been sleeping a few hours a night. She goes out almost every night with her boyfriend, to hang out at the local bar, where she drinks until her boyfriend has to drive her home. She often comes to school dressed in what she slept in, and very rarely brushes her teeth or her hair. She struggles to stay awake during classes, and is failing most of her classes. She works as a waitress 3 days a week, but she has called in sick seven times in the last few months, and has received a final warning from her employer. She spends about 2 hours a day on social media.

She used to spend time walking her dogs every day when she got home from school, but she has stopped doing this. After having a tearful conversation with one of the school counselors, Jessica decides to go visit her primary care physician. During the visit, the doctor determines that Jessica is suffering from depression, and prescribes her an antidepressant. After taking them for 2 weeks, her mother found the prescription bottle and screamed at her "there is no such thing as depression, those pills will kill you!" Since then, Jessica has been hesitant to take the medication and often "forgets" to take it every day.

APPLYING THE DOMAIN SECTION OF THE FRAMEWORK

The domain section of the Framework delineates occupational therapy's focus. Aspects of the domain are interrelated; all are of equal value and contribute to the client's ability to engage in occupations. The *domain* of occupational therapy includes occupations, client factors, performance skills, performance patterns, and contexts. The following sections will use the case of Jessica to illustrate how the domain sections of the Framework apply to mental health practice.

Occupations

Occupations, those "things that people do to occupy their time and attention"[4] or "the everyday activities that people do as individuals, in families, and with communities to occupy their time and bring meaning and purpose to life"[5] are central to our domain. The Framework has identified eight broad categories in which all human occupations lie: activities of daily living (ADL), instrumental activities of daily living (IADL), education, leisure, play, work, sleep/rest, and social participation (Box 4.1). Within each category, there

are specific occupations, with a description of what activities typically are included as part of each occupation. The use of the categories and descriptions helps occupational therapy practitioners use common terminology, as well as serve as a cue for evaluation and intervention. For example, in the case of Jessica, she is showing deficits in personal hygiene and grooming. According to the Framework, this includes removing body hair; caring for fingernails and toenails; washing and caring for skin on face, ears, nose, and eyes; applying deodorant; brushing teeth and flossing; as well as caring for and inserting dental orthotics or prosthetics. To fully assess Jessica's ability to complete hygiene and grooming, the occupational therapy practitioner should evaluate her ability to complete all of those grooming and hygiene activities that are typically part of Jessica's life. This list of specific occupations that lie within each category is a guide for the occupational therapy practitioner, to assure that all areas of occupational engagement are addressed. It also serves to educate those outside of the occupational therapy profession as to what "occupations" are and the scope of those occupations. For example, sexual activity is considered an ADL and is within the scope of occupational therapy. Surprising to many, sleep and rest, an occupation that comprises a large amount of our time as human beings, is also within our domain of practice.

As the occupational therapist evaluates the client, they should gather in-depth information about the range of occupations that the client needs to or wants to engage in. How the client defines each occupation will determine which of the eight categories the occupation falls under. For example, cleaning a car can be home management and maintenance if the car belongs to the client and they see it as part of caring for their material belongings, or it can be considered work, or leisure, depending on the context in which the occupation is occurring. Taking care of a child can be work, social participation, or the IADL of child rearing. This helps the practitioner be more client-centered by understanding the motivations and goals of the client. It also helps the practitioner understand the context where occupational performance will occur, which can affect treatment decisions.

Client Factors

Client factors are characteristics that reside within the client, such as specific body functions and structures as well as the client's beliefs, values, and spirituality. As occupational therapy practitioners, we recognize the influence of client factors on performance of occupations. We address these limitations (or strengths) in our intervention approaches. During the evaluation, we assess the client's client factors and determine the client's strengths and weaknesses as they impact engagement in

BOX 4.1 Occupation Categories and Subcategories[1]

Activities of Daily Living
Bathing, showering
Toileting and toilet hygiene
Dressing
Swallowing/eating
Feeding
Functional mobility
Personal device care
Personal hygiene and grooming
Sexual activity

Instrumental Activities of Daily Living
Care of others
Care of pets
Child rearing
Communication management
Driving and community mobility
Financial management
Health management and maintenance
Home establishment and management
Meal preparation and cleanup
Religious and spiritual activities and expression
Safety and emergency maintenance
Shopping

Rest and Sleep
Rest
Sleep preparation
Sleep participation

Education
Formal education participation
Informal personal educational needs or exploration of interests
Informal personal education participation

Work
Employment interests and pursuits
Employment seeking and acquisition
Job performance
Retirement preparation and adjustment
Volunteer exploration
Volunteer participation

Play
Play exploration
Play participation

Leisure
Leisure exploration
Leisure participation

Social Participation
Community
Family
Peer, friend

CASE STUDY 4.2

Jessica is struggling with several of her occupations. As her occupational therapy practitioner, it would be important to spend time during the evaluation to gain an understanding of the scope of her occupational deficits, as well as which occupations are still successful for her. What occupations have the most meaning for her, and how does she define success in each occupation? Based on the information given, Jessica is struggling with the ADLs of dressing, grooming, and hygiene. She is also having difficulties with the IADLs of care of pets and health management and maintenance. Of grave concern is her deficit in the areas of rest and sleep, with her struggles with sleep participation, as this is most likely impacting her other occupations. Her low grades and difficulty engaging in the classroom show that she is challenged with formal education participation in the category of education. Based on the information in the case study, Jessica used to enjoy walking her dogs, which may have been a leisure activity for her. If so, she is having difficulties engaging in that leisure occupation. The time she spends with her boyfriend is limited to time at the local bar, which may signal that there are issues with social participation on the peer/friend level.

their occupations. For example, a client who has been struggling with taking their medications on time might be having difficulties because of decreased memory, visual acuity, and hand strength. Once the occupational limitations are determined, it is then the occupational therapy practitioner's responsibility to find ways to assure the client overcomes those challenges by adapting the tasks for those client factors that challenge the client (using alarms to remind the client of when to take the medications) or by restoring the client factors (increasing grip strength to open pill bottles). How these client factors relate to intervention will be addressed later in the chapter.

Client factors are features of the client that influence performance, but they are not to be confused with skill level. For example, a client can have the strength, attention, endurance, and body structures conducive to being a good basketball player but still not be skilled at playing basketball. However, a deficit in a body function can negatively impact skill level. Thus it is important to understand the broad range of client factors and how illness or injury impacts body functions, and in turn performance of occupations. This is where it is important for the occupational therapy practitioner to be adept in activity analysis, and be able to determine what client factors are required for an occupation. By understanding the gap between the client's client factors and what is required for an activity, the occupational therapy practitioner can create pointed intervention plans.[6]

Values, Beliefs, and Spirituality

The values, beliefs, and spirituality of the client are those client factors that motivate, inspire, and give meaning to a client's engagement in occupations.[1] *Values* are those "acquired beliefs and commitments, derived from our culture, about what is good, right, and important to do."[1] For example, a client may value spending time with family, and consider that having children is the most important thing a woman can do. What a client values impacts their choice in occupations and puts some occupations as a higher priority than others, based on the client's values. A client's *beliefs* are those things that they believe are true.[1] For example, a client might believe that they will never be able to be independent again. Spirituality is how the client expresses what meaning and purpose there is to life, and how they "experience their connectedness to the moment, to self, to others, to nature, and to the significant or sacred."[7] This includes not only organized religious activities such as praying, going to church, or reading spiritual texts but also spiritual activities such as journaling to search for purpose or meaning in life, meditation, or enjoying nature. Understanding all aspects of our client's values, beliefs, and spirituality helps us understand our client's occupations and occupational choices. Harnessing those aspects of our client's values, beliefs, and spirituality can help motivate our clients, and incorporating those can give our interventions a sense of meaning to the client.

Body Functions and Body Structures

Body functions and structures are the "physiological functions of body systems (including psychological functions) and anatomical parts of the body such as organs, limbs, and their components."[8] Using the International Classification of Functioning, Disability and Health (ICF), the Framework classifies the body functions into the categories of specific mental, global mental, sensory, neuromusculoskeletal and movement-related, muscle, movement, cardiovascular, hematological, immunological, respiratory system, voice and speech, digestive, metabolic, endocrine, genitourinary, reproductive, and skin and related structure functions. Each category has subcategories and a description (Box 4.2). A limitation in a specific client factor does not necessarily mean the client will have difficulties in an occupation that requires that client factor, as performance skill and performance

---

CASE STUDY 4.3

In the case study of Jessica, we see that she values education as well as her family. She enrolled in community college, although her illness is causing her to struggle with her courses. It would be interesting to find out more about Jessica's beliefs about medication, as it appears she is adopting the beliefs of her mother related to antidepressant medication. Further investigation into her values, beliefs, and what spiritual activities Jessica engages in would be helpful to the intervention process, as spirituality can often be a strength and can function as a coping skill.

CASE STUDY 4.4

Jessica's ability to engage in her daily occupations is impacted by limitations in many of her mental functions. Based on the information we have, it appears that her higher-level cognitive functions are impaired, given her poor judgment and insight. Her emotional functions are causing her to have difficulty regulating her emotions, evidenced by crying herself to sleep and expressing that she is feeling depressed. Jessica's global mental function of energy and drive is severely impacted, causing her to have difficulties in getting out of bed, completing her self-care, caring for her dogs, and doing her school work. Her quality of sleep is also impacted. If we were to meet with Jessica for an evaluation, it would be valuable to assess specific mental functions such as her attention, memory, thought, sequencing of complex movement, and experience of self and time, and the global mental functions of temperament and personality (specifically confidence and motivation). Understanding the body functions that are limited with Jessica will help us develop appropriate interventions.

BOX 4.2 Body Functions (AOTA, 2014)[1]

Category	Subcategory	Description
Specific Mental Functions		
	Higher-level cognitive	Judgment, concept formation, meta-cognition, executive functions, praxis, cognitive flexibility, insight
	Attention	Sustained shifting and divided attention
	Memory	Short-term, long-term, and working memory
	Perception	Discrimination of sensations: auditory, tactile, visual, olfactory, gustatory, vestibular, and proprioceptive
	Thought	Control and content of thought, awareness of reality, logical and coherent thought
	Mental functions of sequencing complex movement	Regulating speed, response, quality, and time of motor production
	Emotional	Regulation and range of emotions, appropriateness of emotions
	Experience of self and time	Awareness of one's identity, body, and position in reality and of time
Global Mental Functions		
	Consciousness	State of awareness and alertness, clarity and continuity of wakeful state
	Orientation	Orientation to person, place, time, self, and others
	Temperament and personality	Extroversion, introversion, agreeableness, conscientiousness, emotional stability, openness to experience, self-control, self-expression, confidence, motivation, impulse control, appetite
	Energy and drive	Energy level, motivation, appetite, craving, impulse control
	Sleep	Physiological process, quality of sleep
Sensory Functions		
	Visual functions	Quality of vision, visual acuity, visual stability, visual field, awareness at various distances
	Hearing functions	Sound detection and discrimination, awareness of location and distance of sounds
	Vestibular functions	Sensation related to position, balance, and secure movement against gravity

Continued

BOX 4.2 Body Functions (AOTA, 2014)—cont'd

Category	Subcategory	Description
	Taste functions	Association of taste qualities of bitterness, sweetness, sourness, and saltiness
	Smell functions	Sensing odors and smells
	Proprioceptive functions	Awareness of body position and space
	Touch functions	Feeling of being touched by others or touching various textures
	Pain	Feeling indicating potential or actual damage, generalized or localized pain
	Sensitivity to temperature and pressure	Thermal awareness, sense of force applied to skin
Neuromusculoskeletal and Movement-Related Functions		
	Joint mobility	Joint range of motion
	Joint stability	Structural integrity of joints
	Muscle power	Strength
	Muscle tone	Degree of muscle tension
	Muscle endurance	Sustaining muscle contraction
	Motor reflexes	Involuntary contraction of muscles automatically induced by specific stimuli
	Involuntary movement reactions	Postural reactions, body adjustment reactions, supporting reactions
	Control of voluntary movement	Eye–hand and eye–foot coordination, bilateral integration, crossing of the midline, fine and gross motor control, oculomotor control
	Gait patterns	Gait and mobility as related to daily life activities
Cardiovascular, Hematological, Immunological, and Respiratory System Functions		
	Cardiovascular, hematological, and "immunological systems	Blood pressure, heart rate and rhythm
	Respiratory system	Rate, rhythm, depth of respiration
	Additional cardiovascular and respiratory system functions	Physical endurance, aerobic capacity, stamina, fatigability
Voice and Speech, Digestive, Metabolic, Endocrine, Genitourinary, and Reproductive System Functions		
	Voice and speech functions	Fluency and rhythm, alternative vocalizations
	Digestive, metabolic, and endocrine systems	
	Genitourinary and reproductive functions	Urinary, genital, and reproductive functions
Skin and Related Structure Functions		
	Skin functions	Protection and repair
	Hair and nail functions	

patterns also play a part in performance of an occupation (to be discussed later in this chapter). Occupational therapy practitioners become adept at evaluating each client factor and understanding the interaction between client factors and engagement in occupation. Identifying those client factors which are limiting or supporting participating in occupations is key to establishing effective intervention plans.

Performance Skills

Performance skills are small units of action that make up engagement of an occupation. These are observable skills, goal-directed and developed over time. These are the client's abilities and fall into three categories: motor, process, and social interaction skills (Box 4.3). Under each category, the Framework provides a list of specific skills and a definition of each. Motor skills are "skills observed as the person interacts with and moves task objects and self around the task environment."[4] Process skills are those actions that demonstrate cognitive functioning. Social interaction skills are observed when there is social exchange between the client and others. Body functions and structures impact skill level and skill level can influence body function. It is important to also note that one skill can influence another. One decreased process skill can impact motor or social interaction skills.

Occupational therapy practitioners evaluate the skill level of the client and determine the match between the skill level required of the occupation the client wants to engage in and the skill level of the client. The skill level required of an occupation is influenced by the context in which it takes place.[1] For example, as a person grows and develops, they typically develop the skill level of being able to attend to a task, by engaging in everyday activities such as getting dressed or going to school. However, the required ability to attend is much greater for other occupations, in different contexts, such as in driving a bus full of children up an icy mountain road, where the activity has a high demand for attention, within a demanding environment.

BOX 4.3 Performance Skills (AOTA, 2014)[1]

Motor Skills	Process Skills	Social Interaction Skills
Aligns	Paces	Approaches/starts
Stabilizes	Attends	Concludes/disengages
Positions	Heeds	Produces speech
Reaches	Chooses	Gesticulates
Bends	Uses	Speaks fluently
Grips	Handles	Turns toward
Manipulates	Inquires	Looks
Coordinates	Initiates	Places self
Moves	Continues	Touches
Lifts	Sequences	Regulates
Walks	Terminates	Questions
Transports	Searches/locates	Replies
Calibrates	Gathers	Discloses
Flows	Organizes	Expresses emotion
Endures	Restores	Disagrees
Paces	Navigates	Thanks
	Notices/responds	Transitions
	Adjusts	Times response
	Accommodates	Times duration
	Benefits	Takes turns
		Matches language
		Clarifies
		Acknowledges and encourages
		Empathizes
		Heeds
		Accommodates
		Benefits

CASE STUDY 4.5

To fully understand the skills Jessica is struggling with, we would need to observe her completing tasks. Given the information in the case study, there are several process skills that may be of concern. She is not able to pace herself to complete tasks. She is not attending to or initiating tasks, such as grooming or caring for her dogs. It appears that she has been struggling with continuing tasks and has been terminating tasks prematurely. She is not heeding to instructions given to her in the classroom, or by her doctor to take the medication prescribed. She is not accommodating her actions, based on poor performance in her school work and self-care. It would be helpful to know more about her ability to organize her environments and tasks, as well as her ability to notice/respond to task-related cues. Other process skills, as well as her social interaction skills, may also be impaired and would warrant further assessment.

Performance Patterns

Human beings engage in patterns of performance in everyday life that can either hinder or support engagement in occupational performance. These patterns take form in habits, routines, roles, and rituals. Habits are automatic behaviors or tendencies to perform in a certain way in certain environments and situations.[1] A habit can be useful, such as putting on a seatbelt before driving, or can be dominating and interfere with performance, such as smoking a cigarette every hour. Habits can be impoverished, such as not exercising regularly.

Routines are patterns of behavior, and usually follow a sequence of actions. These routines are part of everyday life, and can be either helpful or damaging.[1] An example of a routine is the sequence of normal morning self-care activities, such as toileting, showering, and dressing. We often engage in daily routines without thought to what we are doing, as the sequence is embedded into our everyday life. Routines are often impoverished with illness or disruption of the physical context, as seen in disaster victims.

Rituals are symbolic actions that reflect the client's culture, values, beliefs, or social identity.[1] Client rituals are often rich with meaning and may have a spiritual component. For example, many people have rituals surrounding holidays, such as specifics around the carving of a turkey on Thanksgiving, or putting decorations on a Christmas tree. Other rituals occur on a regular basis, such a performing a ritual when entering a doorway or meeting someone new.

Roles are part of performance patterns as they are the sets of behaviors that are required as part of the position, title, or responsibility that the client holds. These expected actions or behaviors are set by the culture or society in which the role takes place. For example, the role of a mother has different expectations in different cultures and social contexts. In some cultures, the mother stays at home and her primary responsibility is caring for children and the home. In other cultures, the care of children is completed by a nanny or au pair.

Contexts and Environments

Understanding the environments and contexts in which our clients engage in everyday activities provides us with insights into what contributes to their challenges or successes. Environments (physical and social) surround the client, while contexts (cultural, personal, temporal, and virtual) are within and surround the client. The physical environment includes built and natural structures, physical objects, terrain, plants, or furniture that are in the surroundings of the environment in which the occupation takes place.[1] This also includes sensory aspects of the physical environment, such as sounds and light. The social environment includes people or groups of people that are part of the occupation, either through direct contact or indirectly. The social context includes the support, pressure, or expectations of those surrounding the client, including friends, significant other, coworkers, etc. Understanding the social context gives great insight into our client's social pressures or supports.

The cultural context of the client includes the expectations of the society to which they belong. This includes their belief systems, customs, and expectations for behavior. The cultural context influences activity choices and occupational roles. The personal context relates to the client's age, gender, educational level, and socioeconomic level. It is important to note that the personal context is not associated with medical condition or physical health. The temporal context relates to time and includes duration of an activity, time of day, or stage of life the client is in. The virtual context is where interactions occur without physical contact. This most commonly occurs via the internet or through cell phones, but can also occur through radio transmission or wireless sensors.[1]

To truly understand our clients, we must consider each of their contexts, and understand how each can contribute or inhibit performance. For example, let us consider the occupation of studying for a class. Your physical environment can either inhibit or support studying, based on the noise level, lighting, seating, and availability of space. Your social environment, those who are involved in your daily life, can either support your studying by allowing you time

---

CASE STUDY 4.6

Many of Jessica's performance patterns have become impoverished, while others have become dominating and destructive. Her daily routine of self-care has become impoverished, with her showing up to school in the same clothes she wore the day before, not showering or completing her daily grooming. She no longer engages in her routine of walking her dogs every day. She has not yet developed the habit of taking her medication every day, and thus is missing doses. Her habit of drinking alcohol every night is a dominating and unhealthy pattern. Her role as student and employee are both in jeopardy, as she is struggling to fulfill the requirements of both of those roles. Part of her occupational therapy treatment plan should address these performance patterns, helping Jessica reestablish her healthy routines, extinguish unhealthy habits, and develop new habits that will support occupational performance.

alone, or could inhibit you by trying to distract you from studying. Your cultural beliefs and activity patterns can either promote studying, based on how much your cultural context facilitates studying time, or it can inhibit, by perhaps restricting study time or by a decreased belief in the value of education. The temporal context is often a barrier, as we find we do not have as much time as we would like to be able to study. The greatest challenge to studying for many students is the virtual context, as social media and connecting virtually to others is a luring distractor.

CASE STUDY 4.7

Jessica's physical environments include her home, school, work, and the bar she frequents. Her social environments include her boyfriend, mother, teachers, school counselor, physician, classmates, friends, occupational therapist, and occupational therapy assistant. We do not know much about her cultural context, other than her mother's belief that medication is not effective for depression. Her personal context includes that she is a 22-year-old female. She has been a student for 6 months, has been dating her boyfriend for 2 years, and works 3 days a week, which are all part of her temporal context. Her social media network is part of her virtual context.

THE PROCESS SECTION OF THE FRAMEWORK

The process of occupational therapy includes the evaluation, intervention, and determination of outcomes. All of this is intertwined with the domain of occupational therapy, which we have discussed in the first half of this chapter. Throughout the process of occupational therapy is the therapeutic use of self, clinical reasoning, and activity analysis. Therapeutic use of self is using empathy and a therapeutic relationship to connect with the client. Developing a collaborative relationship by honoring the client's desires is essential to ensuring desired outcomes. Activity analysis is fundamental to the practice of occupational therapy, allowing practitioners to understand and address the skills and external components needed for performance of the activity.[6] This includes understanding the client factors, performance skills, and performance patterns required of the occupation in which the client needs or wants to engage.

Evaluation Process: The Occupational Profile

The evaluation process begins by gathering data about the client's current, past, and future occupations through an unstructured interview called the occupational profile. Information gathered during this interview can include what occupations are important to the client, which occupations are of greatest concern, which are still successful, what are their daily roles, what environments and contexts support or hinder performance, what are their values and beliefs, what are their daily patterns, and how have these changed. What is their occupational history (not life story) and what do they envision for the future? This leads to the final question, which should revolve around understanding what the client's priorities are and what they hope the outcome will be of the occupational therapy intervention.[1] By starting with an occupational profile, the occupational therapy practitioner gains an understanding of the client's perspectives and what is important to them. This helps guide the occupational therapy practitioner, not only in developing goals and outcomes, but in designing meaningful interventions. It also establishes for the client, from the very beginning, the focus of occupational therapy. When every evaluation begins with an occupational profile, no client is confused about the role of occupational therapy. For a free template of an occupational profile, visit: https://www.aota.org/~/media/Corporate/Files/Practice/Manage/Documentation/AOTA-Occupational-Profile-Template.pdf

Evaluation Process: Analysis of Performance

The next step in the evaluation process is to gather data regarding occupational performance. Using information from the occupational profile, the occupational therapist chooses areas to asses, which will help determine current occupational functioning and identify those barriers and supports to performance. This is when specific formal or informal assessments may be chosen to measure specific client factors, performance skills, performance patterns, environments, or contexts, and how they are impacting performance. Data can also be gathered through observation, interview, record review, and direct performance.[1] Using the domain section of the Framework as a guide, occupational therapists should assure they are evaluating all aspects of the client and their occupations.

Intervention Planning: Possible Outcomes

Outcomes are the eventual end result of occupational therapy intervention. Determining what we hope our client achieves should be done in collaboration with the client and their family or caregivers. The end result of our efforts can span across all areas of the domain of the Framework but should ultimately be focused on meaningful occupations. It should also be kept in mind that outcomes can be focused on caregivers or family of the client.[1] The desired outcomes of intervention should be determined in the evaluation stage but can be redefined or refined as the therapeutic relationship develops.

The Framework defines eight outcome categories. The first of these is *occupational performance*. Occupational performance of our clients can be either improved or enhanced. When *occupational performance improvement* is chosen as an outcome, the client is limited in their ability to complete an occupation, and after intervention has an increased ability to participate. *Occupational performance enhancement* is chosen when the client is able to participate in the occupation, but intervention enhances or improves some aspect of participation for the client. An example would be increased confidence and decreased stress in test-taking for a group of students. *Prevention* is an outcome "designed to identify, reduce, or prevent the onset and reduce the incidence of unhealthy conditions, risk factors, disease, or injuries."[1] An example of achievement of this outcome would be reducing the risk of high school drop out in young pregnant women. *Health and wellness* as an outcome includes achieving health (physical, social well-being, and mental health) as well as wellness, which is not just lack of illness but involves the client actively making choices that lead to a thriving existence.[1] *Quality of life* occurs when the outcome of intervention produces a change in the client's perspective on their self-concept, hope, life satisfaction, health, and functioning. An example of this would be if a client with a terminal illness created a daily schedule that included time with each family member. *Participation* as an outcome occurs when the client is able to participate in an occupation to their level of satisfaction, as well as with what is expected within the social and cultural context of the activity. For example, participation for a client with an eating disorder would include eating a meal at a family gathering. *Role competence* is when the client can effectively perform the tasks or behaviors required of a specific role; for example, a student struggling with obsessive-compulsive disorder completing the tasks required of being a student at school despite the compulsions. *Well-being* as an outcome includes the client being content with their self-esteem, health, sense of belonging, and the opportunities available to them. Well-being includes all mental, social, and physical aspects of the human domains.[1] An example of a client achieving well-being would be a homeless person with posttraumatic stress disorder feeling safe and able to help others in the homeless shelter. *Occupational justice* as an outcome occurs when the client has access to and is able to participate in occupations that are meaningful and socially and culturally relevant to the client. This outcome includes assuring access to occupations that meet personal societal and health needs that otherwise would not be available to the client. For example, a woman incarcerated is able to paint her nails and put on makeup as she used to before she was incarcerated.

CASE STUDY 4.8

Multiple outcomes can be chosen for a client, and in the case of Jessica, several would be appropriate. Occupational performance improvement in self-care, pet care, work, and education should be a priority. Another appropriate outcome would be to help her achieve improved health and wellness, addressing her depression and alcohol abuse. Addressing her low self-concept, we can work toward a greater quality of life. Given that her roles of student and employee are suffering, setting goals toward achieving role competency would also be appropriate. Increased sense of well-being would also make a huge impact on Jessica's sense of contentment with life.

Intervention Planning: Choosing Approaches

How the occupational therapy practitioner will approach intervention is reliant on the outcomes chosen, the evaluation data, and evidence that supports approaches to the client's limitations. The approaches are strategies that the occupational therapy practitioner will use to reach the set outcomes and goals. Multiple approaches may be used, and the approaches used inform which frames of reference or models of practice are utilized.[1] How occupational therapy approaches intervention is another unique way our profession is distinctly different from other professions.

The Framework describes five approaches to intervention. The *create/promote* approach is used when there is not a disability present and intervention is designed to improve occupational performance: for example, developing a parenting class for gay men who are adopting children. When the *establish/restore* approach is used, the occupational therapy practitioner works to help the client change a skill or ability that has diminished or has not been developed yet. For example, an occupational therapy practitioner might help a client establish a morning routine that allows them to get all self-care completed and medication taken on time. The *maintain* approach is focused on helping clients continue to keep the gains they have made or preserve their ability to meet their needs. Without the intervention, occupational performance would decrease or the gains they had made would be lost.[1] Using the *modify* approach, occupational therapy practitioners find ways to adapt aspects of the activity or context(s) that will allow the client greater performance. This approach also utilizes compensatory techniques or changes of the tools used to complete the activity. An example would be to modify a client's workspace to decrease noise and visual stimuli that are distracting, therefore allowing the client to perform work more efficiently. The *prevent* approach is used with those with or without a disability, and is focused on preventing barriers to occupational performance. The assumption is that without intervention, the client is at risk for occupational performance problems.[1] For example, occupational therapy sessions might help an older adult client who just experienced the death of her spouse, to prevent social isolation. No one approach is more valuable than another, and they can be used in conjunction with each other. Practitioners should use evidence, their knowledge of the client, the effects of their client's disease or disability, and theoretical principles and models to select which approach to use with each client.

CASE STUDY 4.9

There are many approaches we could take toward Jessica's intervention. There is no one right or wrong choice, therefore the following provides only a few options. Using the establish/restore approach, we could help Jessica reestablish her morning self-care routine, as well as help her return to her pet care activities. We could help her establish a structured schedule to help her chunk tasks and incorporate mindfulness breaks throughout the day. Helping her establish coping mechanisms to replace drinking will also be helpful. Using the modify approach, we adapt her medication compliance regimen, by setting alarms on her phone and setting up daily medication organizers. We can help her modify her study area to help her become more organized. Using the prevent approach, we can address her social context, helping her create a support system which will help her with her drinking problem, possibly connecting her to a support group.

Intervention Types

Implementation of interventions is what invokes change and helps clients reach their goals and expected outcomes. During intervention, the occupational therapy practitioner uses their clinical reasoning skills, evidence, and the needs of the client to choose intervention types that will best help the client reach their goals. The Framework provides a description of five categories of possible intervention types. One or all of the intervention types can be used during a session. Occupations and activities are used as intervention techniques, choosing occupations or activities based on the demands of the activities and the goals of the client. *Occupations* are those daily life activities that are meaningful to the client and will address the goals of the client. For example, a practitioner could have a client go to a grocery store and utilize memory strategies to buy ingredients to make a pie. *Activities* are components of larger occupations.

These activities are meaningful to the client and are chosen to help enhance occupational performance. For example, a client might make a list of ingredients needed to make a pie.

Preparatory methods and tasks are a category of interventions including preparatory methods, splints, assistive technology and environmental modifications, wheeled mobility, and preparatory tasks. This category of intervention is to be used as only part of a treatment session and is to prepare the client for actual engagement in occupations. *Preparatory methods* are modalities or techniques that are often administered to the client (instead of the client doing or being an active participant); for example, providing a hot pack, electrical stimulation, or manual edema control. *Splints* are devices used to immobilize or support body structures. Splints should be used with the intention of enhancing occupational performance. Splints are used in a variety of settings and with multiple conditions, such as carpal tunnel or stroke. *Assistive technology and environmental modifications* are used to change the demands of an activity or environment that will allow the client greater performance. This includes not only assessing the client for the appropriate device or modification but also setup and training. For example, a practitioner would recommend voice recognition software for a client with a learning disability who struggles with typing her papers for school. An occupational therapy practitioner would recommend and train a client to use wheeled mobility devices when the client needs assistance in moving from one place to another. This includes seating and positioning, and any devices that help the client improve mobility and improve occupational performance. Wheeled mobility also addresses reducing the risk of skin breakdown or contractures.[1] *Preparatory tasks* are activities or tasks that simulate components of real occupations or are tasks that address specific client factors but do not have meaning or relevance to the client. An example is having a client squeeze putty to increase hand strength, or have a client role-play how they would advocate for themselves.

Education and training are interventions used in almost every occupational therapy setting. *Education* as an intervention type involves sharing knowledge that will help the client gain needed habits, routines, or behaviors. The information imparted by the occupational therapy practitioner can be related to a health condition or general health behaviors, occupational engagement, or well-being. Education does not require the client to apply the information during the session. With a client who is at risk for social isolation, the practitioner could provide the client with information on resources and health benefits of social connections. *Training* is a technique in which the client is taught specific skills that will help them meet their goals. This is different from education in that training includes actual performance, not just the acquisition of knowledge.[1] For example, a client could be trained to make calls to the pharmacy to refill their medication.

Advocacy interventions are focused on helping clients empower themselves and to promote occupational justice. *Advocacy* occurs when the practitioner advocates for the client. A practitioner might speak to a city board to help raise awareness of the needs of those with mental illness in the community. Intervention focused on *self-advocacy* occurs when the practitioner enables the client to advocate for themselves. A group of war refugees could receive services that would lead them to advocate for needed services.

Group intervention is utilized when social interaction and the dynamics of a group will help facilitate attainment of goals. This can also be seen as a service delivery model as well as an intervention method. Groups can be used to develop social interaction skills, positive choice-making, and to establish self-regulation tools as well as basic skills for social participation. Group interventions can be used in a variety of settings across the lifespan. Group intervention is particularly appropriate for many mental health conditions. A good example is a coping strategies group for teen girls in a substance-abuse clinic.

CASE STUDY 4.10

There are a variety of intervention types that would be appropriate to use with Jessica. Having her engage in meaningful occupations, such a caring for her dogs, will be impactful and meaningful. Activities such as having her create a weekly schedule, including her school assignments, will help her reestablish a routine. She could be introduced to assistive technology strategies, using apps on her cell phone to help her stay focused and organized. Preparatory tasks could include having her role-play how she could talk to her mother about her struggles with depression. Education provided can focus on depression and the effects of alcohol as well as resources available to help her with this. Self-advocacy efforts could be focused on helping her advocate for herself with her mother. Involving Jessica in group sessions focused on coping, depression, or alcohol abuse would also be appropriate.

CONCLUSION

Using the Occupational Therapy Practice Framework to guide intervention allows mental health practitioners to be client-centered and true to the core of the profession's beliefs. It guides us through the domain of our profession, including the broad spectrum of occupations, client factors, performance skills, performance patterns, and contexts and environments. Applying the Framework to mental health practice expands our understanding of our client's world and how they engage in occupations. Occupations are not simply basic daily living tasks, but those complex activities that become very challenging when mental capacity becomes impaired. For example, the role of the occupational therapist in working with those who are homeless and have a mental illness may focus on helping those clients regain the ability to complete instrumental activities of daily living such as home establishment and maintenance, financial management, and meal preparation. When working with those clients, understanding the contexts in which these occupations occur provides input into intervention planning choices, from the physical context to the social and cultural context, as each influence the client's supports and barriers. By recognizing the importance of the client's values, beliefs, and spirituality, the Framework brings to light the importance of recognizing how these factors influence our client's engagement. Especially when our clients are struggling emotionally, utilizing their faith and belief systems can be an effective motivator.

In designing interventions for those with mental illness, incorporating the Framework's performance patterns can also be instrumental in meeting desired outcomes. We need to understand our client's routines, habits, and roles. Routines provide structure to our lives, but if impoverished, it can leave a client lost and occupationally impaired. Investigating other aspects of the client's patterns, such as their habits, rituals, and roles, can contribute to understanding how to help the client. Our clients may engage in rituals or habits that are essential to their self-definition and are incorporated into daily occupations.

The process and social interaction skills are the performance skills most often impaired in clients with mental illness. Using the Framework and activity analysis, we can identify which performance skills are required of the occupations our client needs to engage in, and which are impaired in our client. This serves as a foundation for intervention planning. The mental functions sections of the client factors section also serves in a similar fashion, identifying the areas which are barriers to client success in occupational performance or satisfaction.

The process section of the Framework provides guidance for the evaluation process, selecting outcome measures, approaches to intervention, and intervention types. All of these aspects of the process are intertwined with the domain, with the evaluation process including all aspects of the domain and intervention addressing aspects of the domain. The elements of the process clearly portray how integral mental health is to occupational performance and health and well-being. The Framework demonstrates how to evaluate and provide intervention holistically, incorporating all aspects of the person both mentally and physically, in their contexts and environments.

SUGGESTED LEARNING ACTIVITIES

1. Track all of the activities you do for one day. Download a copy of the Framework from the AOTA website. Using Table 1 of the Framework, identify in which category and subcategory each of your daily occupations lay.

ACTIVITY TRACKING FOR ONE DAY.

Activities per Hour	ADL	IADL	Rest/ Sleep	Leisure	Play	Work	Social Participation
Example:	Bathing, showering Dressing	Health management					Peer
6:00 am							
7:00 am							
8:00 am							
9:00 am							
10:00 am							
11:00 am							
12:00 am							
1:00 pm							
2:00 pm							
3:00 pm							
4:00 pm							
5:00 pm							
6:00 pm							
7:00 pm							
8:00 pm							
9:00 pm							
10:00 pm							
11:00 pm							
12:00 pm							

2. Identify how aspects of each of your contexts and environments either hinder or support your ability to successfully complete your work or schoolwork.

	Hinder	Support
Physical		
Social		
Cultural		
Virtual		
Personal		
Temporal		

REFLECTION QUESTIONS

1. How does understanding a client's values, beliefs, and spirituality contribute to the development of an intervention plan and identify which outcomes or approaches to utilize?
2. Design an intervention session focused on performance patterns—what approach and intervention type(s) would you employ?
3. What are questions that could be asked during an occupational profile that would gather information on all of the domain sections of the Framework?
4. How are the domain and the process sections of the Framework interrelated?
5. Identify one mental illness and using the Framework, identify which client factors and performance skills would impair the person's ability to engage in occupations.

REFERENCES

1. American Occupational Therapy Association. Occupational therapy practice framework: domain and process (3rd ed.). *Am J Occup Ther.* 2014;68(suppl 1):S1-S48.
2. American Occupational Therapy Association. Occupational therapy practice framework: domain and process (1st ed.). *Am J Occup Ther.* 2002;56:609-639.
3. American Occupational Therapy Association. Uniform terminology for occupational therapy (3rd ed.). *Am J Occup Ther.* 1994;48:1047-1054.
4. Boyt Schell BA, Gillen G, Scaffa M. Glossary. In: Boyt Schell BA, Gillen G, Scaffa M, eds. *Willard and Spackman's Occupational Therapy.* 12th ed. Philadelphia: Lippincott Williams & Wilkins; 2014:1229-1243.
5. World Federation of Occupational Therapists. Definition of occupation. 2012. Available at: http://www.wfot.org/aboutus/aboutoccupationaltherapy/definitionofoccupationaltherapy.aspx.
6. Thomas H. *Occupation-Based Activity Analysis.* Thorofare, NJ: Slack; 2015.
7. Puchalski C, Ferrell B, Virani R, et al. Improving the quality of spiritual care as a dimension of palliative care: the report of the Consensus Conference. *J Palliat Med.* 2009;12:885-904.
8. World Health Organization. *International Classification of Functioning, Disability, and Health.* Geneva, Switzerland: Author; 2001.

5

Occupation-Centered Practice Models

Jane O'Brien, Ashley Stoffel, Gail Fisher, and Michael Iwama

LEARNING OBJECTIVES

1. Identify features of specific occupation-centered models.
2. Explain the principles of each occupation-centered model and how to use the principles to guide intervention planning.
3. Describe the techniques and strategies associated with each occupation-centered model that may be used in practice.
4. Apply concepts to case study examples of how to use the occupation-centered models to promote or restore mental health of clients.

INTRODUCTION

Occupational therapy practitioners working in mental health settings create evaluation, intervention, and outcome plans with clients to address a range of occupational challenges and promote engagement in daily occupations (those things that people find meaningful and give them a sense of identity). Occupational therapy practitioners analyze and synthesize information from a variety of sources (e.g., interview, observation, assessment, input from other team members) to create a picture of the client that will guide recommendations for therapeutic intervention. Occupational therapy interventions based on theoretical models have been shown to be effective in improving occupational performance and sense of well-being among individuals with serious mental illness.[1] Occupation-centered models provide structure, terminology, principles, strategies, and techniques that occupational therapy practitioners can use to help clients regain their roles and occupations for improved life satisfaction and quality of life.[2] These models provide a road map for occupational therapy practitioners to follow as they attempt to understand their clients and guide them toward their desired occupational goals. The models guide the thinking process that results in

the selection of occupation-focused evaluation methods to assist the occupational therapy practitioner in understanding the client's strengths, challenges, and goals that can be addressed in therapy. The occupation-centered models provide the base; the intervention plan that is built on that base can include knowledge and techniques from other disciplines and models that are not occupation-centered, such as cognitive-behavioral therapy, psychodynamic theory, sensory modulation approaches, or applied behavioral analysis, but the occupation-centered model provides the underlying context for all interventions. Each model described in this chapter emphasizes the value of focusing on occupation and the multifaceted factors that influence occupational performance, and provides practical tools for the occupational therapy practitioner to employ in their work.

The authors summarize four occupation-centered models used by occupational therapists in mental health settings: Model of Human Occupation (MOHO); Person-Environment-Occupation-Performance (PEOP) Model; Canadian Model of Occupational Performance and Engagement (CMOP-E); and the Kawa Model. The authors describe the principles, assessments, and strategies specific to each model. Case study examples illustrate the interactions between components of the model and the dynamic nature of occupational performance to provide a deeper understanding of the use of the model in mental health practice.

KIELHOFNER'S MODEL OF HUMAN OCCUPATION (MOHO)

Kielhofner's Model of Human Occupation (MOHO) was created in 1980[3-5] to describe the complexities of human behavior for persons with mental health issues. Dr. Kielhofner (1949–2010) refined and expanded the model for over 30 years, responding to feedback from scholars, practitioners, and clients. Dr. Kielhofner and colleagues worldwide created assessments and examined the effectiveness of using MOHO in practice settings and program development. Kielhofner's MOHO[6] includes expanded concepts with research evidence, 15 assessments (covering all areas of the MOHO and age ranges), and over 500 research-based articles supporting its use in practice. The use of MOHO in mental health settings in many cultures and with many populations is supported with evidence suggesting that using MOHO to inform occupational therapy intervention

results in improved outcome for clients; over 300 research articles exist specifically addressing MOHO and mental health assessment or intervention.[7-10] MOHO is designed to complement other frames of reference and offers a client-centered, occupation-focused, holistic, and evidence-based model to evaluate, intervene, and create changes in occupational performance.[11]

Overview

The MOHO is an occupation-centered model of practice that explains human performance as a dynamic interaction between four elements: volition, habituation, performance capacity, and environment (see Fig. 5.1).

Volition is the person's motivations and desires to complete a given occupation; it includes those things that the person finds compelling to complete. Volition is essential for determining those occupations that give someone a sense of identity and meaning. It is a process of thinking and feeling about oneself as an actor and involves anticipating, choosing, experiencing, and interpreting experiences. Volition consists of values, interests, and personal causation. Values are those things people find important, based on family, culture, and experiences. Interests are those things that a

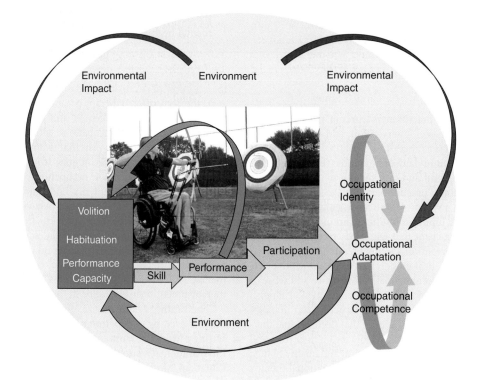

Fig. 5.1 The Model of Human Occupation.[6] (U.S. Navy photo by Mass Communication Specialist 3rd Class, Jake Berenguer/Released)

person finds enjoyable or satisfying. Personal causation includes a person's self-efficacy, defined as one's belief that they have the skills and abilities to perform.

Clients may experience low volition for a variety of reasons. Changes in mental health as a result of loss (physical, psychological, or financial), psychological stress, disease (such as mental health changes or addiction), and circumstantial situations (such as homelessness, incarceration) may affect a person's interests for doing everyday things, their belief in their abilities, and their expectancy for success. This cycle of failure or inability to engage in those things one values may cause a person to feel hopeless or unfulfilled. Understanding the client's past interests, motivations, and occupational history may serve as the first step to designing intervention to produce change.

Habituation refers to the emergence of a pattern of occupation over time and includes a person's habits and roles. Habits are the everyday things that people do that organize the day and includes patterns and timing of activities. "Habits refer to the tendency to respond and perform in certain consistent ways in familiar environments or situations."[12] Roles include the expectations for behaviors and activity associated with a given position with which a person identifies. Roles have a specific set of behaviors, rules, and expectations that can be both internalized and externalized. Internalized expectations are those that the person attributes to the role, whereas external expectations refer to those from other persons or society. MOHO also considers the person's belief that they have the rights associated with the role.

Clients experiencing mental health issues often show dysfunction in habituation; they may lose roles (such as worker, homemaker) and pay less attention to habits that allow them to engage in roles. For example, some clients may forget to perform everyday tasks of grooming, experience sleep disruption, and have no desire to complete regular routines. As one loses the everyday habits and roles, one becomes less able to reengage (low volition), and it becomes a cyclical problem.

Performance capacity refers to a person's mental and physical abilities required to participate in daily activities and the person's *subjective experience* and view of their occupational performance.[11] The objective information (physical and mental components) combined with a person's subjective experience influence what the person is able to accomplish within a given environment.

Clients experiencing mental health issues may forget things, show confusion, have difficulty sequencing tasks, or exhibit emotional lability. The disruption in mental abilities interferes with the person's ability to complete occupations. The person may begin to feel dissatisfied with their own performance, leading to a sense of failure and lack of belief in their own abilities (poor self-efficacy). They begin to believe they are incompetent or unable to perform, and this becomes their reality. Because they feel they are unable to perform, they may stop seeking out the opportunities that may yield enhanced performance over time.

Together the person factors (volition, habituation, and performance capacity) interact with and are influenced by the *environment*, which consists of physical, social, occupational, and cultural contexts.[12] Environment includes physical aspects (space, buildings, objects), social support (relationships, interactions), occupational qualities (activities and their properties), and cultural, economic, and political contexts. The occupational therapy practitioner can consider the immediate environment (home, school, work), the local context (community, social networks), and the global context (social attitudes, job market, policies).[13] The environment can support and provide opportunities or hinder and constrain by placing additional demands on a person that influence occupational performance; this is referred to as *environmental impact*.[12] Clients with mental health issues may face environmental constraints. They may live in a rural area that does not afford them access to transportation to mental health or community agencies that can support them. They may lose housing or work related to disruptions in thought processes and find themselves in unsupportive environments (either physical and/or social). For example, persons with addiction often have difficulty reestablishing healthy relationships and separating from the addictive environment. Modifying the environment can be part of the intervention plan.

MOHO theorizes that human behavior is a result of the interaction of volition, habituation, and performance capacity in a specific environment. It is a dynamic process whereby change in one system affects change in one's thoughts and feelings, and in turn may affect another system. Occupational therapy practitioners using MOHO evaluate all elements (i.e., volition, habituation, performance capacity, environment) and synthesize the information to prioritize how to facilitate change. Box 5.1 lists sample questions associated with each element of MOHO.

Principles

MOHO is a dynamic model of practice that examines the interactions between a person's volition, habituation, performance, and environment to design an occupation-based intervention. Understanding the relationship between these components allows the occupational therapy practitioner to intervene and promote meaningful engagement in occupations for the client that leads to self-efficacy and improved quality of life.[14,15] The principles of the MOHO (Box 5.2) outline human performance and describe how change can result in new patterns of performance.

BOX 5.1 Questions Associated With MOHO	
MOHO Element	**Sample Questions**
Volition	• What things that you do are important to you? (values) • What do you like to do? (interest) • Describe how you do these things? (personal causation)
Habituation	• What does a typical day consist of? (habits) • How do you spend your day? (habits) • What are your most important duties of the day? (roles) • What are the expectations you have for yourself in your day to day life? (role expectation)
Performance capacity	• How do you view your abilities? (subjective experience) • What is difficult for you? (subjective experience) • How has your current situation changed things? (subjective experience) • What are your thoughts regarding your current situation? (subjective experience) • What is difficult or easy for you to accomplish? (skills and abilities)
Environment	• What is your home, work, school like? (immediate–physical & occupational) • Who do you spend time with and what do you do? (immediate–social) • What is the community like where you spend your time? (local–physical) • Do you travel? If so, with whom? (global–physical, occupational, social) • What resources do you have to support you? (occupational supports) • What resources would help you? (occupational needs)

BOX 5.2 Principles of the Model of Human Occupation

• Occupational actions, thoughts, and emotions always arise out of the dynamic interaction of volition, habituation, performance capacity, and environmental context.
• Change in any aspect of volition, habituation, performance capacity, and/or the environment can result in a change in the thoughts, feelings, and doing.
• Volition, habituation, and performance capacity are maintained and changed through what one does and what one thinks and feels about doing.
• A particular pattern of volition, habituation, and performance capacity will be maintained so long as the underlying thoughts, feelings, and actions are consistently repeated in a supporting environment.
• Change requires that novel thoughts, feelings, and actions emerge and be sufficiently repeated in a supportive environment to coalesce into a new organized pattern. (Kielhofner, 2008; O'Brien & Kielhofner, 2017)

Occupational therapy practitioners seek to understand clients holistically so that they can create client-centered intervention plans that allow clients to engage in those things that are meaningful and satisfying. Examination of the client's volition, habituation, performance capacity, and environment allows occupational therapy practitioners to understand the person's actions, thoughts, and emotions to design an intervention. The occupational therapy practitioner synthesizes all the information gained from interview, observation, and assessment to understand the person's occupational performance and make treatment recommendations. This is a dynamic process in which the occupational therapy practitioner continually updates, modifies, and evaluates the client's progress toward the established goals.

Change may be elicited by targeting any aspect of volition, habituation, performance capacity, or environment. The occupational therapy practitioner uses clinical judgement to decide where to prioritize intervention. For example, the occupational therapy practitioner may decide to target a client's habits related to grooming to promote positive interactions among peers (social environment), feelings of self-efficacy, and to engage the client in performing physically. The occupational therapy practitioner may find that targeting grooming is a positive starting point and that the changes reflect in a variety of areas. The occupational therapy practitioner may decide that another client needs to begin with volition by making choices to get up and get dressed. MOHO postulates that change in any aspect (volition, habituation, performance capacity, environment) results in a change in thoughts, feelings, and actions.

The model's principle that volition, habituation, and performance capacity are maintained or changed by what one does and what one thinks and feels about doing, reminds therapists to take the time to encourage and promote both feeling and doing. Change can be elicited by encouraging clients to think about doing things in a different way and also by engaging clients in doing things differently. For example, a client who is trying to establish healthy leisure pursuits may begin therapy by discussing options and later trying some of the options. The occupational therapy practitioner provides a supportive environment to reinforce the client's healthy lifestyle choices and ensures that the client has the performance capacity to engage in the activity in the environment.

The occupational therapy practitioner acknowledges that "change requires that novel thoughts, feelings, and actions emerge and be sufficiently repeated in a supportive environment to coalesce into a new organized pattern." [16] Therefore occupational therapy practitioners who understand the client's volition understand how to promote novel thoughts, feelings, and actions. For example, Hank, a middle-aged client, lacks current interests and expresses no desire to engage in community or family activity. During the initial interview, the occupational therapy practitioner uncovers that in his teen years Hank sang in a band with three friends. After probing, the occupational therapy practitioner learns he sang country songs and even dabbled in writing lyrics. The occupational therapy practitioner uses Hank's past interests in conjunction with new technology and asks him to help a younger peer put words to a beat (country). Hank is encouraged and feels a connection with the teen who is also interested in music. As Hank works with the teen, the occupational therapy practitioner notices his activity level increases and he comes to sessions well groomed. After several weeks, Hank expresses a desire to volunteer to work with teens at the YMCA. Change required that the occupational therapy practitioner help the client reframe his past interests to do things differently.

Assessments Based on MOHO

MOHO includes 15 assessments (see Table 5.1) and three programmatic manuals that address mental health issues: *Work Rehabilitation in Mental Health Programs*; *Work Readiness: Day Treatment for Persons with Chronic Diseases*; and *The Remotivation Process*. These resources are available through the MOHO Clearinghouse (https://www.moho. uic.edu/), which also provides a summary of evidence to support MOHO intervention and several translations of materials. MOHO assessments are easily adapted to a

---

TABLE 5.1 Assessments Based on the Model of Human Occupation (MOHO Clearinghouse, 2018)

Assessment	Reference	Description
The Assessment of Communication and Interaction Skills (ACIS)	Forsyth K, Salamy M, Simon, S., Kielhofner, G. *The Assessment of Communication and Interaction Skills.* [Version 4.0]. Chicago: Model of Human Occupation Clearinghouse, Department of Occupational Therapy. University of Illinois at Chicago; 1998.	An observational assessment that evaluates communication and interaction skills used to accomplish daily occupations.
Assessment of Work Performance (AWP)	Sandqvist J, Lee J, Kielhofner G. *Assessment of Work Performance.* [Version 1.0]. Chicago: Model of Human Occupation Clearinghouse, Department of Occupational Therapy. University of Illinois at Chicago; 2010.	Addresses client's observable work-related skills. AWP assesses 3 skill domains: motor, process and communication, and interaction skills.
Child Occupational Self Assessment (COSA)	Kramer J, ten Velden M, Kafkes A, Basu S, Federico J, Kielhofner G. *Child Occupational Self Assessment.* [Version 2.2]. Chicago: Model of Human Occupation Clearinghouse, Department of Occupational Therapy. University of Illinois at Chicago; 2014.	A self-report that asks young clients to report their sense of competence (how well do they feel they perform) when performing and values (importance) for everyday activities in their home, school, and community.
The Model of Human Occupation Screening Tool (MOHOST)	Parkinson S, Forsyth K, Kielhofner G. *The Model of Human Occupation Screening Tool.* [Version 2.0]. Chicago: Model of Human Occupation Clearinghouse, Department of Occupational Therapy. University of Illinois at Chicago; 2006.	Addresses majority of MOHO concepts, allowing therapist to gain an overview of the client's occupational functioning.

Continued

TABLE 5.1   Assessments Based on the Model of Human Occupation (MOHO Clearinghouse, 2018)—cont'd

Assessment	Reference	Description
The Occupational Circumstances Assessment Interview and Rating Scale (OCAIRS)	Forsyth K, Deshplande S, Kielhofner G, et al. *The Occupational Circumstances Assessment Interview and Rating Scale*. [Version 4.0]. Chicago: Model of Human Occupation Clearinghouse, Department of Occupational Therapy. University of Illinois at Chicago; 2005.	Semi-structured interview that reports on the extent and nature of an individual's occupational participation.
The Occupational Performance History Interview-II (OPHI-II)	Kielhofner G, Mallinson T, Crawford C, et al. *The Occupational Performance History Interview II*. [Version 2.1]. Chicago: Model of Human Occupation Clearinghouse. Department of Occupational Therapy. University of Illinois at Chicago; 2004.	Semi-structured interview that explores a client's life history in the areas of work, play, and self-care performance.
Occupational Self Assessment (OSA)	Baron K, Kielhofner G, Iyenger A, Goldhammer V, Wolenski J. *Occupational Self Assessment*. [Version 2.2]. Chicago: Model of Human Occupation Clearinghouse, Department of Occupational Therapy. University of Illinois at Chicago; 2006.	Reflecting on the uniqueness of each client's values and needs, the OSA is a tool that facilitates client-centered therapy. The OSA self-report and planning forms assist the client in establishing priorities for change and identifying goals. The client reports those things that are important (values) and their ability to complete those things (perceived competency).
The Occupational Therapy Psychosocial Assessment of Learning (OTPAL)	Townsend S, Carey D, Hollins N, et al. *The Occupational Therapy Psychosocial Assessment of Learning*. [Version 2.0]. Chicago: Model of Human Occupation Clearinghouse, Department of Occupational Therapy. University of Illinois at Chicago; 2001.	The assessment uses observation and interviews to evaluate a student's volition (the ability to make choices), habituation (roles and routines), and environmental fit within the classroom setting.
The Pediatric Volitional Questionnaire (PVQ)	Basu S, Kafkes A, Schatz R, Kiraly A, Kielhofner G. *The Pediatric Volitional Questionnaire*. [Version 2.1]. Chicago: Model of Human Occupation Clearinghouse, Department of Occupational Therapy. University of Illinois at Chicago; 2008.	Observational assessment designed to evaluate a young child's volition, including motivation, values, and interests, and the impact of the environment.
Residential Environmental Impact Scale (REIS)	Fisher G, Forsyth K, Harrison M, et al. *Residential Environment Impact Scale* [Version 4.0]. Chicago: Model of Human Occupation Clearinghouse. Department of Occupational Therapy. University of Illinois at Chicago; 2014.	Assessment to evaluate how well a community living environment meets the needs of the resident(s). Strengths and areas for improvement are determined using structured observations and interviews of the resident(s) and caregivers.
Role Checklist	Scott, P.J. *Role Checklist [Version 3.0]. (measure of role participation)*. Chicago: Model of Human Occupation Clearinghouse. Department of Occupational Therapy. University of Illinois at Chicago. 2015.	The newest version of the Role Checklist focuses on current satisfaction with performance and whether the client is satisfied waiting for future opportunities for role engagement or whether they would prefer to engage currently.

TABLE 5.1   Assessments Based on the Model of Human Occupation (MOHO Clearinghouse, 2018)—cont'd

Assessment	Reference	Description
The Short Child Occupational Profile (SCOPE)	Bowyer P, Kramer J, Ploszaj A, et al. *The Short Child Occupational Profile.* [Version 2.2.] Chicago: Model of Human Occupation Clearinghouse. Department of Occupational Therapy. University of Illinois at Chicago; 2008.	SCOPE is an assessment of participation that determines how volition, habituation, skills and the environment facilitate or restrict a child's participation.
The School Setting Interview (SSI)	Hemmingsson H, Egilson S, Hoffman O, Kielhofner G. *The School Setting Interview.* [Version 3.0]. Chicago: Model of Human Occupation Clearinghouse. Department of Occupational Therapy. University of Illinois at Chicago; 2005.	Semi-structured interview that is designed to assess student-environment fit and identify the need for accommodations in the school setting.
The Volitional Questionnaire (VQ)	de las Heras C, Geist R, Kielhofner G. Li Y. *The Volitional Questionnaire.* [Version 4.1]. Chicago: Model of Human Occupation Clearinghouse. Department of Occupational Therapy. University of Illinois at Chicago; 2007.	Observational assessment that evaluates a client's volition, including motivation, values, and interests, as well as the influence of the environment.
Work Environment Impact Scale (WEIS)	Moore-Corner R, Kielhofner G, Olson L. *Work Environment Impact Scale.* [Version 2.0]. Chicago: Model of Human Occupation Clearinghouse, Department of Occupational Therapy. University of Illinois at Chicago; 1998.	Semi-structured interview that evaluates features in the work environment that support or impede occupational performance, and the impact on a person's performance, satisfaction, and well-being.
Worker Role Interview (WRI)	Braveman B, Robson M, Velozo C, Kielhofner G, Forsyth K, Kerschbaum J. *Worker Role Interview.* [Version 10.0]. Chicago: Model of Human Occupation Clearinghouse. Department of Occupational Therapy. University of Illinois at Chicago; 2005.	Semi-structured interview used to evaluate injured workers in the areas of personal causation, values, interests, roles, habits, and perception of environmental support.

variety of clients and include different versions. They are flexible assessments with sound psychometric properties.

Techniques and Strategies

After establishing a rapport and gaining a thorough understanding of the client's circumstances, strengths, weaknesses, and desires, occupational therapy practitioners use a variety of strategies to empower clients to engage in those things they find meaningful. Occupational therapy practitioners use therapeutic reasoning to establish goals and activities tailored to meet the client's needs. The occupational therapy practitioner considers the unique interactions between the MOHO elements (volition, habituation, performance capacity, and environment) to evaluate and determine where to begin and prioritize intervention. In mental health settings, the occupational therapy practitioner facilitates change in the client's thoughts, feelings, and actions so that the client adapts and engages in new or modified occupations. Intervention is aimed at engaging the client in different patterns of doing that will support client success.

The MOHO identifies nine therapeutic strategies (e.g., validating, identifying, giving feedback, advising, negotiating, structuring, coaching, encouraging, and providing physical support) to facilitate change in occupational performance.[17] See Box 5.3 for definitions of each therapeutic strategy. Occupational therapy practitioners use these strategies throughout intervention, reflecting carefully on how the client is progressing toward their goals and the effectiveness of the strategies. Case study 5.1 illustrates how these strategies may be used in a mental health setting.

Specific Intervention Procedures

Along with the strategies detailed above, intervention procedures based on MOHO have been developed for mental health settings to facilitate changes in the client's participation in occupations. This requires that the client shifts their thinking and performance. It is an unfolding process that leads to new or different occupational patterns and responses. If the intervention is not successful, occupational

BOX 5.3 **Therapeutic Strategies**[17]

Therapeutic Strategies	Definition
Validate	Convey respect for the client's experience or perspective.
Identify	Locate and share a range of personal, procedural, and/or environmental factors that can facilitate occupational performance and participation.
Give feedback	Share an overall conceptualization of the client's situation or an understanding of the client's ongoing action.
Advise	Recommend intervention goals and strategies to the client.
Negotiate	Engage in give-and-take with the client to achieve a common perspective or agreement about something that the client will or should do in the future.
Structure	Establish parameters for choice and performance by offering clients alternatives, setting limits, and establishing ground rules.
Coach	Instruct, demonstrate, and cue to teach new skills or abilities to clients.
Encourage	Provide emotional support and reassurance.
Physically support	To use the physical body to support the completion of an occupational form or part of an occupational form when clients cannot or will not use their motor skills or initiative for doing, or to accompany a client somewhere.

CASE STUDY 5.1

Kevin is a 58-year-old man diagnosed with bipolar disorder. He lives in the city alone. When he attends the outpatient intervention session, he is disheveled and has poor hygiene. After completing the Role Checklist (Scott, 2015) and the Occupational Self Assessment (OSA) (Baron et al., 2006) and engaging in conversation with Kevin, the occupational therapy practitioner decides to focus on establishing healthy habits and routines to support Kevin's engagement in social activities within the community.

The occupational therapy practitioner begins the session by *validating* how difficult it may be to live alone in the city and how disruptive mental health issues may be on daily habits and routines. Together they *identify* personal (Kevin enjoys using his smartphone, has good physical skills, and has a college education), procedural (how to facilitate habits and routines consistently), and environmental (apartment, stores nearby, friends who can check in, outpatient therapy support) factors that can facilitate occupational performance. In this case the occupational therapy practitioner and Kevin are working toward independence in completing habits consistently, so that Kevin develops self-confidence to engage in social events again. The occupational therapy practitioner *gives feedback* after each session on Kevin's appearance, and they discuss issues and solutions. The occupational therapy practitioner *encourages* Kevin to use his supports and *coaches* him on routines that ensure success. Over time, Kevin consistently uses his smartphone to schedule hygiene and grooming, sleep schedules, leisure breaks, and medication management. He buys an activity tracker (Fitbit) to ensure he is getting adequate activity and sleep and takes time each day to connect with at least one friend. The occupational therapy practitioner helped Kevin adapt his occupational performance and establish healthy routines that provide him with a new *occupational identity* and sense of satisfaction and quality of life.

Baron, K., Kielhofner, G., Iyenger, A., Goldhammer, V., & Wolenski, J. (2006). *The Occupational Self-Assessment (OSA)* [Version 2.2]. Chicago: Model of Human Occupation Clearinghouse, Department of Occupational Therapy, College of Applied Health Sciences, University of Illinois at Chicago.
Scott, P. (2015). *Role Checklist v.3 (measure of role participation)*. Retrieved from wwww.rolechecklist.com

therapy practitioners reevaluate and revise intervention. MOHO provides the structure, assessments, and sample intervention procedures and strategies to assist occupational therapy practitioners working in mental health settings. The following paragraphs describe intervention approaches used with MOHO.

Evaluation Doubling as Intervention

The process begins with the evaluation, where the occupational therapy practitioner develops a rapport with the client and empowers the client to share, discuss, and make decisions. Allowing clients to tell their story and frame their experiences is therapeutic and part of mental health intervention.

Participation in Meaningful Occupations

Clients engage in meaningful occupations (whereby the occupational therapy practitioner grades the challenges so the client is successful). Clients may need encouragement or structure to participate, and they may need emotional and physical support. Participating in meaningful occupations can help them discover strengths, past interests, and new interests and allow clients to reinvent their story. Through meaningful occupations, clients may discover a new or reimagined identity and sense of self, possibly enabling them to adapt to situations more easily and develop coping skills.

Facilitation of Exploration

Sometimes clients experience loss in their interests, activities, and skills. They may not have the problem-solving skills or resources (physical, emotional, or cognitive) to identify new ways to engage in the community. Occupational therapy intervention may help clients begin exploring options and empower them by engaging them in the process.

Occupational Consulting

Occupational therapy practitioners may help clients problem-solve, negotiate, and develop occupational identity and competence. This requires a client-centered consultation approach where the occupational therapy practitioner engages in a conversation with the client and helps identify occupations that may fulfill the client's needs. Occupational therapy practitioners have unique knowledge of the skills and abilities required to complete daily activities, and they also are able to make modifications to ensure success. Case study 5.2 provides an example of occupational consulting.

MOHO-Based Skills Teaching

Some clients may need to learn specific MOHO-based skills so they are able to engage in their desired occupations. For example, a client may need to identify their values, interests, and beliefs in their skills. It may be important for clients to establish habits to complete daily activities safely. Some clients with mental health issues may need to develop coping skills that can be taught or practiced within an occupational therapy intervention session. MOHO can also be used with other frames of reference, such as cognitive behavioral therapy, coping, or sensory modulation.

Peer Support Educational Groups

Peer groups may be beneficial to provide clients with support and education. For example, grief support groups may help clients relate to peers who understand. Peer groups may provide resources and education on specific topics, such as local activities, financial management, leisure, and coping with mental illness.

Occupational Self-Help Groups

Self-help groups focus on helping clients work through issues that allow them to engage in desired occupations. The group may have a common theme (e.g., independent living or return to work) that they work on together. Occupational self-help groups empower members to support each other and cooperate to create strategies for success. These groups may serve as networking possibilities for clients in the community.

CASE STUDY 5.2

Cassie is a 29-year-old woman admitted to an inpatient mental health hospital after a suicide attempt. The occupational therapist completes a thorough evaluation and hypothesizes that Cassie has not established a firm occupational identity. Cassie's boyfriend recently broke up with her and she does not have a steady job or friends close by. She states her boyfriend left her because she does not "party" anymore. Cassie has been sober for 6 months. The therapist provides *occupational coaching*, by exploring work, leisure, and healthy options within the community. The therapist engages Cassie in the Worker Role Interview[18] to find out how she sees her work-related skills and what supports and training she needs to succeed. The therapist asks probing questions to *encourage* Cassie to think closely about her values and beliefs (volition), and they spend time examining her strengths (personal causation) to see if they can match occupations to her values and interests. This *structure* makes it easier for Cassie to identify options. She creates a "vision board" and applies for several positions. The therapist *validates* her decisions and *coaches* her on the next steps. Over the course of therapy, Cassie engages in some work-related tasks, job shadows, explores a variety of work options, and role plays interviewing. The therapist *advises*, *gives feedback*, and *encourages* Cassie on interviewing and work expectations. The intervention focused on occupational consulting regarding the worker role. Using MOHO as the model, the therapist helped Cassie establish a strong *occupational identity* by exploring work that was volitionally motivating and promoted healthy habits and routines within a positive environment for which she perceived she had adequate skills and abilities (self-efficacy).

Social Groups Education

Some clients may benefit from social groups where the occupational therapy practitioner addresses habits (e.g., grooming, hygiene), routines, and skills to engage in social activities. Oftentimes, therapists use role-play, community outings with reflection, and discussion to educate clients on social expectations. They may coach clients, validate the difficulty of the situations, give feedback, and advise clients.

Environmental Management

Occupational therapy may emphasize restructuring the environment so the client is successful and safe. This may involve educating clients on the resources available to them in the environment and how to access the resources. It may also involve helping clients develop safe living situations (such as managing their home).

Occupational Role Development and Habit Change

Occupational therapy practitioners help clients establish new roles or regain previous roles (e.g., friend, family member). The therapist provides structure to model roles and routines, and reinforces occupational development through coaching, providing feedback, validating, and advising. As the client develops abilities and changes their performance, the therapist encourages and provides positive support that may lead to a new or modified occupational identity. Case study 5.3 provides an example of facilitating occupational role development and habit change.

CASE STUDY 5.3

Margie is a 60-year-old woman who experiences episodes of severe depression leading to difficulty engaging in work, household, and community activities. She lives alone in a city apartment and states she has close friends who live nearby. She enjoys spending time with her friends, going out for coffee, visiting local festivals, and cooking together. Margie works close by at a jewelry store, where she has been employed for 10 years. She has been hospitalized several times for depression. She is currently in an inpatient psychiatric setting to manage her medications and develop an outpatient intervention plan. Margie was admitted after missing work for 10 days and not answering her phone. She was found lying on her bed in her apartment and crying. Table 5.2 summarizes the findings of her initial interview using the Occupational Performance History Interview-II (OPHI-II).[19]

The occupational therapy practitioner summarized that Margie's environment provides support for her, she has medical insurance, friends, food, and entertainment nearby. She does not have to drive to have her occupational needs met and has access to green spaces. Margie's volition and habituation are low currently, secondary to clinical depression. This interferes with her ability to work and engage in leisure. She is at risk for losing her job due to frequent absences. Margie has a history of engaging in a variety of leisure and social activities; however, Margie exhibits slow movements and difficulty initiating tasks at the current time.

The occupational therapy practitioner and client determine that Margie would benefit from a structured routine (habituation) to promote medication management (performance capacity) and increase her motivation to engage in work and social activities. The therapist hypothesizes that engaging in a routine will help Margie become more active until she is feeling motivated to participate in her daily occupations. In this scenario, engaging Margie in daily occupations (grooming, dressing, and preparing for work) may facilitate feelings of competency and success. This is an example of "doing" to improve one's abilities at doing (the occupation as a means and end). Afraid that Margie may lose her job, which may result in financial difficulties and lack of the worker role (one she values) and may lead to a low sense of self-efficacy (volition), the therapist begins the session by encouraging Margie to call her boss. The therapist *coaches* Margie and together they develop a script. The therapist *gives feedback* to Margie and *validates* Margie's anxiety about calling her boss. After Margie makes the phone call, they discuss the outcome. Margie is relieved and able to smile that she has kept her job. The therapist reinforces Margie's strengths by asking her to restate why she thinks her boss did not fire her for missing work. Margie is able to identify that she is a good employee who is loyal, good with customers, and consistent, when she is feeling well (this means taking her medications consistently). Together, the therapist and Margie develop a plan (*provide structure*) to help Margie maintain her occupational roles, which Margie identifies as friend, worker, renter, community member, and person with mental health issues. Again, the therapist *validates* Margie's assessment and together they develop a plan. Margie has established strategies to maintain her occupational identity and continue to engage in her valued occupations. This example highlights the complex nature of occupational behaviors on which MOHO provides insight.

TABLE 5.2 Summary of Margie's Occupational Profile	
Volition	Past: Margie enjoys work and spending time with friends, going to coffee shops, cooking meals together, and going to local festivals. Current: She states there is nothing she wants to do, she is bad at everything and she can't do her job well. Margie is tearful and sullen with low energy.
Habituation	Past: Margie works 5 days a week from 9–4 and has weekends free. She gets up at 7:00 am, grooms, dresses, has breakfast, walks to work, returns, prepares dinner, and relaxes before bedtime. Weekend routine: Margie cleans her apartment, goes grocery shopping, and socializes. Current: Margie has not worked in 2 weeks or socialized with friends. She states she may have already lost her job. She is not caring for herself. She has not bathed or groomed, has not eaten consistently, and has stopped taking her medications. There was no food in the house and it was not well kept.
Performance capacity	Past: Margie lived independently, managed her health (medications, diet, exercise), and socialized on a regular basis with friends. She worked a steady job where her boss stated she was pleasant with customers, knowledgeable, and on time (unless she is experiencing a severe depression episode as she has in the past). Because she is a valuable employee, her boss allows the absences and checks up on her. He states Margie is pleasant and shows a nice sense of humor with familiar people and customers. Current: Margie was difficult to engage in conversation and answered questions with short one-word responses. She walked slowly. Margie spoke softly and did not make eye contact with the therapist. She had difficulty following multistep directions.
Environment	Margie lives in an apartment in a city. She walks to work and has easy access to stores (grocery, drugstore, clothing) and leisure activities (festivals, shops, theater). The environment has outdoor areas (a walking path along a river and park). Margie has lived in the city for 20 years and has many friends nearby. Margie has disability insurance that covers her expenses and medical costs when she is not able to work. Current: Margie has not left her apartment in 10 days and is not caring for herself. Her friends checked up on her when she would not return calls.

PERSON-ENVIRONMENT-OCCUPATION-PERFORMANCE (PEOP) MODEL

The Person-Environment-Occupation-Performance (PEOP) Model was developed in the 1980s and first published in 1991.[20] The PEOP Model was updated in 1997,[21] 2005,[22] and most recently in 2015[23] in recognition of advancements in knowledge within occupational therapy practice and within other biomedical and sociocultural fields. The PEOP Model was conceived from knowledge within occupational science, neuroscience, environmental science, and other biological and social sciences to identify, clarify, and emphasize the unique contributions of occupational therapy to the health, participation, and well-being of individuals, populations, and organizations.[23] The PEOP Model makes explicit occupational therapy's role in supporting occupational performance through the intersection of person, environment, and occupation factors. The model emphasizes using a client-centered approach and collaboration with the client and team, regardless of the occupational therapy practitioner's setting or level of care, the client's age, life stage, diagnosis, or occupational performance challenge.

Overview

The PEOP Model includes four parts that are key to understanding the occupational performance of individuals, organizations, and populations: the narrative, person factors, occupation factors, and environment factors (see Fig. 5.2). The PEOP Model describes the narrative as "the past, current, and future perceptions, choices, interests, goals, and needs that are unique to the Person, Organization, or Population."[23] The narrative (personal story) is the start of the occupational therapy process, guides the development of an occupational profile, and provides understanding of the client's perspective regarding their own occupational performance challenges, needs, and values. The narrative provides the occupational therapist with information about the past, current, and future needs, desires, and goals from the client perspective. The PEOP Model describes aspects of the narrative for

PEOP: Enabling Everyday Living

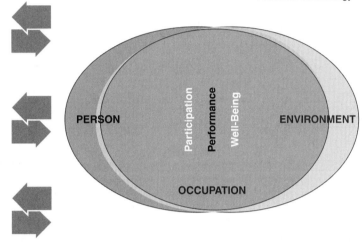

THE NARRATIVE	PERSON	OCCUPATION	ENVIRONMENT
The past, current, and future perceptions, choices, interests, goals, and needs that are unique to the Person, Organization, or Population	• Cognition • Psychological • Physiological • Sensory/Perceptual • Motor • Spirituality/Meaning	• Activities, Tasks, Roles • Classifications	• Cultural Environment • Social Support • Social Determinants and Social Capital • Health Education and Public Policy • Physical and Natural Environment • Assistive Technology

Personal Narrative
• Perceptions and Meaning
• Choices and Responsibilities
• Attitudes and Motivations
• Needs and Goals

Organizational Narrative
• Mission and History
• Focus and Priorities
• Stakeholders and Values
• Needs and Goals

Population/Community Narrative
• Environments and Behaviors
• Demographics and Disparities
• Incidence and Prevalence
• Needs and Goals

PERSON — Participation Performance Well-Being — ENVIRONMENT

OCCUPATION

The **performance** of occupation (doing) enables the **participation** (engagement) in everyday life that contributes to a sense of **well-being** (satisfaction).

Fig. 5.2 Person-Environment-Occupation-Performance Model. (From Baum CM, Bass JD, Christiansen, CH. The Person-Environment-Occupation-Performance (PEOP) Model. In CH Christiansen, CM Baum, JD Bass eds., *Occupational Therapy: Performance, Participation, and Well-Being*, 4th ed., pp. 49-55. Thorofare, NJ: SLACK Inc; 2015.)

individuals, organizations, and populations (see examples in Box 5.4).

The PEOP Model identifies factors that come together to support performance, participation, and well-being. The occupational therapy practitioner, in collaboration with the client, identifies the personal capabilities or constraints (person factors) and the environmental enablers or barriers (environment factors) that will guide the intervention process and ultimately support the client's participation in meaningful occupations. Table 5.3 describes the person, occupation, and environment factors that are utilized in the PEOP model.

Principles

The PEOP Model proposes the following key principles for occupational therapy practitioners to use when planning and implementing interventions: client-centered, evidence based, ethics and advocacy, communication, culture,

professional lifelong development, business fundamentals, and therapeutic use of self. The PEOP Model outlines several aims, including that the model values collaboration, is focused on occupational performance, emphasizes a systems perspective, and supports client-centered practice.[23]

Collaboration: The model values and requires client input to guide decision-making, goal setting, and intervention planning. The PEOP Model stipulates that occupational therapy intervention with a client may be direct intervention with an individual (e.g., patient, child, adult, family), in collaboration with other professionals (e.g., health care team members), or with an organization or entire community.

Occupational performance: The PEOP Model emphasizes the active (*doing*) component of occupational performance and defines occupational performance as "the doing of meaningful activities, tasks, and roles through complex interactions between the person and environment."[23] The model is based on the premise that

BOX 5.4   **Examples of Aspects of the PEOP Occupational Therapy Process Narrative**

Person-Centered Narrative	Population-Centered Narrative	Organization-Centered Narrative
• Individual's interests, goals and concerns • Client's perceptions of their own strengths and challenges • Roles and responsibilities	• Characteristics of the population or community (e.g., demographics, geographic area, values, preferences) • Priorities, goals, and concerns • Stakeholders • Disparities • Environments	• Organization mission and vision • Goals • Funding sources • Stakeholders

TABLE 5.3   **Person, Occupation, and Environment Factors: Examples and Questions**

Factors	Examples	Questions to Consider*
Person Factors		
Cognition	Attention Memory and learning Social awareness (theory of mind) Communication and social skills Executive functions Awareness (insight)	How do cognitive factors interact with the whole person in context? How do cognitive factors influence capacity to perform occupations? How might personal and environmental resources be maximized to support performance and participation for given cognitive status?
Psychological	Identity Self-concept Self-esteem Self-efficacy Mood Emotional regulation Motivation Coping	How do narratives help understand psychological factors? What is the relationship between psychological factors and well-being and life balance? How do interventions for psychological factors enable skills for daily life?
Physiological	Physical fitness Nutrition Sleep Stress Pain Skin integrity	How do tissues, organs, and systems support biological function? How does adequate physiological functioning support the capacity for daily functioning? How does performance in physical activity support physiological functioning?
Sensory	Vision Audition Olfactory and gustatory Tactile Proprioception Vestibular Multisensory	How do sensory factors support occupational performance? What populations or conditions may have impairments in sensory factors? How are sensory factors evaluated using standard measures?
Motor	Motor control Motor learning Strength Muscle tone Balance and postural control Coordination	How does practice and feedback support motor learning in occupational performance? What motor behaviors are associated with specific conditions? How do task-oriented approaches support occupational performance?

Continued

TABLE 5.3 Person, Occupation, and Environment Factors: Examples and Questions—cont'd

Factors	Examples	Questions to Consider*
Spirituality	Meaning Mind–body connections Motivation Values and beliefs	How do personal life stories provide information on a person's spirituality and meaning? How do beliefs, values, and goals influence occupational performance? How are spiritual practices related to occupational performance?
Occupation Factors		
Activities, tasks, and roles	Habits and routines Lifestyle and life balance Time use	How does development and stage of life impact participation in meaningful activities? What routines and patterns of daily occupations influence health and well-being?
Environment Factors		
Culture	Values Beliefs Customs Norms Communication Standards Power Decision-making Practices Shared ideas	Why do individuals have multiple cultural identities? How does culture influence perceptions of occupational therapy and occupational performance? How are client-centered care and culturally sensitive care similar?
Social determinants	Social cohesion Social connectedness Structural factors Health disparities Health inequalities	How do the circumstances in which one is born and live influence performance, participation, well-being? Why are there inequalities/disparities in occupational performance? What occupational therapy intervention approaches are recommended to address social determinants?
Social support and social capital	Informational, tangible, and belonging Community and societal cooperation	Who can provide positive and helpful support to the client? How is the client's occupational performance influenced by their neighborhood or community?
Education and Policy	Access Utilization Advocacy Costs Policies Procedures Systems	How does public policy influence occupational therapy services? What is the relationship between policy and performance, participation, and well-being? What key policies affect individuals who receive occupational therapy services?
Physical and Natural	Space Products Built environment Climate, terrain, and population density	What barriers in the physical and natural environment affect performance, participation, and well-being? What is meant by person–environment fit? How do interventions that address the physical and natural environment change performance?
Assistive Technology	Accessibility Universal design Ergonomics Seating and mobility	How does well-designed technology support performance? How is the functionality of technology evaluated? What are the evaluation components that are important in determining technology needs?

*Questions contributed by Carolyn Baum, Theresa Carroll, and Ashley Stoffel.

occupational performance supports and enables participation in everyday life, which contributes to overall well-being (health, satisfaction, and quality of life).[23]

Systems perspective: The PEOP Model acknowledges the reciprocal relationship between person, environment, and occupation factors. Occupational therapy practitioners using the PEOP Model recognize the dynamic nature of occupational performance and utilize this reciprocal relationship to influence occupational outcomes. For example, a change in a client's capacity, occupational choices, or environmental aspects could result in a change in occupational performance. It is important to recognize that the client determines the outcomes that are important to them.[23]

Client-centered practice: The PEOP Model supports client-centered practice and emphasizes the importance of the partnership between the client and practitioner. The client's choices, interests, and context drive decision-making, goal-setting, and intervention planning. The collaborative

relationship allows occupational therapy practitioners to elicit a client's narrative, which is used to set meaningful goals for participation and well-being.

The fourth edition of the PEOP Model includes the PEOP Occupational Therapy Process (see Fig. 5.3), which is intended to guide occupational therapy practitioners through all the steps of implementing the PEOP Model.[23] The PEOP Occupational Therapy Process includes the narrative, assessment/evaluation, intervention, and outcome.

Assessments

The PEOP Occupational Therapy Process begins with eliciting the client's narrative through conversation and observation. The *narrative* assists in developing the client's occupational profile. The client and occupational therapy practitioner decide together if the client's needs and goals align with occupational therapy interventions and will proceed with the PEOP Occupational Therapy Process if

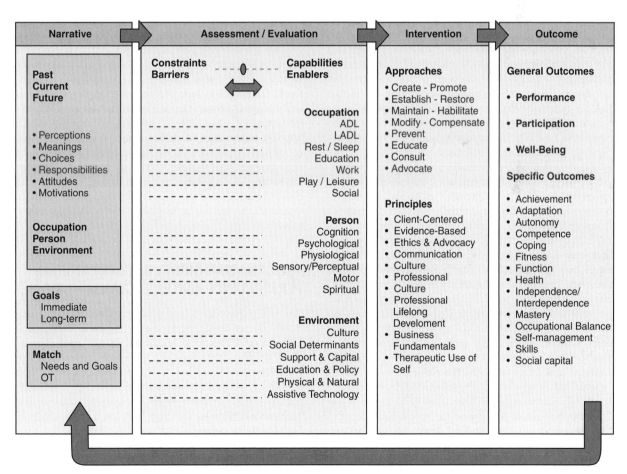

Fig. 5.3 Person-Centered PEOP Occupational Therapy Process.

there is a match, or make appropriate referrals if not.[23] The PEOP Model provides the PEOP Occupational Therapy Process as a guide to occupational therapy assessment and evaluation, and the authors explicitly encourage the occupational therapist to use readily available assessments with this model. The Activity Card Sort, 2nd ed.[24] is an example of an assessment that is based on PEOP principles. The activity card sort includes institutional, recovering, and community-living versions and can be used to support the development of the person-centered narrative as part of the PEOP Occupational Therapy Process. The client describes their participation in instrumental, leisure, and social activities by viewing and sorting photographs of adults performing various activities. An occupational therapist can partner with the client to understand the client's level of participation in activities and determine if activities have changed and why. This information, paired with additional assessment and evaluation results, supports the occupational therapist in developing a client-centered intervention plan that addresses the activities most meaningful to the client. The assessment and evaluation phase of the PEOP Occupational Therapy Process includes utilizing formal assessments with strong measurement characteristics and psychometric properties in order to ground this phase in evidence and provide a baseline for intervention planning. The occupational therapist uses assessments and information from the narrative to determine the factors that are constraints/barriers or capabilities/enablers.

In the PEOP Occupational Therapy Process, a continuum scale (see Fig. 5.3) is used to show the relationship between factors (i.e., which factors are strengths and which are potential problems for the client) and the client's overall status. The continuum scale is also used to represent change over time. For example, consider a 5-year-old child who was initially referred to occupational therapy by her parents due to concerns with self-regulation and difficulty participating in family gatherings and social events. As the occupational therapist developed an occupational profile for the child and family, it was revealed that the child's personal narrative included having been adopted by the current family after being in three different foster care placements due to removal from the birth home at 8 months of age after multiple traumatic experiences, including physical abuse. In this scenario, the personal narrative provided important foundational information to the occupational therapist in understanding the child's occupational performance challenges and strengths. The occupational therapist observed that the child had developed a solid attachment to the adoptive mother and looked to her for comfort and encouragement but showed signs of fear and hesitation around her adoptive father. Further evaluation of the child's capabilities and environment revealed that the child responded fearfully to all men in any setting whether or not that person was familiar to the child.

Using the PEOP Occupational Therapy Process Assessment/Evaluation continuum scale, the occupational therapist might place a marker closer to constraints/barriers on the psychological person factor and the social participation occupation factor. The occupational therapist might place a marker more toward capabilities/enablers for the social support environment factor due to the child being adopted by a highly invested and involved family.

Techniques and Strategies

The PEOP Model focuses on occupational performance and thus requires the use of a top-down client-centered strategy. The occupational therapy practitioner collaborates with the client to determine the client's perceptions around the important occupational performance challenges that are limiting participation and causing difficulties in carrying out the tasks and activities that are central to the client's roles. The PEOP Model includes a variety of intervention approaches that closely align with the intervention approaches used in the Occupational Therapy Practice Framework, 3rd ed.[26]: create-promote; establish-restore; maintain-habilitate; modify-compensate; prevent; educate; consult; and advocate. The overall outcomes of the PEOP Model include performance, participation, and well-being. Outcomes are essential to measuring the effectiveness of the PEOP Occupational Therapy Process. Specific outcomes and assessment choice for outcome measurement are driven by the client's perceptions of their occupational performance challenges and strengths. Case study 5.4 demonstrates the use of the PEOP Occupational Therapy Process: narrative, assessment/evaluation, intervention, and outcome. Case study 5.5 applies PEOP to address organizational change to benefit a child.

THE CANADIAN MODEL OF OCCUPATIONAL PERFORMANCE AND ENGAGEMENT (CMOP-E)

The Canadian Model of Occupational Performance (CMOP) was developed by the Canadian Association of Occupational Therapists as part of the national association's effort to create practice guidelines. A series of five consensus guidelines led to the publication of a book detailing the model and its application.[29] The CMOP emphasized the core concepts of enablement, social justice, and environment in the first iteration of the model.[29] *Enablement* is viewed as "a model of helping that promotes *empowerment*" and "as the positive form of the term *disablement*."[30] Social justice is the "vision and

CASE STUDY 5.4 Person-Centered PEOP Occupational Therapy Process: Anthony and Family

Anthony was 4 years old when his parents requested an occupational therapy evaluation. Anthony's preschool teachers brought up concerns to the parents that included inattention at circle time, aggressive behavior toward peers such as pushing, and difficulty making friends. During the initial evaluation, the occupational therapist used discussion and observation to discover Anthony's occupational history and profile (*person-centered narrative*). Anthony's parents and paternal grandmother all attended the initial evaluation at an outpatient clinic. Anthony is part of a bicultural and bilingual family. Both Spanish and English are spoken in the home. Anthony's mother is from Mexico and the family frequently visits relatives in Mexico. Anthony's father grew up in an urban setting in the USA. Anthony has a younger sister. Anthony's parents shared that they appreciate his preschool teachers alerting them to the concerns but they are not sure what to think about his behavior. His mother shared that she feels some of Anthony's behaviors are "normal for a Latino boy" and her parents have told her not to be worried. Anthony's paternal grandmother was a former preschool teacher and she expressed concerns that Anthony would not be able to learn and develop friendships as he was not able to sit still, attend to tasks, or have a conversation with another child. The occupational therapist used the Spanish version of the Preschool Activity Card Sort[27,28] to identify occupational performance challenges and strengths of Anthony and his family and to assist in setting meaningful goals. Formal assessments were also used to further understand Anthony's personal capabilities and constraints.

Using the PEOP Occupational Therapy Process Assessment/Evaluation continuum scale, the occupational therapist and Anthony's family marked the following toward the constraints/barriers: occupations of play, education, and social participation; person factors of sensory and psychological; and environment factors of culture, education, and policy. Toward the capabilities/enablers: occupations of activities of daily living (ADL) and sleep; person factors of physiological and motor; and environment factors of culture and social support were marked. It was interesting to note that Anthony's family reported culture as both a barrier and an enabler to their son's occupational performance, participation, and well-being. *Intervention* using the PEOP Occupational Therapy Process included modifications to both the home and community (e.g., church) environments by providing sensory aids (e.g., tactile cushion) to support Anthony's ability to remain seated and attentive during mealtimes and story time at Sunday school (*modify intervention approach*). Education regarding self-regulation strategies and sensory processing and the impact on participation was also provided to the parents and both the maternal and paternal grandparents (*educate and advocate intervention approaches*). Utilizing Anthony's strong social support and social capital (*environment factors*), his sister and neighbor children were included in intervention sessions to promote Anthony's social skill development. Later, sessions were provided at Anthony's home and a community park to enhance generalization. After 6 months of occupational therapy, example *outcomes* of the PEOP Occupational Therapy Process included Anthony independently seeking out a play opportunity with a neighbor child and Anthony's parents being able to advocate for their son and educate other caregivers and Anthony's teachers about his strengths and needs.

CASE STUDY 5.5 Organization-Centered PEOP Occupational Therapy Process: Anthony's School

When Anthony was in first grade, his parents reached out to the occupational therapist again. At this time, Anthony's occupational history and profile (*person-centered narrative*) revealed that he had no friends at school, his teacher reported difficulty engaging Anthony in school-related tasks, and the school principal discussed with the family that the private school was concerned about being able to provide continued supports for Anthony in second grade.

The occupational therapist collaborated with Anthony's family and school personnel to address both Anthony's needs and school-wide interventions. The *organization-centered narrative* included gaining an understanding of the private school's mission, values, funding, and stakeholders[25] and revealed that the private school principal was highly interested in learning how to support all children, including Anthony, who were experiencing mental health challenges such as self-regulation difficulties, anxiety, and depression that impacted academic and social performance at school. The occupational therapist completed observations in various classroom and school environments (e.g., playground, bus drop-off, physical education gym) and conducted semi-structured interviews with teachers and staff as part of the *assessment and evaluation*.

Continued

CASE STUDY 5.5   **Organization-Centered PEOP Occupational Therapy Process: Anthony's School—cont'd**

The PEOP Occupational Therapy Process Assessment/ Evaluation continuum scale for the organization (i.e., Anthony's private school) revealed environment factor barriers (education and policy), such as a need for teacher and administrative training to support participation of diverse learners in mainstream classrooms, and environment factor enablers (social support and capital), such as a highly supportive parent base and community, in addition to funding streams to support bullying prevention and positive social engagement for all children in the school. The occupational therapist used the *promote and prevent* and *educate and consult* intervention

approaches to develop and provide professional development training to the teachers, staff, and administrators at the school. The occupational therapist collaborated with teachers to implement a school-wide positive behavior and bullying prevention program based on evidence from occupational therapy interventions. An example of the organization-centered *outcomes* that were measured included using parent, student, and school personnel knowledge change surveys and having the teachers and administrators complete an action plan to determine changes in inclusivity and receptivity within the school environment.

---

everyday practice in which people can choose, organize, and engage in meaningful occupations that enhance health, quality of life, and equity in housing, employment, and other aspects of life."[29] Social justice is viewed as being linked to empowerment and enablement. Environment is considered broadly and includes "cultural, institutional, physical, and social elements that lie outside of individuals, yet are embodied in individual actions."[29] Spirituality is viewed as the essence of the self and encompasses purpose and meaning, a central focus in understanding human occupation.[31]

Principles

This model emphasizes client-centered practice as a collaborative partnership between the therapist and the client that would facilitate enabling occupation.[29] In 2007, the CMOP model was expanded to include engagement as the desired outcome, becoming the Canadian Model of Occupational Performance and Engagement (CMOP-E).[32] Fig. 5.4 illustrates the CMOP-E. The goal of creating the CMOP-E was to expand on the CMOP to include elements of performance that had not been explicit in the first model, such as the level of importance the performance holds for the person and satisfaction with performance. The expanded model reflects a broader scope of practice, one more focused on creating supportive environments and advancing a vision of health, well-being, and justice.[33]

In the CMOP-E, the authors emphasize *occupational engagement* and experience, which includes a broader understanding of cognitive and emotional involvement in performance.[32,34] Occupational performance is an active means to engagement. However, "humans frequently engage in occupations without performing them,"[32]

such as passively watching a sporting event or engaging in a theatrical or musical experience. Occupational performance and engagement are elaborated as the ultimate goals of therapy.[35]

Assessments

The Canadian Occupational Performance Measure (COPM)[36] is the only assessment tool developed along with the CMOP. This assessment, widely used as a screening tool and outcome measure, breaks occupational performance down into three occupational areas that are commonly known as self-care, productivity, and leisure. However, the rating process has not been revised since 2005[36]; therefore it has not included the CMOP-E's more recent emphasis of occupational engagement.

The COPM incorporates several principles of the CMOP-E, such as client-centeredness. By determining the areas that the client considers most important but is least satisfied with, the occupational therapist can tailor the therapy goals and intervention focus to address those identified areas of greatest concern. Calculating a change score reflects improvement, or lack thereof, between the first assessment and subsequent reassessments, a very useful metric for therapists measuring outcomes of intervention.

The COPM has some limitations, as it cannot be used with nonverbal clients or those who lack insight in their areas of dissatisfaction. It cannot be used with young children, although caregivers can be used as proxy informants. Studies have been conducted to evaluate the utility of the COPM.[37,38] A systematic review by Parker and Sykes found 64 journal articles on the COPM and more have been published since that time.[39] They concluded that there may be

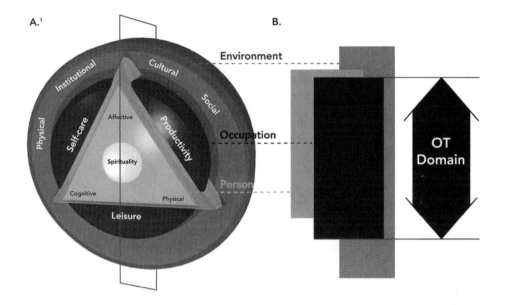

A.[1] Referred to as the CMOP in *Enabling Occupation* (1997a, 2002) and CMOP-E as of this edition
B. Trans-sectional view

Fig. 5.4 Canadian Model of Occupational Performance and Engagement. (From Polatajko HJ, Townsend EA, Craik J. Canadian Model of Occupational Performance and Engagement. In Townsend EA, Polatajko HJ, eds. *Enabling Occupation II: Advancing an Occupational Therapy Vision for Health, Well-being, and Justice Through Occupation.* Ottawa: CAOT ACE, 2007.)

difficulties using the COPM with clients with significant cognitive deficits or acute mental illness,[39] as individuals with mental illness may have trouble articulating areas of difficulty. This does not mean it cannot be used in a psychosocial context, but extra time may be needed to perform the assessment. In some instances, individuals may need to complete the COPM after acute symptoms have subsided.

The COPM has been translated into 25 languages and used in 40 countries. Training materials cover administration, scoring, and reassessment and include video examples and sample materials (www.thecopm.ca).

Techniques and Strategies

The CMOP-E's *Canadian Practice Process Framework* describes a step-by-step process for implementing the model. The *Canadian Model of Client-Centered Enablement* presents core skills for enabling occupation (Box 5.5),[32] emphasizing the importance of the start and closure of the therapeutic relationship as depicted in both the framework and model listed above. Terry Krupa described the three aspects of the model as the "Canadian Triple Model Frame-

work for Enabling Occupation."[31] Over 60 occupational therapists have contributed to the development of the CMOP-E triple model framework to advance the application of the ideals of health, well-being, and justice through occupation.[31] The CMOP-E provides guidelines for the usage of the three components in organizations and communities, and is useful in the growing trend of occupational therapists working with communities and populations.[35]

An occupational therapist using the CMOP-E focuses on *enabling* occupation through identifying gaps between desired and actual occupational participation, such as with the use of the COPM as it identifies performance and satisfaction scores.[36] *Collaboration* with the client is a key component, and goal setting is viewed as an opportunity to set priorities together. Therapeutic approaches to bridge the gaps that prevent optimal occupational performance include *establishing/restoring* ability or skill, and *modifying* the task or activity demands to promote *compensatory strategies*.[26] Assisting clients to maintain their level of performance or to prevent secondary conditions are also relevant to this model, as are health promotion

BOX 5.5	Canadian Model of Client-Centered Enablement: Skills for Enabling
Key skills	**Selected Examples of Related Enablement Skills**
Adapt	Accommodate, adjust, break occupations into components, observe, tailor
Advocate	Challenge, champion, enlighten, lobby, promote, raise consciousness, strategize
Coach	Encourage, guide, expand choices, listen, mentor, motivate, reflect, reframe
Collaborate	Communicate, cooperate, facilitate, form alliances, mediate, negotiate, partner
Consult	Advise, brainstorm options, confer, recommend, synthesize, summarize
Coordinate	Arrange, document, integrate, allocate resources, link, manage, network
Design/build	Conceive, construct, create, develop, fabricate, plan, strategize, visualize
Educate	Demonstrate, enlighten, instruct, inform, promote learning, teach, train, tutor
Engage	Build trust, develop readiness, involve, optimize potential, spark hope
Specialize	Facilitate body function, apply hands-on techniques and specialized frameworks

approaches.[26] The use of *environmental adaptation*, including the modification of the environmental context or task demands to support performance, is emphasized in the CMOP-E.

To build *client-centeredness*, the occupational therapist can use questions that aim at creating a relationship that is based on collaboration and justice, such as, "Am I providing real choices when I work with this person?" and "Do I truly listen to what my clients are sharing, looking beyond their words at the meaning they are trying to convey?[40] The occupational therapist could ask for feedback to assess whether the client is having a positive emotional experience of therapy as part of the client-centered approach.[35]

The Canadian Model of Client-Centered Enablement identifies six enablement foundations that the occupational therapy practitioner can incorporate. These foundations stress the importance of considering choice, risk, and responsibility and emphasize collaboration to share a vision of possibilities and change with our clients.[32] Injustice is often faced by people with disabilities, and reflecting on diversity and equity is also a part of this model.[32] In the psychosocial context, where many individuals experience stigma and discrimination, this model provides support for occupational therapy practitioners to intentionally address these experiences and enable clients to address their feelings and perceived barriers. Case study 5.6 illustrates the use of CMOP-E in practice.

CASE STUDY 5.6 Maria

Maria recently moved from a nursing-care facility into a new apartment at age 28. She sustained a traumatic brain injury in a car accident, 2 years prior to her move, and lived in a nursing home after being released from inpatient rehabilitation. She received intensive therapy initially, but little therapy after the first 3 months of her stay. She was diagnosed with depression after 6 months, due to her prolonged recovery and her limited social interactions in the nursing facility, as the residents were primarily older adults with dementia. Maria went to a presentation by a disability advocacy organization, which helped her to make the transition back to independent living with financial, logistical, and social support. Maria used a wheelchair for long distances but was ambulatory in her apartment. A week after her move, she was referred for home-based occupational therapy by the local community mental health agency that was assisting Maria with transitioning to independent

living. The caseworker at the agency was concerned about Maria's ability to manage in her new environment, especially with her history of depression.

Upon meeting Maria, the occupational therapist used her enablement skills to *collaborate* with Maria and *coach* her through the challenges with her new living situation. The occupational therapist administered the COPM to *identify* the priority areas of occupation that Maria wanted to address. While the occupational therapist wanted to address some of Maria's residual cognitive deficits, Maria did not want to focus on cognition. Since the CMOP-E uses a *client-centered* approach, the occupational therapist followed Maria's lead on the priorities that were most important to her. One of Maria's priorities was to go out into the neighboring business district and access stores and restaurants, but she was anxious about her ability to communicate with

CASE STUDY 5.6 Maria—cont'd

others due to her slow rate of speech as a result of her brain injury. She had also encountered physical barriers when attempting to go out in her wheelchair, as there was no fully accessible restroom in one of the businesses she visited. She tried to ask for help from the staff, but they were impatient with her and she was not able to clearly articulate her needs. She became very anxious and upset and returned to her apartment, giving up on the idea of venturing out. She recently became more reclusive and withdrawn.

The occupational therapist was guided by the philosophy of the CMOP-E of *promoting self-advocacy and social justice*, and focused on building Maria's ability to *advocate* with the local businesses for disability accommodations, such as installing a door opener on the restroom, altering the entrance to the restroom, or providing physical assistance to navigate the heavy door. She *engaged* Maria in developing a plan of action to address her limited access to the community and her anxiety about asking for disability accommodations. The occupational therapist *educated* Maria on her disability rights and role-played situations with her to build her confidence.

They went together to visit local businesses, where Maria introduced herself as new to the neighborhood and asked if their physical facilities were accessible to wheelchair users, presenting a card with written information that she and the occupational therapist created in case the staff had limited time or difficulty understanding her. If the facility was not accessible, Maria provided information on resources to improve accessibility and the occupational therapist left her contact information for follow up if needed. The occupational therapist *consulted* with Maria after each visit to assess her level of comfort and anxiety and to offer encouragement and strategies if Maria requested this.

Two months later, Maria reported that a coffee shop that she and the occupational therapist visited had improved accessibility and was very welcoming and supportive. She visited there every morning and was getting more confident with requesting help if needed. The occupational therapist readministered the COPM and noted that Maria's satisfaction rating improved in that area, and that she identified some new priorities to address transportation resources so she could venture further from her apartment. The occupational therapist's role in *enabling occupation* was guided by her knowledge of the CMOP-E, and she confidently approached this new challenge in collaboration with Maria.

KAWA MODEL

The Kawa Model,[41] developed by Michael Iwama and a team of occupational therapists in Japan, explores clients' narratives of their daily life experiences as the basis for occupational therapy intervention.[42] The Kawa Model originated from East Asian cultures and views the person from their own perspective, as explained by the person in their own words and on their own terms. This reversal of hierarchical structure between therapist and client presents a paradigm shift in how models are used in occupational therapy practice. Whereas established occupational therapy models have followed the familiar pattern of application in which one grand narrative or framework (including the model's concepts and principles) is applied universally to all clients regardless of diversity and uniqueness, the Kawa Model elevates the client's unique narrative, which then forms the basis of the uniquely informed occupational therapy intervention that follows. It allows occupational therapy practitioners to gather data and engage clients in the process of identifying their unique needs.

Kawa is the Japanese word for river. The Kawa model uses the metaphor of a river to describe one's life journey. As occupational therapy practitioners use the metaphor of the river to represent the client's past, present, and future experiences and needs, they help clients understand and work through a variety of life issues. The model explains that as the river flows, so do a person's life experiences; sometimes there are rocks (obstacles and challenges) that disrupt the flow from place to place, from instance to instance. Occupational therapy practitioners try to enable, assist, restore, and maximize their client's life flow.[43]

Overview

The Kawa Model allows clients to construct their own narrative as a way to inform occupational therapy intervention and as such, the Kawa Model considers the client's culture (their own personal social phenomena). As the client engages in a conversation related to viewing their life as a river, the therapist and client learn the directions to take in therapy. Importantly, the therapist does not attribute meaning to the client's narrative, but rather encourages the

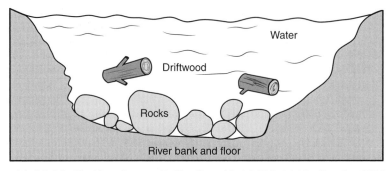

Fig. 5.5 Kawa Model. (Modified from Iwama, H. *The Kawa Model*. Philadelphia: Elsevier; 2006. p. 144).

client to express the meaning and direction. The Kawa Model (see Fig. 5.5) uses the metaphor of a river to identify five interrelated constructs:

- *River flow* represents life flow and priorities.
- *River banks* refer to environments and contexts (social and physical).
- *Rocks* represent obstacles and challenges.
- *Driftwood* is the influencing factors in one's life.
- *Spaces* include opportunities for enhancing flow. Spaces have often been interpreted by Western occupational therapists to be synonymous with *occupations*.

The Kawa Model uses these constructs to engage clients in assessing their lives by asking questions related to each construct. The interview is dynamic and allows the occupational therapist to probe and return to earlier concepts. The subjective information gained from the interview helps determine supports and resources (internal and external) that can be used to create occupational therapy intervention.

The interview is used as an assessment tool to gather information from the client. The intent in using the Kawa Model is to better understand clients by getting them to identify their issues and problems, and explain their meaning. This allows the occupational therapist to plan intervention. It is not important for the client and therapist to agree on whether something is a rock or driftwood.[43] By learning more about the client's experiences and the meaning attached, occupational therapy practitioners are better able to design meaningful intervention based on the person's day-to-day activities.

Culture

The Kawa Model was developed to provide a different cultural viewpoint of evaluating and assessing occupational performance. The Kawa Model views culture as "relative to each individual within their environment, based on the discourse of his or her society."[41,44] The model asserts that occupational therapists view the meaning and contexts of

occupations in the same lens as the client, rather than ascribing one's own values and meanings to their client's performance.

The key features of this model include a focus on a *decentralized self*, which differs from Western culture, which places importance on individuals. The decentralized self views a person as part of a social collective that influences individual actions, choices, and meaning. The value of human performance is based on the need to contribute to the *collective whole*, rather than to establish personal or individual competency. Instead of valuing "doing," the Kawa Model suggests that "belonging" is more valued in a collective society (such as in Eastern and indigenous cultures). Since individuals view themselves as part of a collective group, they value dependence on others (a concept opposing Western cultural values and often perpetuated in occupational therapy practice). Consequently, identity and meaning are ascribed in light of the collective, rather than the individual. Occupation is made up of the self and the environment.[41] The Kawa Model views the person as an inseparable part of the environment and nature. The model views nature and her resources as key to occupational engagement, not as separate entities.

When the self is considered as inseparably embedded in nature, the concept or sensation of time is affected. The concept of time in Eastern culture is focused on the "here-and-now" with less attention being placed on future outcomes. When the world and self are imagined as one, and constantly changing, the rational boundaries between past, present, and future can easily blur. The prospect of future success and achievement is a "hope" embedded in collective factors rather than on individual and independent will. Thus through the Kawa Model perspective, each person's life experience (or river) is uniquely constructed and lived, and warrants an occupational therapy intervention that is similarly uniquely configured and delivered.

It is up to the occupational therapist to determine how the person views their own actions. The factors of environment, life circumstances, personal assets and liabilities, and instance in time and place set the stage for occupational therapy intervention.[45] The aim of occupational therapy in the context of the Kawa Model is to increase life flow.

Principles

The Kawa Model is based on Eastern principles and defines occupation as life flow; occupational therapy practitioners facilitate life flow.[41] The principles of the Kawa Model can be summarized as follows:

- Client's viewpoint is the ultimate perspective and it is gathered by using the metaphor that life is a river.
  - Decentralized self is an Eastern value (individuals are part of a collective) as opposed to the centralized self (individual, autonomy) that is prevalent in Western cultures.
  - Belongingness and interdependence are valued in Eastern and indigenous cultures, whereas individualism and independence are Western values.
- Using a metaphor of a river to describe one's life journey allows clients to think more deeply about their life circumstances and reflect on concepts that form parts of the metaphor (such as rocks, driftwood, river banks, water, spaces).
- All elements in nature are profoundly connected, and people seek ways to live in harmony with nature and circumstances. Therefore the metaphor of a river resonates with clients and helps them discover things about themselves to help them engage in life.
- Environment is part of the person (not a separate entity).
  - The therapist examines the environment as part of the person, rather than something acting on them or simply influencing them.
  - The person is the river and an essential part of the environment.
- Disability is a collective experience. It affects the environment and the people surrounding the person with disability. Finding out the person's viewpoint of their disability informs occupational therapy intervention. For example, some clients may view disability as an obstacle (rock), whereas others may view disability as a turn in the river (or a different stream). In the latter case, disability becomes the person's new identity.
- The strategy for rehabilitation is not to confront the perceived problems directly and rationally, but rather to bend, flex, and adapt one's circumstances to the circumstances of the surrounding environment.[41]

- How occupational therapy practitioners work with their clients will be largely dependent on the clients' values. How clients perceive themselves will then influence their expectations of what they would like to get out of their occupational therapy.

Strategies and Techniques

The strategies and techniques of the Kawa Model focus on engaging the client in a therapeutic discussion and reflection process, and therefore it is based on honoring the client, trusting their emergence, and examining the client's identity (centralized and decentralized self) (see Box 5.6 for specific techniques). Once the therapist understands the client's narrative through the process of engaging in river flow, intervention focuses on removing obstacles (rocks), facilitating river flow by adding resources (driftwood), and promoting environmental supports (widening river banks). Occupational therapy practitioners may use traditional methods to make changes.

The occupational therapist examines the client's viewpoint of themselves by exploring the following concepts related to the centralized and decentralized self (see Box 5.7). A client's viewpoint informs the occupational therapy approaches that may be most effective. For example, clients who perceive themselves to be on their own and are seeking "meaning" and wishing to succeed exhibit centralized

---

> **BOX 5.6 Techniques to Engage Clients in Process Using Kawa Model**
>
> - Be ready to discard all universal assumptions about the relevance and appropriateness of this model, start working with your client from a clean, objective slate.
> - If the model and the metaphor on which it is based fail to resonate with either the client or occupational therapist, it should be modified or placed aside in exchange for a more appropriate and relevant model.
> - The client's narrative becomes the model on which we base the occupational therapy process. Trust that the client's narrative will emerge through a process of enabling them to do so.
> - Be aware of your own cultural lens. Competent therapists will appreciate not only the culture embodied within the client but also the cultures at play within themselves, with the occupational therapy they have learned and experienced, and the institutional conditions that set the mandate and structure for the therapeutic process.
>
> From Teoh JY, Iwama MK. *The Kawa Model Made Easy: A Guide to Applying the Kawa Model in Occupational Therapy Practice.* 2nd ed. 2015. Available at: www.kawamodel.com.

BOX 5.7	Kawa Model Concepts of Self		
Concept	**Definition**	**Questions**	**Diagram**
Decentralized self	Clients who perceive themselves to be integrated into a larger whole might appreciate values like balance, co-existence, and harmony more.	Does the client experience the self as an integrated part of a greater entity?	Clients who experience the self as integrated parts of a whole frame will regard the entire diagram of the river as embedded in the environment and circumstance, with occupation embedded into the river as well.
Centralized self	Clients who perceive themselves as distinct from the environment might be more appreciative of values like autonomy, independence, and control.	Does the client experience the self as separate from the environment?	Clients who experience the self as separate might draw themselves on a boat on the river.

From Teoh JY, Iwama MK. *The Kawa Model Made Easy: A Guide to Applying the Kawa Model in Occupational Therapy Practice.* 2nd ed. 2015. Available at: www.kawamodel.com.

self. The occupational therapy practitioner works to help them achieve skills and abilities to engage in their desired occupations. Clients who value centralized self believe in independence and autonomy. Conversely, a client who believes her role as part of her family is to take care of her children may benefit from learning ways to accomplish tasks more quickly or with help from others, as this allows clients to depend on others. This represents a decentralized self where the client values interdependence and the collective whole.

Assessment

The Kawa Model is a subjective assessment of the client's life experiences. Occupational therapists engage clients in an interview using the metaphor of life as a river (with flow to beginning, middle, and end). The therapist asks guiding questions to explore and understand the five underlying constructs and delves into the meaning by probing and asking "how" and "why" questions. The author provides suggested guiding questions for each of the four constructs (river flow, rocks, river banks, driftwood), but encourages occupational therapists to develop their own (see sample guiding questions Table 5.4).

The final construct, *spaces*, is created after examining the four constructs and identifying opportunities for enhancing flow. Every space in the client's river where the water is flowing has potential to flow more powerfully.[43] Occupational therapy intervention can be used to create or widen the spaces for water to flow. For example, rocks can become smaller, river banks can be widened, or the client can use driftwood to overcome obstacles (i.e., push away rocks).

The results of the subjective assessment with the Kawa Model may indicate further assessment measures. The occupational therapist interprets data from the interview, observations, and engagement in the Kawa Model to create an intervention that identifies spaces for flow. The therapist develops short-term and long-term goals based on a synthesis of assessment data. Rocks are addressed based on *driftwood* and *environments* with the intention of enhancing the client's life *flow* (occupational therapy outcome).[43]

Specific Intervention Procedures

The occupational therapist creates a welcoming environment to conduct the interview and makes the client feel relaxed. The practitioner conducts the interview in an inviting manner using guiding questions and probing for insight into the client's feelings regarding their occupational performance abilities. The client's narrative is central to this model. The therapist engages the client in describing their narrative and making connections to past, present, and future. After examining the findings of the interview, the therapist and client create priorities for occupational therapy intervention. The narrative informs occupational therapy with no preconceived notions of the linkages and hypotheses. The Kawa Model is intended to be interpreted and applied in relation to a person's culture (which is defined as shared meanings). The occupational therapist establishes goals (with input from the client and in alignment with the setting). The occupational therapist conducts the intervention session and evaluates the client's progress towards the established goals. Case study 5.7 provides an example applying Kawa Model in a mental health setting.

TABLE 5.4	Sample Guiding Questions for the Kawa Model	
Kawa Model Construct	**Sample Questions**	**Notes**
• River flow (life flow and priorities)	• If your life was a river, what does your river look like? How would you describe the flow of your river right now? • What do you enjoy doing? Why do you enjoy it? • What makes you happy? How does it make you happy? Why?	• Questions take past, present, and future into consideration. • Include questions regarding work history, medical history, life roles, processes, self-care, and leisure. • River flow can comprise many little streams and include flow of significant persons in client's life.
• Rocks (obstacles and challenges)	• Are you having any difficulties right now? What are they? Why do you think (those things) are difficult for you? How is it difficult? • Is there anything in your life right now that you would like to change? What is it? Why? How would you like things to change? If things were better, what do you think would be different?	• Rocks can typically be categorized into (but are not restricted to) occupational performance difficulties, fears, and concerns, inconvenient circumstances out of occupational therapy's control, and impairments or medical concerns. • The rocks of significant persons in the client's life should also be considered and incorporated where relevant.
• River banks (Physical and social environment)	Who are you currently living with right now? • Who do you typically spend most of your time with? How do you spend your time with them? What do you usually enjoy doing together? • Can you describe to me the place where you live/work? How do you find your ability to get around there?	Social environment can represent friends and family, classmates, colleagues, lovers, pets, deceased relatives, acquaintances, or any social supports that the client considers significant.
• Driftwood (Personal resources that can be assets or liabilities)	• How do you see challenges in life? • How would you describe yourself? • How do you typically cope with stress?	• Driftwood can be personal traits or characteristics (such as personality or attitude). • Driftwood includes special skills, abilities, and experiences. • Driftwood can represent beliefs, values, and principles. • Driftwood can represent material and/or social capital (such as finances, social connections).

From Teoh JY, Iwama MK. *The Kawa Model Made Easy: A Guide to Applying the Kawa Model in Occupational Therapy Practice.* 2nd ed. 2015. Available at: www.kawamodel.com.

CASE STUDY 5.7   Application of The Kawa Model: Jamie (Courtesy Alison O'Brien)

Jamie is 19 years old and in her first semester of college. She enjoys going out socially and is on the girls' rugby team. Jamie is taking a full course load this semester as she works toward her business degree, and her schedule keeps her busy. During one rugby practice, Jamie gets lightheaded and has to sit out. Concerned, a few teammates invite Jamie to dinner to keep an eye on her. During the meal Jamie explains that she has been staying up late at night to keep up with her course load. One of her teammates suggests that she drop a class, but Jamie shoots this idea down

Continued

CASE STUDY 5.7   Application of The Kawa Model: Jamie (Courtesy Alison O'Brien)—cont'd

while pushing some of her food around the plate. She likes being busy and she needs to keep on track with her degree.

As the semester continues, Jamie continues to push herself through the workload and rugby practice. By the time the first game comes around, most of the team has forgotten about Jamie's lightheadedness until she ends up passing out on the field after a tackle. Jamie recalls feeling as if she might vomit before she collapsed. The medical team on standby gets Jamie off the field. They place her in the shade and give her water, then ask her questions and check her for a concussion. Jamie insists that she is fine and "just needs a moment" but she passes out again. The medical team transports her to the hospital, where a doctor determines that she is significantly dehydrated and malnourished. She is transferred to the hospital's inpatient eating disorders unit, and the occupational therapist evaluates her as part of the interprofessional team.

The occupational therapist used the Kawa Model to engage Jamie in reflective exercises to develop awareness for change. Through the process, Jamie showed greater understanding of how her personal river reflects her life journey and how the rocks are symbolic of her stresses. She is able to articulate her assets and strengths (driftwood and spaces), in that she has a supportive friend group, many interesting life activities, and is doing well in school. She identifies her obstacles (rocks) within her river as representing her poor body image, low self-confidence, financial stress, and adolescent trauma (abuse by family friend). Together, the therapist and Jamie prioritize developing self-confidence and coping strategies to improve life flow. The psychologist will target discussion and coping with regard to past traumatic experiences. Fig. 5.6 illustrates Jamie's river as summarized by the occupational therapist.

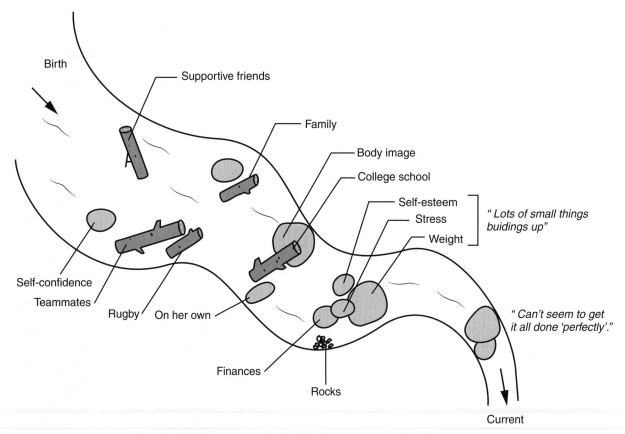

Fig. 5.6 Jamie's river as summarized by the occupational therapist and Jamie.

Jamie's Occupational Therapy Intervention Guided by the Kawa Model

Water. The goal of occupational therapy intervention is to maximize Jamie's life flow. This requires removing rocks and elements that interfere with flow and maximizing channels or spaces where the water currently flows.[41]

Rocks. Identify the rocks and work with Jamie to reduce these obstacles: Jamie is overscheduled with little time to reflect and relax. She is taking a full course load, is on the rugby team and is a freshman in college who is social and enjoys a variety of activities. This is her first time away from home and she is the youngest of four children, so she is experiencing some home sickness.

The therapist will work with Jamie to help her develop coping skills to accept less than "perfection" in school and athletics. The therapist will introduce mindfulness techniques to help Jamie be present in the "here and now," which may allow her to enjoy life events and develop self-confidence. The occupational therapist will collaborate as a member of the interprofessional team to address Jamie's issues related to her eating disorder (to empower Jamie to engage in a balance of healthy eating and physical activity). Jamie has not been sleeping and this presents an obstacle to her overall well-being and learning. The occupational therapist and Jamie will develop a sleep hygiene routine together. Addressing the obstacles will allow for more life flow.

Spaces/channels. Identify spaces and the context of her river, while determining areas most important to Jamie. Occupational therapy intervention will maximize spaces by utilizing Jamie's desire to succeed in college and athletics to establish healthy lifestyle habits (balance between physical and nutritional activities). The therapist will engage Jamie in activities to maximize the support of her close friends, teammates, and family so that Jamie is empowered to ask for support and also realize that others care. Jamie is doing well in college and enjoys spending time with her many friends. The therapist will use cognitive behavioral therapy to develop Jamie's self-confidence, coping skills, and healthy patterns of eating and physical activity. Reinforcing the supports that exist (both internal and external) will increase the river flow.

River bed and sides. Widen the river sides and deepen the river bed, through advising Jamie to seek counseling at school. Encourage Jamie to participate in a college support group for athletes. This will help Jamie realize she is not alone and provide her with additional support. Jamie may have outpatient visits with a sports nutritionist and/or psychologist to monitor her nutrition and weight gain. The occupational therapist will work with Jamie so she can develop healthy habits (physical, mental, and social) and routines to support her desired activities at college. Jamie will reach out to family, friends, and college resources to continue progress once discharged from the hospital.

The therapist will work with Jamie and the interprofessional team to establish healthy eating and physical activity habits with the goal that Jamie gain weight and enough endurance to complete one hour of physical activity.

Driftwood. Identify aspects of Jaime's character and attributes that may enhance her life flow. Examine her sociocultural context to understand factors that may help or hinder her health, recovery, and well-being. Enhance the positive aspects, like Jamie's friendliness, organization, sense of humor, intelligence, athleticism, and her determination to succeed. Work with her rugby coach to support Jamie's health (focus on performance and strength, not weight). Recommend that Jamie work with the college counselor to help her explore underlying psychological issues (related to childhood trauma).

The Kawa Model provides a client-centered holistic model to structure Jamie's occupational therapy evaluation and intervention. This creative approach allows Jamie to articulate her narrative and explore areas in her life that she can address to improve her overall health and well-being. Helping Jamie make sense of her own narrative and empowering her to make changes provides her with lifelong coping skills. Furthermore, the model highlights the person's strengths and resources as a way to influence and change those things that are challenging, difficult, and interfering with life flow.

CHOOSING AND COMBINING MODELS

Each of these four occupation-centered models have unique principles and strategies for implementation. Therapists can choose the model that matches their values, setting, and population served, and more fully explore the application of the model through reading primary sources, reviewing updated application examples, and consulting clinicians and clients who have used the model of choice. If the therapist can apply more than one of the occupation-centered models competently, selecting the model to use for a particular client may depend on the client's needs, culture, challenges, and strengths, as well as the supports and barriers in the environment.

It is recommended that occupational therapy practitioners consider the occupation-centered model they choose to use as their foundational or organizing model as described by Ikiugu and colleagues[46] and further illustrated by Wong and Fisher.[35] If additional assessments and interventions are needed, they can be considered complementary models. For example, if a psychosocial program uses the cognitive-behavioral model, it would be considered a complementary model, with one of the occupation-centered models driving the assessment and intervention process, as well as the therapist's view of the client's areas of concern and goals. Implementing the occupation-centered models will keep practitioners grounded in occupational therapy principles and guide them in collaborating with the client to enact the client's goals through occupation-based interventions.

SUGGESTED LEARNING ACTIVITIES

1. Apply each of the models to the same case study example of a person with mental health dysfunction. Compare and contrast the intervention process.
2. Describe specific assessments that help measure client's performance according to each occupation-centered practice model.
3. Describe the occupational therapy process based on one selected occupation-centered practice model as used with a client who has mental health issues. (Instructor's Note: Have students each select a different occupation-centered practice model so the class can engage in discussion.)

REFLECTION QUESTIONS

1. What are the specific features of each occupation-centered practice model?
2. What are the principles of each occupation-centered model and how do the principles guide intervention planning?
3. What specific techniques and strategies are associated with each of the occupation-centered practice models?

REFERENCES

1. Ikiugu MN, Nissen RM. Intervention strategies used by occupational therapists working in mental health and their theoretical basis. *Occup Ther Ment Health*. 2016;32(2):109-129.
2. Fisher AG. Occupation-centred, occupation-based, occupation-focused: Same, same or different? *Scand J Occup Ther*. 2013;20:162-173.
3. Kielhofner G. A model of human occupation: part 2: ontogenesis from the perspective of temporal adaptation. *Am J Occup Ther*. 1980a;34:657-663.
4. Kielhofner G. A model of human occupation: part 3: benign and vicious cycles. *Am J Occup Ther*. 1980b;34:731-737.
5. Kielhofner G, Burke J. A model of human occupation: part 1: conceptual framework and content. *Am J Occup Ther*. 1980;34:572-581.
6. Taylor R. *Kielhofner's Model of Human Occupation*. 5th ed. Philadelphia: Wolters Kluwer Health/Lippincott Williams & Wilkins; 2017.
7. Asmundsdottir EE. Creation of new services: collaboration between mental health consumers and occupational therapists. *Occup Ther Ment Health*. 2009;25:115-126.
8. Kramer J, Walker R, Cohn E, et al. Striving for shared understandings: therapists' perspectives of the benefits and dilemmas of using a child self-assessment. *OTJR*. 2012;32(1):S48-S58.
9. Lee S, Forsyth K, Morley M, Garnham M, Heasman D, Taylor R. Mental health payment-by-results clusters and the model of human occupation screening tool. *OTJR*. 2013;33(1):40-49.
10. Smith J, Mairs H. Use and results of MOHO global assessments in community mental health: a practice analysis. *Occup Ther Ment Health*. 2014;30:381-389.
11. Taylor R, Kielhofner G. Introduction to the Model of Human Occupation. In: Taylor R, ed. *Kielhofner's Model of Human Occupation: Theory and Application*. 5th ed. Philadelphia: Wolters Kluwer Health/Lippincott Williams & Wilkins; 2017.
12. Yamada T, Taylor R, Kielhofner G. The person-specific concepts of human occupation. In: Taylor R, ed. *Kielhofner's Model of Human Occupation: Theory and Application*. 5th ed. Philadelphia: Wolters Kluwer Health/Lippincott Williams & Wilkins; 2017.
13. Fisher G, Parkinson S, Haglund L. The environment and human occupation. In: Taylor R, ed. *Kielhofner's Model of Human Occupation: Theory and Application*. 5th ed. Philadelphia: Wolters Kluwer Health/Lippincott Williams & Wilkins; 2017.
14. Cahill SM, Bowyer P, O'Brien JC, Munoz L, Kielhofner G. Applying MOHO in pediatric practice: working with children with sensory processing, motor, medical, and developmental issues. In: Taylor R, ed. *Kielhofner's Model of Human Occupation: Theory and Application*. 5th ed. Philadelphia: Wolters Kluwer Health/Lippincott Williams & Wilkins; 2017.

15. Kramer J, Bowyer P. Applying the model of human occupation to pediatric practice. In: Solomon J, O'Brien J, eds. *Pediatric Skills for Occupational Therapy Assistants*. St. Louis: Elsevier; 2016.

16. O'Brien J, Kielhofner G. The interaction between the person and the environment. In: Taylor R, ed. *Kielhofner's Model of Human Occupation: Theory and Application*. 5th ed. Philadelphia: Wolters Kluwer Health/Lippincott Williams & Wilkins; 2017.

17. de las Heras C, Parkinson S, Pepin G, Kielhofner G. Intervention process: enabling occupational change. In: Taylor R, ed. *Kielhofner's Model of Human Occupation: Theory and Application*. 5th ed. Philadelphia: Wolters Kluwer Health/Lippincott Williams & Wilkins; 2017.

18. Braveman B, Robson M, Velozo C, Kielhofner G, Forsyth K, Kerschbaum J. *Worker Role Interview*. [Version 10.0]. Chicago: Model of Human Occupation Clearinghouse. Department of Occupational Therapy. University of Illinois at Chicago; 2005.

19. Kielhofner G, Mallinson T, Crawford C, et al. *The Occupational Performance History Interview-II*. [Version 2.1]. Chicago: Model of Human Occupation Clearinghouse. Department of Occupational Therapy. University of Illinois at Chicago; 2004.

20. Christiansen C, Baum C. *Occupational Therapy: Overcoming Human Performance Deficits*. Thorofare, NJ: SLACK Inc; 1991.

21. Christiansen C, Baum C. *Occupational therapy: enabling function and well-being*. 2nd ed. Thorofare, NJ: SLACK Inc; 1997.

22. Christiansen C, Baum C. *Occupational Therapy: Performance, Participation, and Well-Being*. 3rd ed. Thorofare, NJ: SLACK Incorporated; 2005.

23. Baum CM, Christiansen CH, Bass JD. The person-environment-occupation-performance (PEOP) model. In: Christiansen CH, Baum CM, Bass JD, eds. *Occupational Therapy: Performance, Participation, and Well-being*. 4th ed. Thorofare, NJ: SLACK Inc; 2015:49-55.

24. Baum CM, Edwards DF. *Activity card sort (ACS): test manual*. 2nd ed. Bethesda, MD: AOTA Press; 2008.

25. Bass JD, Baum CM, Christiansen CH. Intervention and outcomes: The Person-Environment-Occupation-Performance (PEOP) occupational therapy process. In: Christiansen CH, Baum CM, Bass JD, eds. *Occupational Therapy: Performance, Participation, and Well-being*. 4th ed. Thorofare, NJ: SLACK Inc; 2015:57-79.

26. American Occupational Therapy Association. Occupational therapy practice framework: domain and process. 3rd ed. *Am J Occup Ther*. 2014;68(suppl 1):S1-S48.

27. Berg C, LaVesser P. The preschool activity card sort. *OTJR: occupation, participation, health*. 2006;26(4):143-151.

28. Stoffel A, Berg C. Spanish translation and validation of the preschool activity card sort. *Phys Occup Ther Pediatr*. 2008;28(2):171-189.

29. Canadian Association of Occupational Therapists. *Enabling occupation: an occupational therapy perspective*. Ottawa, ON: CAOT Publications ACE; 1997.

30. Polatajko HJ. Muriel Driver Lecture 1992, Naming and framing occupational therapy: a lecture dedicated to the life of Nancy B. *Can J Occup Ther*. 1992;59(4):189-200.

31. Krupa T. Canadian triple model framework for enabling occupation. In: Krupa T, Kirsh B, Pitts D, Fossey E, eds. *Bruce & Borg's Psychosocial Frames of Reference: Theories, Models and Approaches for Occupation-based Practice*. 4th ed. Thorofare, NJ: SLACK Inc; 2016.

32. Townsend EA, Polatajko HJ. *Enabling Occupation II: Advancing an Occupational Therapy Vision for Health, Well-being, & Justice Through Occupation*. Ottawa, ON: CAOT Publications ACE; 2007.

33. Polatajko HJ, Davis J, Stewart D, et al. Specifying the domain of concern: occupation as core. In: Townsend EA, Polatajko HJ, eds. *Enabling Occupation II: Advancing an Occupational Therapy Vision for Health, Well-being, & Justice Through Occupation*. Ottawa, ON: CAOT Publications ACE; 2007.

34. Turpin M, Iwama M. *Using Occupational Therapy Models in Practice: A Fieldguide*. Edinburgh: Elsevier; 2010.

35. Wong S, Fisher G. Comparing and using occupation-focused models. *Occup Ther Health Care*. 2015;29(3):297-315.

36. Law M, Baptiste S, Carswell A, McColl MA, Polatajko H, Pollock N. *Canadian Occupational Performance Measure*. 4th ed. Ottawa, ON: CAOT Publications ACE; 2005.

37. Colquhoun H, Letts L, Law M, MacDermid J, Edwards M. Routine administration of the Canadian Occupational Performance Measure: effect on functional outcome. *Aust Occup Ther J*. 2010;57(2):111-117.

38. Larsen AE, Carlsson G. Utility of the Canadian Occupational Performance Measure as an admission and outcome measure in interdisciplinary community-based geriatric rehabilitation. *Scand J Occup Ther*. 2012;19(2):204-213.

39. Parker DM, Sykes CH. A systematic review of the Canadian Occupational Performance Measure: a clinical practice perspective. *Br J Occup Ther*. 2006;69(4):150-160.

40. Sumsion T, Law M. A review of evidence on the conceptual elements informing client-centered practice. *Can J Occup Ther*. 2006;73:153-262.

41. Iwama M. *The Kawa Model: Culturally Relevant Occupational Therapy*. Edinburgh: Churchill Livingstone-Elsevier Press; 2006.

42. Iwama MK, Thomson NA, Macdonald RM. The Kawa model: The power of culturally responsive occupational therapy. *Disabil Rehabil*. 2009;31(14):1125-1135.

43. Teoh JY, Iwama MK. *The Kawa Model Made Easy: A Guide to Applying the Kawa Model in Occupational Therapy Practice*. 2nd ed. 2015. Available at: www.kawamodel.com.

44. Winch P. Understanding a primitive society. *Am Philos Q*. 1964;1(4):307-324.

45. Gregg BT, Howell DM, Quick CD, Iwama MK. The Kawa River Model: applying theory to develop interventions for combat and operational stress control. *Occup Ther Mental Health*. 2015;31(4):366-384.

46. Ikiugu MN, Smallfield S. Ikiugu's eclectic method of combining theoretical conceptual practice models in occupational therapy. *Aust J Occup Ther*. 2011;58(6):437-446.

6

Psychosocial Theories

Nancy Carson

LEARNING OBJECTIVES

1. Understand the theoretic basis of the psychodynamic, cognitive-behavioral, humanistic, and developmental approaches.
2. Discuss the influence and contributions of the psychodynamic, cognitive-behavioral, humanistic, and developmental approaches to the practice of occupational therapy.

3. Review some of the assessment and treatment implications of the psychodynamic, cognitive-behavioral, humanistic, and developmental approaches to the practice of occupational therapy.

INTRODUCTION

Occupational therapy's roots are in the mental health domain; therefore psychosocial theories have contributed to therapeutic approaches and are essential in understanding how to approach the client. It would be impossible to provide an in-depth review of all the theories that have contributed to the development or practice of occupational therapy; therefore a brief overview of some of the theories and how they contribute to occupational therapy practice is provided in this chapter.

The profession grew out of moral treatment for individuals with mental illness.[1] The humanitarian movement strove to move the mentally ill from confinement and provide individuals with meaningful activity. Occupational therapy emerged as a means of fulfilling this humanitarian mission with the focus on both the activity aspect and the human relationship aspect. From the beginning, the early therapists understood what is now referred to as "therapeutic use of self." They understood the importance of connecting with the patient in an appropriate, empathetic manner and embodied humanitarian principles in psychiatric practice.[2] The founders viewed the profession as a humanistic-scientific practice.[3] William Rush Dunton embraced the philosophy of the moral treatment era and saw similarities to occupational therapy in valuing a humanistic approach to the mentally ill through

the use of therapeutic occupation.[4] He believed in science, along with occupation, and he maintained a holistic view with a focus on mind and body.[3]

Modern-day humanistic psychology is also congruent with the concept of occupational therapy as a client-centered profession. It is different from the humanitarian movement in that it arose from dissatisfaction with behavioral and psychodynamic approaches used by the psychiatric profession during the early 1900s. Although occupational therapy has continued to embrace humanistic values through a client-centered approach and concern for the individual as a human being, other approaches have also influenced the development of the profession and contribute to professional practice.

Psychodynamic Approach

The psychodynamic approach is based on the work of Sigmund Freud. Freud is the father of psychoanalysis, which he founded in the 1890s.[5] Psychoanalysis seeks to treat psychological problems by bringing unconscious thoughts and beliefs into the conscious realm for the individual, thus providing insight into personal behavior. Unresolved issues during development or repressed trauma in early life are considered likely causes of psychological distress. The purpose of psychoanalysis therapy is to release repressed emotions and experiences and, in making the unconscious

conscious, the individual progresses. Core assumptions include the following: most psychological processes take place outside conscious awareness; early life experiences strongly influence personality development and behavior; and all thoughts, feelings, and behaviors arise from identifiable psychological processes.[5,6]

Freud viewed the personality as being composed of three parts—the id, the ego, and the superego. The id is the unconscious part of the psyche present at birth. It operates to satisfy basic needs and is driven by a desire for immediate gratification. The ego develops from the id and operates in both the conscious and unconscious realms of the psyche to deal with reality. The ego works to satisfy the id and works on the basis of delayed gratification and socially acceptable behavior to satisfy needs. The superego is the part of the psyche responsible for our sense of right and wrong—our conscience.[7]

In the psychodynamic approach, what is in the unconscious mind can have a strong influence on behavior and can direct people to behave in certain ways. When the unconscious mind directs a behavior, the reason for the behavior is not clear to the individual, and this can lead to anxiety, frustration, guilt, or some level of discontent. Defense mechanisms are the unconscious strategies directed by the ego to protect a person from these negative feelings.[6,8,9] Every person uses defense mechanisms and they serve a valuable purpose to protect the ego but, when excessive use of defense mechanisms is employed, psychological distress escalates, resulting in increased anxiety and decreased ability to function. Defense mechanisms can be categorized as primitive or mature.[10] Defense mechanisms that are more adaptive or helpful are mature mechanisms, and those that are learned early in life are referred to as primitive. Some defense mechanisms are somewhere in between and can be effective and noneffective, depending on how they are used. Mature defense mechanisms are the most effective and can be learned with practice. Primitive defense mechanisms can be very effective at first but are usually not effective in resolving anxiety or distress over time. Individuals who do not have effective coping mechanisms for stress and anxiety tend to resort to primitive defense mechanisms to cope.

Being aware of how an individual may be using defense mechanisms can provide insight into occupational behavior. With some individuals, exploring the use of defense mechanisms appropriately can be beneficial. It can complement and enhance clinical reasoning and reflective practice for the occupational therapy practitioner. A list of defense mechanisms with definitions is provided, along with examples for occupational therapy of selected mechanisms.

Primitive Defense Mechanisms

Acting Out

Acting out occurs when the individual is not able to express highly charged emotions in a mature manner.[10–12] Instead, the individual who is angry at another person or angry over a situation engages in behaviors that are extreme, such as punching a hole through a wall. The person may report feeling better afterward through the physical release of tension.

Example: A patient may not be able to perform a desired occupation such as mixing food together in a bowl when preparing a meal. Instead of verbalizing frustration, the patient throws the bowl across the room. The practitioner can facilitate discussion with the patient to help them learn how to verbalize future frustrations and to help the patient identify an appropriate tolerance level in future therapy sessions. The patient or practitioner may be setting unrealistic goals, and the practitioner may need to adapt or downgrade the activity to offer the most appropriate challenge.

Avoidance

Deciding not to do something because it is anxiety provoking is avoidance.[11] Although avoidance can serve as an escape from a stressful event, it does not deal with the cause of the stress. It may just delay the inevitable, which can then create more stress, or avoidance may be a permanent choice not to deal with a problem—for example, not confronting a friend who lied or not applying for a new job because it is anxiety provoking. Avoidance may protect the individual from acute stress but it does not remove the stress that results from unfinished business or unfulfilled dreams.

Example: A patient who has been out of work due to illness may be anxious about returning to work and avoids going back to work for a variety of unsubstantial reasons. On discussing return to work with the patient, the practitioner realizes that the patient is avoiding returning to work due to anxiety. The practitioner assists the patient in addressing the anxiety by identifying appropriate modifications or alternative ways to return to work successfully and supports the patient in exploring options.

Conversion (Conversion Reaction)

This is a process whereby the anxiety caused by unconscious feelings or thoughts that are repressed become apparent as a physical symptom or somatic complaint.[12] Some examples of conversion reaction include paralysis, dystonia, psychogenic nonepileptic seizures, amnesia, motor tics, and hallucinations. Conversion reaction is a type of somatization that is the expression of psychologic problems through physical symptoms. Somatization ranges from preoccupation with mild symptoms to the development of real pain, discomfort, or dysfunction.

Example: Following the death of his wife from a house fire, a 60-year-old man, who survived the fire with second-degree burns, experiences psychogenic nonepileptic seizures over the course of the next few months. He is being seen by an occupational therapist for treatment of his injuries. The occupational therapist provides opportunities for him to talk about his wife and to express his feelings in a nonthreatening environment.

Denial

This is the refusal to accept reality; the individual protects the self from a painful situation or fact by refusing to accept its validity.[7,8,9–12] Denial can occur after a traumatic event or after being informed of horrific news as a defense mechanism to protect the self from emotional pain.

Example: A classic example of denial is the person who is a heavy drinker or drug abuser yet denies a substance use problem because of perceived satisfactory functioning in their job and with their family. The occupational therapy practitioner can use motivational interviewing to explore ambivalence to change and attempt to elicit motivation to address the substance abuse.

Displacement

This is the redirection of feelings about one person onto another person or object.[9–12] Displacement may occur when the individual does not feel comfortable expressing feelings safely to the other person. Expressing anger at a boss or coworker may result in retribution; therefore those feelings may be redirected toward family or friends or onto an object.

Example: A client being seen by the occupational therapy practitioner expresses anger toward the therapist, who is aware that the client is angry with his physician over the course of treatment. The client is not able to express his feelings directly to his physician because he is dismissive and the client is uncomfortable talking to him and feels very frustrated. The practitioner provides opportunities for the client to express his feelings during therapy sessions and gradually provides support for him to talk directly to his physician.

Dissociation

Dissociation allows the person to cope with uncomfortable situations by separating the self mentally from the present.[10,12] The individual loses track of time and self and becomes disconnected from the outside world and is instead in a place that is free of unbearable thoughts or feelings. The individual may appear to be daydreaming to others and may require prompting to return to reality. Dissociation may occur as a result of childhood abuse or trauma.

Projection

Projection is the process of attributing the feelings that a person is having to another person.[7–12] These may be undesired thoughts, feelings, or impulses that are considered unacceptable for the person to express. Projection often stems from a lack of personal awareness and insight into one's own motivations and feelings. It allows the person to deny personal weaknesses or mistakes and protects self-image.

Example: A mother is told that her child needs to continue school-based therapy for another year and she blames the therapist for not providing adequate therapy. The practitioner calmly provides her specific reasons and examples for the child needing continued therapy and engages in active listening of the mother's concerns. The practitioner remains empathetic and supportive in talking with the mother.

Reaction Formation

Reaction formation is the converting of unconscious and unwanted thoughts or feelings into conscious thoughts and feelings on which the person acts.[7,9,10,12] A woman may have feelings for another woman's husband and, deeming this socially unacceptable, she exhibits contempt for him instead.

Regression

Regression is the return to an earlier stage of development when faced with unacceptable thoughts or feelings.[7,9–12] The stress and anxiety of adult life may lead a person to seek the security and associated behaviors of previous happier times.

Example: A young adult with severe anxiety attends the community mental health center. She prefers to spend her free time watching TV shows that she watched as a young child and continues to live at home with her mom, who supports her and takes care of her. The practitioner encourages her to make goals toward independence and to identify age-appropriate occupations and relationships.

Mature Defense Mechanisms
Acceptance

Accepting an undesirable situation that cannot be controlled or changed is one way to deal with anxiety or negative feelings caused by the situation.[12] Acceptance is usually not easy and requires the person to make the intentional choice to accept the situation.

Example: The practitioner assists a patient who can no longer participate in a specific occupation due to health issues to accept the situation by focusing on participation in other occupations.

Anticipation

Planning ahead for an emotionally painful or potentially stressful event is a technique called "anticipation."[12] This defense mechanism may involve mentally rehearsing possible outcomes of an upcoming event and convincing oneself that it will not be that bad or that it can be managed successfully.

Example: A caregiver for a spouse with a terminal disease may use anticipatory grief to prepare for the spouse's death. The practitioner can encourage the caregiver to prepare by finding ways to say goodbye, by finalizing any necessary plans, and by encouraging the caregiver to consider how to transition from a caregiver role to roles that are meaningful when the time comes.

Altruism

Altruistic behavior involves doing something kind or helpful for another person.[11,12] It can be used as a defense mechanism when used toward a person who the individual has difficulty getting along with or dislikes. By being kind and helpful, the situation or feelings are diffused, and the individual also experiences self-gratification. It may also help relieve personal distress by upholding a view of the self as kind, empathetic, and selfless.

Example: The practitioner may assist the patient with role-playing in nonconfrontational ways to respond to individuals when an argument ensues, and other methods of assertive behavior have not resulted in resolution or positive feelings.

Compensation

Compensation is a process whereby a person strives to overcome a perceived weakness or undesirable personal trait by emphasizing a perceived strength or trait.[7,10,11] The person may strive for overachievement to offset the perceived deficit. By focusing on one's strengths, there is the recognition that one cannot be successful or the best at everything. When done appropriately and not obsessively, compensation serves to reinforce a person's self-image and self-esteem.

Example: As part of treatment, the occupational therapy practitioner supports the individual in identifying strengths and in modifying occupations for success.

Humor

Humor is a mature defense mechanism that allows one to deal with painful thoughts or situations with less stress or anxiety.[11,12] Acknowledging the humorous aspect of a situation in which the individual does not have control can be a way to exert control over the perspective of the situation and allows the person to deal more effectively with it.

Identification

Identification occurs when a person admires or fears another person and aspires to be like that person by adopting similar qualities or attributes.[8,12] This may be done to appeal to a person who is perceived to be a threat; by use of identification, the goal is to appease the person and reduce personal anxiety. This may also be done to gain favor of someone who is highly respected by the individual. Identification may also occur with a group of people, such as a new group of social or work peers to gain acceptance. Identification helps the person avoid self-devaluation.

Sublimation

This defense mechanism is the process of refocusing unacceptable impulses and thoughts into more personally and socially acceptable channels.[7,9–12] The unacceptable impulses or thoughts may be of a sexual, aggressive, or anxiety-provoking nature. Refocusing may be achieved through appropriate physical or creative outlets; as such, it helps a person channel energy into productive use and decreases anxiety. The use of humor and fantasy are also specific types of sublimation that can be used appropriately as a form of coping with a situation.

Example: A client who has difficulty dealing with anger is encouraged to participate in therapeutic media sessions and is provided with resistive activities such as woodworking and expressive activities such as painting and journaling. The client is encouraged to express feelings through the use of media. The client is also encouraged to engage in physical exercise on a daily basis.

Substitution

When a person values another person or object that is unavailable, the choice may be made to replace that person or object with another person or object that is available and is similar to the original, although less desirable than the original.[11] This is a defense mechanism referred to as "substitution"; it helps the person achieve goals while minimizing disappointment

Example: A client can no longer participate in a valued occupation due to health deficits. The practitioner assists the client in modifying the activity or identifying similar occupations that are meaningful and within the client's abilities.

Suppression

This is the conscious or semiconscious decision not to think about something that is anxiety provoking; it may be a memory, idea, desire, or emotion that is the focus.[7,11,12] The person may try to think of something else or may engage in an unrelated task to avoid thinking the unpleasant thoughts. An individual may also have feelings of love or hate toward another individual that they suppress, and they do not treat the individual any differently than other people.

Other Defense Mechanisms

The following defense mechanisms can be considered primitive or mature, depending on how they are used and the context in which they are used.[13] It can be beneficial for the practitioner to consider if a client is using any of these approaches in dealing with emotional distress. Awareness of which defense mechanisms the client is using to deal with emotional pain and facilitating the use of mature, appropriate defense mechanisms can be a useful approach in enabling occupational performance.

Fantasy

Fantasy is used to escape from reality when life is distressing or the person is unhappy.[11] Fantasizing about a better life or situation can be helpful in exploring potential changes, but unrealistic expectations based on fantasy alone can lead to losing touch with reality and making irrational choices.

Idealization

Idealization is an ideal recollection or awareness of a person, place, object, event, or situation.[12] This occurs by emphasizing the positive attributes and ignoring or diminishing the negative ones. Idealization affects the perception that the individual has of the world and can influence judgments, so that idealized concepts are supported. Some examples include memories from childhood or memories of people who were highly regarded. Negative memories or attributes are diminished, and excuses may be made for any suggested difficulties or failures.

Intellectualization

Intellectualization occurs when there is a distressing emotional attachment or reaction to a situation or event. By intellectualizing and focusing on the nonemotional aspects of the situation or issue, the person protects the self from dealing with painful emotions. Instead, the person focuses on the factual information and logistics to explain the situation or event and ignores the emotional aspects.[7,10,11,12]

Rationalization

Rationalization is making excuses for oneself or someone else to justify behavior that would otherwise be considered unacceptable or would damage one's self-concept.[7,9–12] The person attempts to explain or create excuses for a situation or behavior in rational terms and thereby avoids accepting the true cause or reason for the current situation. Rationalization helps a person cope with the inability to meet goals or certain standards.

Repression

This is the process in which an individual's mind unconsciously subdues painful or anxious feelings, emotions, and memories to protect the person's emotional stability.[7,9–12] Freud believed that repressed feelings were represented in symbolic dreams and unexplained patterns of behavior and that repressed memories would need to be recalled and, with emotional support, accepted by the individual to achieve emotional wellness.

Projective Assessments

The psychodynamic approach in psychiatry led to the development of projective assessments, first in psychiatry and then in occupational therapy. Projection is the process of transferring emotions, feelings, or thoughts onto an object or material in the environment or through a form of media.[14] Projective assessments and techniques emerged in the 1940s and 1950s and, in occupational therapy, they served to formalize projective techniques. Expressive media, which allowed for creative expression and emotional reactions, was most often used in developing projective tools. These developed naturally with the activity focus of occupational therapy and served to elevate the use of expressive media beyond recreational or diversional use. The use of expressive media allowed the therapist to view the patient in a more intimate way through various expressions that fostered deeper understanding and communication.[15] There are many types of expressive media used by occupational therapy practitioners, such as clay, drawing, painting, mosaics, enameling, beadwork, creative writing, drama, and music. Any activity that can be used for self-expression can be used as a projective medium.

The Azima Battery, developed in the 1950s, was the first occupational therapy projective assessment.[16,17] It consists of drawing, finger painting, and making an object out of clay. The Goodman Battery is another projective assessment, which consists of a tile task, spontaneous drawing, figure drawing, and clay task.[16] The Lerner Magazine Picture Collage is an example of a projective assessment that could be completed in a group setting.[18,19] Clients are instructed to select pictures from magazines and are given 30 minutes to complete a collage. They are asked to explain why they selected the pictures and what meaning the pictures hold for them. Additional projective assessments were developed in occupational therapy during this time using various media as the focus of the assessment.

With the emergence of other approaches to psychiatric care, such as cognitive-behavioral therapy (CBT), the use of projective assessments and the psychodynamic influence in occupational therapy practice has diminished. Additionally, the subjectivity of projective assessments has been overshadowed by objective evaluations, which are more suitable for establishing reliability and validity. Evaluator skill in administering and interpreting projective assessments has also been questioned. Potential client resistance to projective assessments is cited as a limitation because some clients do not resonate with the use of expressive media. It can also be time-consuming to administer some of the projective assessments considering the setup of materials, implementation of assessment, and time to interpret and report results. All these factors have contributed to the decline in the use of projective assessments in occupational therapy.[20]

Despite this decline, there continues to be value in using projective media for assessment and therapeutic reasons. Occupational therapists can benefit from knowledge of the psychodynamic approach in understanding client behavior. Projective assessments can reveal deficits in activity performance and can identify relational difficulties. They also support a recovery-oriented approach to evaluation, in which the client gives personal meaning to the expressive media. As the mental health recovery movement continues to gain momentum, the importance of subjectivity and the lived experience gives renewed value to the use of projective assessments and approaches in mental health.[20]

There are many reasons for the occupational therapy practitioner to use expressive media as a form of treatment. Engaging in expressive media allows the client to relax and focus on activity outside of the self. In doing so, this can allow for a therapeutic rapport to develop between the client and therapist. Meaningful conversation often flows after the client has been engaged in expressive media. Observing a client working with media also provides the practitioner insight into many aspects of the client's persona. Personal strengths and weaknesses, as well as likes and dislikes, may be revealed in a different context as compared to verbal discussion alone. Observations of visual spatial abilities, task management, and cognitive abilities can also be observed. Engagement in expressive media provides a rich context for understanding the client's internal world.[14,20]

COGNITIVE-BEHAVIORAL THERAPY

CBT draws on both behavioral and cognitive theory and techniques. Behavior therapy emerged in the early 1900s from the work of Ivan Pavlov and his study of the learning process, which became known as "classic conditioning."[17,21]

Classic conditioning occurs when two stimuli are repeatedly paired together. One stimulus previously evoked a specific response, whereas the second stimulus did not evoke that response. Following pairing, the second stimulus now evokes that response without the first stimulus being present. This is classic conditioning.[21] BF Skinner further studied the learning process and the influence of positive and negative consequences on reinforcing behavior, a process he named "operant conditioning."[22] The focus of behavioral therapy is on the environment, and behavior is changed through reinforcement and learning strategies; it does not rely on insight as in the psychodynamic approach. In behavioral therapy, the focus is on reinforcing desirable behaviors and eliminating maladaptive behaviors. Behaviors that result in desirable consequences are more likely to occur again, whereas behaviors resulting in negative consequences are less likely to be repeated.[17,21]

There are two basic types of reinforcement that influence behavior—positive and negative reinforcement.[22] Positive reinforcement occurs when something is provided for the purpose of increasing the response in the future. Negative reinforcement occurs when something is removed for the same purpose of increasing the response in the future. For example, giving a student an A for a job well done on a project is positive reinforcement. Exempting the final examination for a job well done on a project is negative reinforcement. A mental health example for reinforcement is getting praise from others when practicing stress management techniques; this is positive reinforcement. Negative reinforcement would be feeling less anxiety afterward. The removal or reduction in stress reinforces the behavior to practice stress management techniques. Reinforcers include tangible and nontangible rewards—for example, money, candy, praise, getting out of unwanted work, social participation opportunities, and engagement in fun activities. The occupational therapy practitioner can benefit by considering how reinforcement can support learning and behavior in treating clients. Two commonly used examples of behavior therapy are token economies and extinction.[21]

Token economies use reinforcement to modify behavior.[21] Individuals earn tokens, such as coins or stickers, which can be redeemed for prizes or privileges. This strategy is often used by parents and teachers to reinforce positive behaviors. Extinction is the removal of reinforcement to eliminate a behavior.[21] An example is a time-out in which a person is removed from a situation that provides reinforcement and required to sit in isolation, without attention or other forms of reinforcement.

In 1957, Albert Ellis introduced rational emotive behavior therapy (REBT), which purports that irrational beliefs lead to emotional distress.[23] The focus of REBT is on changing irrational beliefs into rational beliefs, thus leading to healthier emotions and adaptive behaviors versus maladaptive behaviors.[23] RET focuses on the irrational belief of an individual who demands that others and life circumstances be exactly as the person wants them to be. For example, "I must get that promotion; you must invite me to participate; my vacation must be perfect." If these beliefs are not fulfilled, the individual has little tolerance and becomes noticeably frustrated and agitated. The view that events are catastrophic if they don't occur in a certain way or people are awful if they don't act in a certain way is a common theme disrupting occupational functioning. Examples of irrational values or beliefs held by some individuals include the following[17]:

- The need to be loved and approved by everybody
- The need to be perfect to be worthwhile
- The belief that some people are bad and must be punished
- The belief that a person's unhappiness is caused by other people or events that are out of that person's control.

Irrational beliefs can also be explained within the ABC model.[24] An A refers to an activating event, B refers to the belief that the individual has about the event (in this case an irrational belief), and C refers to the consequences of that belief (in this case an unhealthy consequence). Ellis referred to this as the ABC model. In this model, activating events do not cause unhealthy consequences, such as negative emotions or behaviors; it is the irrational beliefs that cause the consequence.[24] It is how these activating events are cognitively processed and evaluated—in other words, the formation of beliefs—that determines the consequences.[25]

Cognitive theory was developed by Aaron Beck and states that an individual's thoughts, or personal view of the world, affects how situations are perceived.[17,26] Distressing or unrealistic thoughts lead to negative interpretations and feelings, and these can result in negative actions or behavior. When this is a pattern for the individual, psychological distress ensues, and occupational functioning is affected. Cognitive therapy uses a scientific method to identify and test personal beliefs. The therapist helps the patient identify personal thoughts or beliefs and consider alternate behaviors that are healthier.[26]

Beck identified three levels of cognition—core beliefs, dysfunctional assumptions, and negative automatic thoughts.[27,28] Core beliefs are those beliefs that are usually formed early in life and are firmly ingrained regarding the world, self, and others. Dysfunctional assumptions are unrealistic thoughts that frame how one lives and functions in the world. Negative automatic thoughts emerge in the face of daily tasks and new situations and have a theme of pessimism or defeat. This thought process results in what is

referred to as "cognitive distortions." Examples of cognitive distortions include overgeneralization, jumping to conclusions, black-and-white thinking, blaming, global labeling, catastrophizing, and always being right.

REBT has similarities with Beck's cognitive theory approach, and both contributed significantly to the development of CBT. CBT seeks to change the thoughts believed to result in negative perceptions and behaviors. Four characteristics of CBT that are unique from other psychotherapeutic approaches are as follows: a focus on the present; a collaborative process between therapist and client; problem-focused; and usually is a time-limited process.[29]

There are a variety of cognitive and behavioral techniques that can be used in therapeutic settings to assist the person in changing nonproductive thoughts and negative beliefs and therefore change behavior.[28] Occupational therapy practitioners can use these techniques with clients who they believe are having difficulty progressing in occupational therapy due to distorted thinking. A list of techniques and potential occupational therapy examples is provided here.

Cognitive Techniques

Guided discovery[26,27] uses a form of questioning that is referred to as "Socratic questioning" because it is modeled after the manner in which Socrates, the classical Greek philosopher, used to guide his students in resolving questions. Socratic questioning can be used to understand and ultimately resolve complex questions. The questions focus on clarification and probing assumptions, evidence, viewpoints, perspectives, implications, and consequences. It involves trying to understand the client's view of the situation and helps the client explore personal assumptions. Examples of questions include the following:

- "What could you assume instead?"
- "What could be an alternative way to look at this?"
- "What are the strengths and weaknesses of . . . ?"
- "What are the consequences of that assumption?"

Guided discovery can be embedded into a therapy session when clients struggle with occupational performance and the therapist suspects it to be more of a cognitive perception of ability or task performance as opposed to skill level and potential. Assumptions about what people with disabilities, and ultimately self, can and cannot do may be a factor in how therapy is progressing. Exploring the client's assumptions and helping the individual explore underlying assumptions and alternative perspectives and potential solutions for self can be very beneficial. This may also be referred to as "logical or rational analysis"[26,27] of an assumption or belief and can help dispute irrational beliefs.

Targeting dysfunctional assumptions[26,27] is an approach whereby the client is asked to provide evidence that supports or does not support personal assumptions. If the assumption is that the client cannot be independent in cooking, the client is asked to provide specific evidence that supports this assumption. If the client is unable to provide specific evidence, or it does not hold up to scrutiny and discussion with the therapist, it can help the client rethink the assumption and consider alternatives to being successful. Additionally, if the thought or belief is true, what would it mean for the client? This is referred to as "vertical descent."[26] The therapist guides the client in a process of conceptually exploring in a downward direction:

- If the client cannot be independent in cooking, then how will meals be prepared?
- What options are available?
- What does this mean for the client?

This can help alleviate fears and challenge the underlying assumption: "If I cannot cook (or do another occupation) independently, then I am a burden to others," and so forth. Some individuals with disabilities, both of a physical and mental nature, have this assumption, which interferes with their quality of life and personal well-being.

The double-standard dispute[26,30] is a technique in which the therapist asks the client if they would hold another person they know to the same standard. For an individual with mental illness who sees self as flawed or unlovable, the therapist would ask that person how others with similar diagnoses or occupational performance limitations should be viewed. Are others held to the same standard? If not, why not? This can be helpful for individuals who think that their illness or performance deficits are weaknesses that prevent them from obtaining any quality of life or happiness. It can help the client address core beliefs about self and ultimately become less rigid in the view the client has of self.

The catastrophe scale[30] is a technique in which the client is asked to rate something that has been anxiety-provoking or has been the focus of negative energy for the individual. If the client fears rejection due to the stigma of mental illness from a friend or family member, the client is asked to rate how that would feel on a scale of 1 to 100. Other items are added to the scale to put it into perspective[26]; in other words, what would be worse than this? As more items are listed, the rating of the feared item is adjusted accordingly. The client can objectively see how these compare to other potential occurrences, and the opportunity for adjusting the negative assumption is presented.

Similarly, the client can be asked to rate the degree of belief in the negative thought or assumption and rate the degree of emotion associated with the thought or assumption.[26] Any scale can be used, such as a 10-point rating scale. The client can rate the degree of belief and emotion in a variety of differing scenarios with varying environmental contexts and different people. For example, if the client has a belief of being disliked by others because of body image concerns, the individual is asked to rate this belief and associated emotion in a variety of contexts.

Reverse role-playing[26,30] provides a method for the client to argue against the negative assumption or belief that the client possesses. The therapist plays the role of the client, and the client becomes the therapist. The conversation follows, with the client working to convince the therapist of the irrationality of the belief or assumption. For example, if the client believes that independent living is not possible, the client will argue to convince the therapist that it is possible. The client must understand and buy into this exercise for it to be successful. If the client is willing to participate, the opportunity to identify different assumptions and perspectives is useful for the client.

Reframing[30] is a technique whereby the therapist works with the client to consider all aspects of a situation:

- Is there a positive side to the negative situation?
- Is something that is considered unbearable able to be reevaluated as uncomfortable?
- If the client cannot resume a former occupation, does this allow for participation in another occupation of interest?

The occupational therapy practitioner works with the client to brainstorm and identify other interests and occupations for participation and personal satisfaction

Behavioral Techniques

Graded task assignments[26,27] involves rating activities based on complexity, level of skill needed, and/or pleasure to make the task manageable and increase the client's success. Occupational therapy practitioners are trained to grade and adapt activities; therefore this is a natural part of the therapeutic process in occupational therapy. The emphasis in CBT is the collaboration with the client to enhance personal awareness and skills in breaking down activities into manageable steps and engaging the client cognitively to affect behavior. This fits well with the client-centered approach in occupational therapy, and it assists clients in dealing with difficult issues related to occupational performance. For the client with mental illness, engaging in previous activities that have been neglected by beginning with the least difficult and progressing to more complex tasks can be beneficial.

Additionally, activity scheduling[26,27] is a behavioral technique that involves planning routines and tasks in advance to promote success. Again, this is a core concept in occupational therapy practice. Teaching clients to understand the impact of routines and habits on occupational performance can help reduce negative beliefs related to occupational performance by reestablishing daily routines and increasing participation in pleasurable activities.

Behavioral experiments[27] can be used to test predictions that certain behaviors will be catastrophic or disastrous. At times, the client will avoid a certain behavior because of the belief that it will not result in success or pleasure. The client is guided in gathering evidence to the contrary. For example, if a client is fearful of going to public places for fear that something awful will happen, evidence is collected to counter this belief. Evidence might include talking to other people about the safety of public places and experimenting with short trips during nonpeak times. If the fear is grounded in decreased functional abilities or emotional tolerance, identifying ways to adapt needed skills and experimenting in low-stress situations can be beneficial. Specific techniques that can be used in behavioral experiments include targeted exposure, planned risk taking, and hypothesis testing.[27]

Modeling[26] is a behavioral technique in which the therapist or another person demonstrates the desired behavior to the client. The behavior may be something that clients do not believe they can do, such as putting on a shirt with one arm or manipulating an assistive device. The person then imitates the behavior, modifying it as needed until successful. Behavioral rehearsal[26] or role-playing can also be used and works well in situations in which a client is struggling with verbal interaction, such as in being assertive with someone. Practicing what to say and how to say it can be helpful and can break down negative assumptions regarding personal ability. Coaching can also be part of the process to encourage and support new behaviors, as can scripting, the process of writing a script for handling a difficult upcoming situation.[26]

Brief techniques that can be helpful include teaching the client to use thought-stopping techniques.[26] An example is the use of a rubber band on the wrist that the client snaps every time a negative thought emerges. Teaching a client to use new self-statements[26] is also a brief simple technique that can be used effectively. For example, the client can be encouraged to create self-statements such as "I am assertive" or "I will accomplish my goal for today" and write the self-statement on a card, placing it where it will be seen multiple times throughout the day. The client can also practice saying the goal out loud frequently. Positive self-statements provide an opportunity for learning to believe in oneself; what is heard is more likely to develop into a belief.

There are many types of relaxation skills that are behavioral techniques for clients to learn in managing anxiety and addressing negative assumptions about personal ability to handle stressful situations. Progressive relaxation training[27] is a relaxation approach in which the individual is taught to focus on one muscle group at a time, tense the muscle group, and then release the tension, relaxing that muscle group completely. The individual moves through different muscle groups, focusing on tensing and relaxing each group. Progressive muscle relaxation creates awareness of the feeling of tension versus relaxation throughout the body; it is based on the idea that mental calmness is a result of physical relaxation. It is relatively easy to learn and can be completed in about 10 to 20 minutes.[27]

Breathing exercises[27] are also easy to learn and implement. There are different ways to focus breathing exercises to reduce anxiety and focus the mind on the body. One way is deep breathing, in which the intent is to breathe in as deeply as possible. Lying down or in a sitting position, the individual breathes in through the nose while one hand is on the stomach. The stomach should move as the lungs fill with air to ensure a deep breath. If the chest and shoulders are rising more than the lungs, then the breath is too shallow. Most people have a tendency toward shallow breathing. Once the person is comfortable with deep breathing, it is practiced for several minutes at a time. At least three deep breaths at a time are encouraged. Additionally, focusing on peaceful images while deep breathing, imagining stress and tension being released when exhaling, and counting while breathing in and out to regulate breathing can be useful. This is a very easy and quick technique to encourage clients to use when feeling anxious. It can easily be taught and practiced in a treatment session and should be reinforced regularly. Breathing exercises can be implemented prior to any activity that is anxiety-provoking.

There are many behaviors that people can engage in to manage negative beliefs related to anxiety and self-perception. Identifying ways to protect self from stress, such as biofeedback and listening to soothing music, is referred to as "stress inoculation."[26] The therapist can encourage the client to develop skills to use when needed. Guided imagery, yoga, and mindfulness are additional tools that people can learn to feel calmer, grounded, and more self-aware. Other skills such as assertiveness training and communication skills training can also benefit the client in addressing core beliefs and assumptions.[26] Each client is unique, and the therapist must collaborate with the client to identify the most appropriate strategies.

An important element of CBT is cognitive homework.[26] Having the client engage in experiential activities and practicing skills at home and in daily life are important for learning to use behavioral techniques. Bibliotherapy, the provision of appropriate articles or books to read, can be beneficial. Clients can learn to engage in rational self-analysis to evaluate assumptions that they have about everyday occurrences. Clients can then discuss their homework experiences with the therapist for further understanding of their beliefs and assumptions and how they affect their occupational performance.

Assessments

There are a variety of assessments that can be considered as learning or behavioral assessments. A brief description of selected tools is provided here, and the reader is referred to the reference list for an in-depth discussion of each assessment.

Comprehensive Occupational Therapy Evaluation

The comprehensive occupational therapy evaluation (COTE),[31] developed in 1975, is a behavior rating scale that is designed to be used by occupational therapists in short-term, acute care psychiatric settings. It is used to identify general behaviors, interpersonal behaviors, and task behaviors that affect occupational performance. There are 26 behaviors defined, and each one is rated on a five-point scale. The scale can be used as an initial evaluation or as a record of patient progress. The COTE scale serves as a guide for the assessment of behaviors that affect occupational performance. It can be completed in as little as 5 minutes, and usually no more than 20 minutes is required.

Kohlman Evaluation of Living Skills

The Kohlman Evaluation of Living Skills (KELS)[32] was developed in 1977; it was initially intended for use in short-term psychiatric units. The KELS assesses a person's ability to function in basic living skills. Following evaluation, recommendations for living as independently as possible are made; 13 living skills in the following five areas are tested: self-care, safety and health, money management, transportation and telephone, and work and leisure. The fourth edition is appropriate for use with many populations and in many settings. It is easily administered in approximately 45 minutes through interview questions and task performance.

Bay Area Functional Performance Evaluation

The Bay Area Functional Performance Evaluation (BaFPE)[33] was developed in 1977 and revised in 1987; it was developed for inpatient and outpatient mental health facilities. It assesses functioning needed for daily living and includes the task-oriented assessment (TOA) and social interaction scale (SIS). The TOA looks at the person's ability to act on the environment in goal-directed ways and includes five tasks: (1) sorting shells by size, shape, and color; (2) calculating the amount of money needed to buy certain items; (3) drawing a home floor plan; (4) duplicating a block design; and (5) drawing a person doing a task. The SIS assesses the ability to relate to other people in five different social settings: (1) one-to-one interview; (2) mealtime; (3) unstructured group situation; (4) structured activity group; and (5) structured discussion-focused group. It can be completed in 30 to 45 minutes.

Performance Assessment of Self-Care Skills

The Performance Assessment of Self-Care Skills (version 4.0; PASS)[34,35] is designed to measure occupational performance of daily life tasks. It consists of 26 tasks in 4 domains: 5 functional mobility tasks, 3 basic activities of daily living (ADL) tasks, 14 instrumental ADL tasks with a cognitive emphasis, and 4 instrumental ADL tasks with a physical emphasis. It can be used in a variety of settings and is a performance-based observational tool. There are two versions, a clinic version and a home version. Selected items can be used alone for assessment. Items are scored on a four-point ordinal scale resulting in scores for task independence, task safety, and task adequacy. PASS was developed by occupational therapists Joan Rogers and Margo Holm. Practitioners can access all materials at the following link by completing a brief survey—http://www.shrs.pitt.edu/ot/about/performance-assessment-self-care-skills-pass.

HUMANISTIC PSYCHOLOGY

By the 1950s, psychologists who were interested in a more humanistic vision for the practice of psychology, different from the psychodynamic and behavioral approaches, met to discuss the humanistic approach. It was referred to as the "third force" behind psychoanalysis and behaviorism.[36] There were perceived limitations of these two approaches in that behaviorism did not take into account the subjective elements of consciousness in behavior because it did not lend itself to scientific study and understanding, and psychoanalysis focused primarily on the unconscious mind.[37] Humanistic approaches instead focus on the subjective meaning of behavior and the innate motivation of the individual to engage in personal growth and fulfillment.[37]

It was at this time that the Association for Humanistic Psychology was formed.[38] Humanistic psychology values a person's subjective perception and understanding of the world more than objective reality. It offers a set of values for understanding human nature, such as the capacity to develop personal competence and self-respect. Independent dignity, the worth of human beings, and the interaction of the body, mind, and spirit are emphasized. The core values of the Association for Humanistic Psychology include the following[38]:

- A belief in the worth of persons and dedication to the development of human potential

- An understanding of life as a process—change is inevitable
- An appreciation of the spiritual and intuitive
- A commitment to ecologic integrity
- A recognition of the profound problems affecting our world and a responsibility to hope and constructive change

The contributions of humanistic psychology can be summarized as providing a different perspective toward understanding human nature, focusing on qualitative approaches for scientific inquiry of human behavior, and expanding the repertoire of effective approaches in counseling clients. The focus of behavior is considered from the perspective of the meaning that the client has for that behavior. Humans are believed to be inherently good and motivated toward personal positive growth and self-exploration. A holistic view of the person is supported; this is necessary for effective collaboration and therapeutic outcomes.[38]

Prior to the formal development of humanistic psychology, Abraham Maslow developed a hierarchic theory of human motivation and subsequent "hierarchy of human needs." This theory proposed that an individual is motivated to meet basic physiologic needs before other needs can be met. The order of needs to be met move from physiologic to safety, followed by a sense of belonging, then esteem, and finally self-actualization.[39,40] Maslow stated that the inability to have needs met within the levels of the hierarchy could result in the development of mental health issues. For example, the failure to have safety needs met could result in the occurrence of posttraumatic stress disorder, or the failure to feel belongingness or love could result in depression or anxiety. Motivational theory can be applied to rehabilitation by helping structure a process whereby the patient can prioritize lower-level goals that need to be achieved as progress toward independence in functional activities is achieved.[40]

Carl Rogers, one of the early leaders of humanistic psychology, is credited with the introduction of person-centered therapy in the 1960s. Person-centered therapy focuses on a therapeutic relationship in which the therapist collaborates with empathetic understanding and provides unconditional positive regard. In 1962, Carl Rogers stated, "An assumption unusual in psychology today is that the subjective human being has an important value which is basic; that no matter how he may be labeled and evaluated he is a human person first of all and most deeply."[38]

The collaboration between practitioner and client is the central element in the occupational therapy process, as depicted in the Occupational Therapy Practice Framework.[41] Therapeutic use of self is a therapeutic agent essential to the practice of occupational therapy, and it is to be used consistently with all clients. The use of narrative and clinical reasoning, empathy, and collaboration are necessary components of the interaction between the practitioner and client.[42] Connecting with clients at an emotional level and assisting clients to identify their needs, priorities, and goals by facilitating the sharing of life experiences and personal perspectives support the collaborative process. This allows clients to find meaning in their current situation and identify personal meaningful goals for the future. Occupational therapy is congruent with the value orientation of humanistic psychology. Through knowledge of occupational engagement and therapeutic use of self, occupational therapy practitioners support clients' health, participation in everyday living, and quality of life.

The influence of humanism has grown and is not isolated as a specific approach. For example, elements of humanism are reflected in the recovery model as part of personal empowerment and growth. Examples of techniques that embrace a humanistic approach include mindfulness, sensory awareness, spirituality, and strength-focused therapies. An emphasis on greater self-awareness and personal growth toward self-actualization is emphasized. Humanism is reflected in occupational therapy through the development of the occupational profile and the collaborative process that drives treatment.

Humanistic psychology focuses on the subjective and qualitative aspects of the individual. Assessments that engage the client through the use of a narrative approach or life history review reflect a humanistic orientation. Qualitative interviews that are unstructured work well to elicit the subjective nature of the individual. The therapist should develop a list of topic questions to guide the interview and then develop additional questions in response to the information provided by the patient during the interview. Semistructured interview assessments, such as the Canadian Occupational Performance Measure (COPM), allow for the patient to provide subjective, qualitative information.[43]

Through the therapeutic use of self, a humanistic approach is always present in therapy sessions with clients. Examples of Maslow's hierarchy of needs also provide insight into the influence of humanism in occupational therapy. Examples of populations at risk for fulfilling the needs at each level are provided in Box 6.1.

DEVELOPMENTAL APPROACH

In this section, the focus is on various aspects of adult psychosocial development. There are many models, each with their own perspective and approach to understanding how individuals develop and change throughout adulthood. A brief overview of selected models is provided, with considerations for occupational therapy practitioners.

BOX 6.1 Maslow's Hierarchy of Needs

Level	Needs	Populations at Risk
Self-actualization	Realizing personal potential, creativity, spontaneity, lack of prejudice, happiness, self-fulfillment	Individuals with depression and anxiety Substance abusers
Esteem	Self-esteem, confidence, achievement, respect, recognition, status	Individuals with depression and anxiety Individuals who hear distressing voices
Love, belonging	Friendship, family, intimacy belongingness, love, affection, family, friends, relationships	Individuals with poor social skills Dysfunctional families Individuals with personality disorders
Safety	Safety, shelter, security, law and order, employment, health, stability	Victims of abuse Prisoners Individuals experiencing psychosis
Physiologic	Food, water, sleep air, food, water, shelter, warmth, sleep	Homeless individuals Low SES populations

SES, Socioeconomic status.

Perhaps the most well-known model is Erik Erikson's psychosocial theory consisting of eight stages throughout the life span.[44] Erikson focused on the importance of social interaction in development and proposed a stage theory consisting of eight stages, each with a defined developmental task. Each stage is characterized by a psychosocial crisis of two conflicting forces with a resulting outcome, or virtue, if the forces are reconciled appropriately. The last four stages cover the period from adolescence to late adulthood and are presented in Box 6.2. Transitioning from stage to stage may create tension as the individual works toward resolving the psychosocial crisis, and unresolved tasks may be carried forward. Challenges may result from unresolved tasks of previous stages creating tension for the individual.

Robert Havighurst was a psychologist and one of the primary contributors to the Developmental Tasks Theory.[45] According to this theory, development occurs in stages throughout the life span, with specific tasks identified for each stage. It is a biopsychosocial model of development in that tasks are influenced by many factors, such as genetics, physiology, personal values, interests, and cultural norms. For an individual to progress from one stage to the next stage, developmental tasks must be successfully mastered in a somewhat sequential manner. There is a sense of pride and satisfaction, both by the individual and social community, when tasks are completed or skills are mastered. Progression to the next stage is facilitated, and development continues successfully. Failure to accomplish developmental tasks results in dissatisfaction with self, and negative coping mechanisms and behaviors may emerge. There may be disapproval by the individual's social community as well.

Havighurst identified six major periods of development, the last three stages occur in adulthood and are young adulthood from approximately 19 to 29 years; middle adulthood from approximately 30 to 60 years; and later maturity from approximately 60 years to end of life. Age ranges are not rigid, but significant variations would indicate problems in successful development for the individual. A summary of Havighurst's developmental tasks is provided in Box 6.3.

Vaillant, a psychiatrist, also focused on adult development and identified six adult life tasks to be successfully accomplished for a person to mature as an adult.[46] The focus is on tasks, as opposed to stages, because "task" reflects an active intentional process, not merely a stage to be passed through automatically. These tasks are as follows:

1. Developing an identity. The adolescent establishes a personal identity defined by values, passions, and beliefs that allows for separation from parents. This includes living

BOX 6.2 Lifespan Stages: Adolescence Through Late Adulthood

Stage	Psychosocial Crisis	Virtue
Adolescence	Identity versus role confusion	Fidelity
Early adulthood	Intimacy versus isolation	Love
Middle adulthood	Generativity versus stagnation	Care
Late adulthood	Integrity versus despair	Wisdom

BOX 6.3 Developmental Tasks of Adulthood	
Stage (years)	**Task**
Early adulthood (19–29)	Selecting a life partner Learning to live with a life partner Starting a family Raising children Managing a home Engaging in an occupation of choice Developing civic interests and responsibility Establishing role within a social group
Middle adulthood (30–60)	Assisting children to become successful adults Fostering equality in spousal relationship Achieving career satisfaction and success Supporting economic standard of living Developing adult leisure time activities Accepting the physiologic changes of middle age Achieving adult social and civic responsibility Adjusting to aging parents
Later maturity (≥60)	Adjusting to decreases in physical health Adjusting to retirement and reduced income Adjusting to death or illness of spouse Maintaining relationships with one's age group Adjusting to declining social and civic obligations Maintaining satisfactory living quarters

apart from one's parents or guardians and establishing one's own independence economically and socially.

2. Development of intimacy. The person expands the sense of self and becomes involved intimately with a partner in an interdependent, reciprocal, and committed relationship.

3. Career consolidation. The person identifies a career that is meaningful and valuable to self and society. A career is defined as providing contentment, compensation, competence, and commitment.

4. Generativity. This task involves giving to others or society in an unselfish manner, such as providing mentorship to others. The focus is on caring for the next generation and may take the form of community building through coaching and guiding others in society.

5. Becoming keeper of the meaning. Linking the past to the future is the purpose of this task. Traditions are passed on as a means of preserving the culture in which one lives.

6. Achieving integrity.

The last task is centered around achieving a sense of peace about the life one has lived and being at peace with the world; wisdom in the life one has lived is apparent.[46]

Carl Jung, a psychiatrist and psychoanalyst who is regarded as the founder of analytic psychology, contributed to the understanding of adult development, particularly what is referred to as "middlescence."[17] He was an early follower of Freud and shared some of his ideas regarding the unconscious mind. He valued the older adult but, unlike Freud, believed that there is substantial developmental work for the adult to achieve to reach full potential. He identified four expressions of the adult psyche that he saw as creating tension in the unconscious mind and that needed to be explored and resolved for optimal growth and development. These expressions exist on a continuum and include the following[17]:

- Introversion, focused on the self, versus extroversion, focused on others
- Tangible seeing versus intuition
- A desire for material comfort versus spirituality
- Femininity versus masculinity

Jung believed that attitudes or behavior are expressed on one end of the continuum and that attention needed to be provided to explore attitudes and behaviors on the other end of the continuum. Those latent qualities needed to be developed and be allowed expression in a person's life. This process is referred to as "individuation." He referred to these opposing expressions as "polarities" or "forces" in the psyche. A major task of middle adulthood is to explore these polarities and integrate them satisfactorily, a process called "transcendence." To achieve transcendence is the primary goal of adulthood. Jung saw middle age as a time of significant individual growth that could last well into older adulthood. He put great value in older adults and valued the wisdom that can be achieved as one approaches the end of life.[17]

In more recent years, a new life stage has been identified. The age in between adolescence and young adulthood was identified in the 1990s as emerging adulthood.[47] This stage is identified by difficulty in leaving adolescence and moving to a state of personal independence and responsibility. There is difficulty in severing the ties of dependence on parents and difficulty with establishing personal identity and independence. This time from the end of adolescence to the young adult responsibilities of a stable job, relationship, and children is a newer phenomenon in this country, which has developed in response to social and economic changes. Five features define this stage[47]:

1. Identity exploration as the individual focuses on what is desired out of relationships and work
2. Instability due to frequent moves between college, job transitions, and relationships
3. Self-focus as time is invested in different experiences prior to committing to marriage, children, and a career
4. Feeling in between, despite taking responsibility for themselves
5. Optimistic that life will be satisfying in both work and relationships

Research has indicated that emerging adults have high expectations for satisfying, well-paying careers and long-lasting happy relationships and may be setting themselves up for unhappiness. Times have changed in that 50 years ago, the median age for marriage was 22 years for men and 20 years for women. Now, the median age for marriage is more than 28 years for men and 24 years for women. Greater opportunities to attend college or receive post–high school training have delayed career and marriage. Additionally, more women attend college and strive for careers than previously, and they delay marriage and children. Advances in birth control have allowed women more control in delaying childbearing as well. Relaxed attitudes toward sexual relationships outside of marriage have also delayed the commitment of marriage by many young adults. Finally, young adults have more choices than in previous years and are therefore exploring many different paths on their way to adulthood.[47]

Interestingly, this has created challenges for many young adults. More opportunities mean less structure and predetermined paths to follow. For some young adults, this can be difficult to navigate. Practitioners may find it difficult to distinguish between emerging adults who are having normal identity issues with those who are having more serious issues. National survey data have revealed that it is common for about half of all young adults to feel anxious and one-third to feel depressed.[48] The instability can be frustrating, and many young adults may not have adequate social support. The survey data noted that half rely on social media for social support. Young adults who are struggling to progress through this stage could benefit from occupational therapy services to help them transition into new roles and routines. Many emerging adults who face problems becoming independent have faced past challenges meeting developmental tasks for one reason or another. Occupational therapy practitioners gather information during the occupational profile and interview that provides insight into developmental task performance. Understanding the context and meaning of developmental tasks relevant to the client's age or developmental progression overall will determine if unsuccessful task implementation is negatively affecting occupational performance.

SUMMARY

This chapter has provided a brief overview of various psychosocial approaches that have contributed to the practice of occupational therapy, not just in mental health settings but in all practice areas. Looking at the client using different theoretic approaches can allow for a greater understanding of what drives human behavior. Understanding the different approaches broadens the treatment approaches as well and provides more tools for the occupational therapy practitioner to embrace. Understanding occupational performance is a complex, multifaceted process that benefits from a broad base of knowledge regarding human behavior. The practitioner is encouraged to learn more about these and other approaches that contribute to practice.

SUGGESTED LEARNING ACTIVITIES

1. Ask a friend or family member to create a collage that is a representation of their self. Reflect on the personal meaning of the completed collage, as well as their use of materials, approach to the task, and organizational skills. What did you learn about the person that you did not already know? What did the individual "project"

onto the collage that you might not have learned from an interview alone?

2. Identify a negative thought or belief that you personally recognize about yourself. Apply a cognitive behavioral approach to elicit a change in your thoughts and/or beliefs. Potential approaches to apply include thought-stopping techniques such as wearing a rubber band on your wrist and "snapping" it when the thought is present or engaging in making positive self-statements throughout the day to replace the negative thoughts. This may include writing positive statements and posting them on your mirror or carrying it with you to read throughout the day. After a week, reflect on whether this

has made a difference in your thoughts and beliefs. If yes, why? If no, try another approach such as journaling (expressive media) to see if it makes a difference. Reflect on how these approaches could be used with clients.

3. Interview someone you know well, preferably a family member or close friend, who is between the ages of 40 and 65 years and someone you know well who is older than 65 years. Use the developmental tasks for their age range as a guide for the interview, and identify which tasks they are currently addressing. Ask them to reflect on their successes and challenges in addressing developmental tasks from young adulthood. Reflect on everything you have learned about each person that you did not previously know.

REFLECTION QUESTIONS

1. What are some commonly used defense mechanisms that you may observe in clients?
2. How can a cognitive-behavioral approach be integrated into occupational therapy treatment sessions?
3. What elements of humanistic psychology are present in occupational therapy practice today?
4. How is an understanding of adult development relevant to the practice of occupational therapy?

REFERENCES

1. Peloquin SM. Moral treatment: contexts considered. *Am J Occup Ther.* 1989;43(8):537-544.
2. Solomon AP. Occupational therapy; a psychiatric treatment. *Am J Occup Ther.* 1947;1(1):1-9.
3. Schwartz KB. Reclaiming our heritage: connecting the founding vision to the centennial vision. *Am J Occup Ther.* 2009;63(6):681-690.
4. Dunton WR. History of occupational therapy. *Mod Hosp.* 1917;8(6):380-382.
5. McLeod SA. Psychoanalysis. www.simplypsychology.org/humanistic.html.
6. Bornstein R. The psychodynamic perspective. In: Biswas-Diener R, Diener E, eds. *Noba Textbook Series: Psychology.* Champaign, IL: DEF; 2018.
7. Daniel MA, Blair SEE. An introduction to the psychodynamic frame of reference. In: Duncan E, ed. *Foundations for Practice in Occupational Therapy.* 5th ed. Churchill Livingstone, Elsevier; 2012.
8. Cramer P. Defense mechanisms: 40 years of empirical research, *J Pers Assess.* 2015;97(2):114-122.
9. McLeod SA. Defense Mechanisms. Available at: www.simplypsychology.org/defense-mechanisms.html.
10. Grohol J. 15 common defense mechanisms. Available at: https://psychcentral.com/lib/15-common-defense-mechanisms.
11. Burgo J. *Why Do I Do That? Psychological Defense Mechanisms and the Hidden Ways they Shape our Lives.* Chapel Hill, NC: New Rise Press; 2012.
12. Vaillant GE, Bond M, Valliant CO. An empirically validated hierarchy of defense mechanisms. *Arch Gen Psychiatry.* 1986;73:786-794.
13. Blackman J. Defense mechanisms in the 21st century. *Synergy.* 2011;16(2):1-7.
14. Zafram H, Tallant B. "It would be a shame to lose them": a critical historical, scoping, and expert review on the use of projective assessments in occupational therapy, part I. *Occup Ther Ment Health.* 2015;31(3):187-210.
15. Reynolds F. Expressive media used as assessment in mental health. In: Hemphill-Pearson BJ, ed. *Assessments in Occupational Therapy Mental Health. An Integrative Approach.* 2nd ed. Thorofare, NJ: Slack Inc; 2008:81-96.
16. Azima H, Azima FJ. Outline of a dynamic theory of occupational therapy. *Am J Occup Ther.* 1959;13(5):215-221.
17. Ikiugu MN. *Psychosocial Conceptual Practice Models in Occupational Therapy: Building Adaptive Capability.* St. Louis, MO: Elsevier; 2007.
18. Lerner C, Ross G. The magazine picture collage: development of an objective scoring system. *Am J Occup Ther.* 1977;31(3):156-161.
19. Lerner C. The magazine picture collage: its clinical use and validity as an assessment device. *Am J Occup Ther.* 1979;33(8):500-504.
20. Zafram H, Tallant B. "It would be a shame to lose them": a critical historical, scoping, and expert review on the use of projective assessments in occupational therapy, part II. *Occup Ther Ment Health.* 2015;31(4):328-365.
21. Cherry K. What is behavioral therapy? Available at: https://www.verywellmind.com/what-is-behavioral-therapy-2795998.
22. Cherry K. Positive and negative reinforcement in operant conditioning: how reinforcement is used in psychology. Available at: https://www.verywellmind.com/what-is-reinforcement-2795414.

23. Altrows IF. A man for all reason: Albert Ellis and rational emotive behavior therapy. *Synergy*. 2011;16(2):8-10.
24. Sarracino D, Dimaggio G, Ibrahim R, Popolo R, Sassaroli S, Ruggiero GM. When REBT goes difficult: applying ABC-DEF to personality disorders. *J Ration Emot Cogn Behav Ther*. 2017;35(3):278-295.
25. Oltean HR, Hyland P, Vallieres F, David DO. An empirical assessment of REBT models of psychopathology and psychological health in the prediction of anxiety and depression symptoms. *Behav Cogn Psychother*. 2017;45(6):600-615.
26. Leahy RL. *Cognitive Therapy Techniques: A Practitioner's Guide*. 2nd ed. New York: Guilford Publications; 2017.
27. Fenn K, Byrne M. The key principles of cognitive behavioural therapy. Available at: https://journals.sagepub.com/doi/full/10.1177/1755738012471029
28. Leahy RL. *Practicing Cognitive Therapy: A Guide to Interventions*. Lanham, MD: Jason Aronson; 1997.
29. Creek J. Cognitive approaches to intervention. In: Bryant W, Fieldhouse J, Bannigan K, eds. *Creek's Occupational Therapy and Mental Health*. 5th ed. Edinburgh: Churchill Livingstone; 2014:50-71.
30. Froggart W. A brief introduction to cognitive-behaviour therapy. Available at: https://www.rational.org.nz/prof-docs/Intro-CBT.pdf.
31. Brayman SJ. The comprehensive occupational therapy evaluation (COTE). In: Hemphill-Pearson BJ, ed. *Assessments in Occupational Therapy Mental Health: An Integrative Approach*. 2nd ed. Thorofare, NJ: Slack; 2008.
32. Kohlman L, Robnett R. Kohlman evaluation of living skills. 4th rev ed. *American Occupational Therapy*: 2016, Bethesda, MD.
33. Klyczek JP, Stanton E. The Bay Area functional performance evaluation. In: Hemphill-Pearson BJ, ed. *Assessments in Occupational Therapy Mental Health: An Integrative Approach*. 2nd ed. Thorofare, NJ: Slack; 2008.
34. Holm MB, Rogers JC. The performance assessment of self-care skills (PASS). In: Hemphill-Pearson BJ, ed. *Assessments in Occupational Therapy Mental Health: An Integrative Approach*. 2nd ed. Thorofare, NJ: Slack; 2008.
35. Rogers JC, Holm MB. Performance Assessment of Self-Care Skills (PASS). Available at: https://www.ono.ac.il/wp-content/uploads/PASS-Home-Test-Manual.pdf.
36. Maslow AH. *Toward a Psychology of Being*. 2nd ed. New York: Van Nostrand; 1968.
37. Glassman W, Hadad M. *Approaches to Psychology*. 5th ed. New York: McGraw-Hill; 2008.
38. Association for Humanistic Psychology. What is humanistic psychology? Available at: https://www.ahpweb.org/item/8-humanistic-psychology-overview.html.
39. McLeod SA. Humanism. Available at: www.simplypsychology.org/humanistic.html.
40. Stineman MG, Kurz AE, Kelleher D, Kennedy BL. The patient's view of recovery: an emerging tool for empowerment through self-knowledge. *Disabil Rehabil*. 2008;30(9):679-688.
41. American Occupational Therapy Association. Occupational therapy practice framework: domain & process 3rd. ed. *Am J Occup Ther*. 2014;68(Suppl 1):S1-S51.
42. Taylor RR, Van Puymbroeck L. Therapeutic use of self: applying the intentional relationship model in group therapy. In: O'Brien JC, Solomon JW, eds. *Occupational Analysis and Group Process*. St. Louis, MO: Elsevier; 2013:36-52.
43. Baptiste S. Client-centered assessment: the Canadian Occupational Performance Measure. In: Hemphill-Pearson BJ, ed. *Assessments in Occupational Therapy Mental Health: An Integrative Approach*. 2nd ed. Thorofare, NJ: Slack; 2008.
44. Erikson EH. *Identity and the Life Cycle*. London: W.W. Norton; 1980.
45. Gallaue DL, Ozmun JC, Goodway JD. *Understanding Motor Development: Infants, Children, Adolescents, Adults*. 7th ed. New York: McGraw-Hill; 2012.
46. Vaillant GE. *Aging Well*. New York: Hachette Book Group; 2002.
47. Arnett JJ, Žukauskiėn R, Sugimura K. The new life stage of emerging adulthood at ages 18–29 years: implications for mental health. *Lancet Psychiatry*. 2014;1:569-576.
48. Arnett JJ, Schwab J. The Clark University poll of emerging adults: thriving, struggling, and hopeful. Available at: http://www2.clarku.edu/clark-poll-emerging-adults/pdfs/clark-university-poll-emerging-adults-findings.pdf.

Cognitive Approaches

Nancy Carson

INTRODUCTION

Cognition is a complex process necessary for effective occupational performance. Everything a person does in daily life requires some aspect of cognition. Consider the activities that make up a typical day, and consider the skills needed for completing these activities. A cognitive process or skill is required to some degree for successful completion of all daily activities and tasks.

> The American Occupational Therapy Association (AOTA) asserts that occupational therapists and occupational therapy assistants, through the use of occupations and activities, facilitate individuals' cognitive functioning to enhance occupational performance, self-efficacy, participation, and perceived quality of life. Cognition is integral to effective performance across the broad range of daily occupations such as work, educational pursuits, home management, and plan and leisure.[1]

Cognition is defined as a range of mental processes or thinking skills that enable people to learn and function in daily life. These skills are needed for processing information and problem-solving at home, in the community, and in relationships.[2] This includes a broad range of processes such as attention, decision-making, problem-solving, behavioral regulation, memory, and language.[3] Most psychiatric disorders include some degree of cognitive dysfunction, and there is evidence suggesting that cognitive deficits may predispose individuals to developing the psychiatric disorder.[3]

COMPONENTS OF COGNITION

Cognition can be categorized into four broad processes: attention, memory, executive function, and social cognition. Within these broad areas are more specific processes as well as cognitive abilities and skills necessary for occupational performance. Skills and abilities vary in level of complexity and certain ones will be needed for certain activities. Everything we do requires specific cognitive skills for us to be successful.

Attention

Attention is the ability to stay focused on a task for a prolonged period of time despite distractions.[4] Most people can identify times and situations when it was difficult to pay attention. The demands of daily life and the amount of stimulation in our environment can be challenging to our ability to attend to a task or an activity. Imagine reading directions as you are assembling a small item. The directions require multiple steps and there are multiple parts to assemble. You have difficulty attending to the task, as there are people talking in the room, music is playing in the background, and the phone is ringing. There is a storm developing and you can hear thunder rumbling outside. The lights blink off and on, and you notice you are cold and stop to put on a sweater. You eventually give up on assembling the item because it is too frustrating with the auditory, visual, and tactile stimuli present. You can't focus your attention on the task.

An individual experiencing challenges with attention may present in a variety of different ways besides not being able to complete a task. Other examples include not being able to recall several items off a list just read, having trouble learning simple tasks, difficulty concentrating when reading, losing track of time, or appearing absentminded. While the environment contains a broad array of useful and interesting information, it also contains a multitude of distractions. It is impossible to attend to everything that is present in our environment. Effective attention involves figuring out what is important to respond to for satisfactory occupational performance and figuring out how to block out stimuli that are not relevant for the current task at hand. There are constant competing challenges throughout the day for our attention. How we deal with them affects our overall functioning.[5]

There are different types of attention that may be used in different situations. *Sustained attention* is the ability to concentrate or focus attention on one activity for a prolonged time without being distracted.[4,5] Being sufficiently aroused and being alert are supporting elements of sustained attention. Being able to read an article without being distracted is an example of sustained attention. *Selective attention* is the ability to suppress unwanted stimuli and filter distractions that are not relevant, instead focusing on what is desired and relevant for task completion or engagement.[4,5] The ability to focus on one person when at a social gathering and attend to what that person is saying despite the background noise is an example of selective attention. The ability to shift the focus of attention between two or more different tasks is referred to as *alternating attention*.[4] Switching between activities can be demanding, as each activity has its own cognitive demands that are required for success, and alternating back and forth requires additional energy to process the different demands of the activity.[5] Consider alternating between cooking when using a new recipe and listening to the news. At first the focus may be on preparing the ingredients and starting the cooking process. Attention may be shifted to the news while waiting for the stove or oven to heat the food, with the intent to shift back to cooking within a certain length of time. Depending on the content of the news and the cognitive resources used to absorb the information, there may be a delay in shifting the focus back to cooking. Perhaps the food began to burn or overflow before attention was shifted. The ability to effectively alternate attention between two or more tasks can be cognitively demanding and can be difficult for some people to do so effectively. *Divided attention* is the opposite of alternating attention. It is the ability to share attention between two activities simultaneously.[4] This is often referred to as multitasking. An example would be walking on a treadmill while reading a book or listening to music while studying. The more complex the cognitive demands, the more difficult it is to multitask. Many people continue to text while driving, mistakenly thinking they can perform both activities simultaneously without difficulty; however, research has found that this is not true.[6] It can be difficult for the individual to accurately assess the cognitive demands of both activities, therefore divided attention can result in decreased occupational performance.

Memory

Memory can be categorized into three types: short-term memory, long-term memory, and working memory. *Short-term memory* refers to the ability of the human mind to hold a limited amount of information temporarily, generally for a few seconds to a few minutes.[7] *Long-term memory* refers to the storage of information over a longer period of time, anywhere from an hour to decades.[7] Short-term memory and long-term memory differ primarily in this duration of time and also in capacity. Capacity refers to the number of items stored at one time, and this is limited in short-term memory. Research conducted in the 1950s suggested that approximately seven items can be held at one time for processing in short-term memory, and that multiple items can be combined into a larger unit or chunk with a capacity limit of three to four units or chunks.[8] This is referred to as chunking information into groups or categories based on some association in order to remember the information. An example is a grocery shopping list that is organized into small groups based on food group categories such as fruits, vegetables, grains, and dairy. The key is to look for meaningful ways to connect the items by considering what they have in common and then chunk them accordingly. Other strategies for chunking items include making associations with the items: for example, you may remember that you need to buy milk, bread, and eggs if you associate them with making a favorite food such as French toast. Another way to chunk items is to use mnemonics. If you need to remember to buy soap, toothpaste, envelopes, and pens you can create a word out of the first letters of each item you need, in this case it is the word STEP. Recall of this word facilitates recall of the items represented by each letter of the acronym.

Long-term memory is the individual's knowledge base. Long-term memory can be categorized as declarative (explicit) memory and nondeclarative (implicit) memory.[9] Declarative memory is the conscious recollection of knowledge. There are two major types, semantic memory and episodic memory. Semantic memory is the storage of facts. Episodic memory refers to the ability to recall a specific autobiographical event in its original context. Nondeclarative memory refers to several forms of memory that are not declarative; it includes procedural knowledge, simple forms of conditioning, priming, and perceptual learning. *Procedural* knowledge refers to skills and habits, or skill-based information. This includes skills such as tying your shoe and making a cup of coffee. Skills that have been learned in the past are embedded into a procedure that guides behavior when needed. There is not a focus on how to do the procedure, therefore the knowledge is implicit. Habits such as walking the same route when walking a dog or donning clothing in a specific order are also behaviors that are more implicit. *Priming* is another form of an experience-dependent behavior that is implicit. Priming refers to the increased ability to classify or detect an item due to recent exposure with the same or similar item. "The unconscious status of nondeclarative memory creates some of the mystery of human experience. Here arise the habits and preferences that are inaccessible to conscious recollection, but they nevertheless are shaped by past events, they include our current behavior and mental life and they are a fundamental part of who we are."[9]

Working memory functions to keep information available over brief periods of time for use in directing purposeful behavior. Maintaining that information involves the interaction of a selective attention process, short-term memory storage, and long-term memory representations.[10] When multiple tasks are in progress, working memory functions to coordinate these tasks and guide behavior by relying on the relevant information that is maintained. This allows for the planning and execution of cognitive tasks as needed, therefore working memory is essential to our everyday functioning.[11,12]

Executive Function

Executive function is a neuropsychological construct that refers to the ability to form, maintain, and change mental frameworks for reasoning and making plans. It involves taking the time to think before acting and the ability to meet novel, unanticipated challenges. It includes the ability to focus, as well as the motivation to follow through with goals and make changes as needed. Defining executive function includes a focus on its purpose such as making choices to engage in purposeful, goal-directed, future-oriented behavior. It can also be defined by focusing on the skills that are needed (including problem-solving, planning, and organization) and the neurocognitive processes that are the foundation of executive function (including working memory, sequencing, inhibition, initiation, and response selection).[13]

The use of executive function requires effort to complete a task in a different manner than previously attempted. It is tempting to rely on previous behaviors to progress through the day instead of considering a different approach to daily tasks. There are three generally accepted core executive functions: inhibition, cognitive flexibility, and working memory. Inhibition includes self-control or behavioral inhibition in which the individual can resist temptations and resist impulsive behavior. It also includes interference control, which involves selective attention and cognitive inhibition. Cognitive flexibility includes creative thinking and being able to see different perspectives of a situation or task. It involves mental flexibility in quickly adapting to changing circumstances. Working memory, the third core function, has been discussed already in relation to short-term and long-term memory. The ability to use executive function skills is essential for mental and physical health and overall success in life.[14]

Metacognition

Metacognition refers to the ways in which one monitors and directs one's own cognitive processes.[15] It is sometimes defined as thinking about one's own thinking processes.[16] Generally, people are capable of evaluating their own cognitive abilities and can recognize their mistakes. Metacognition allows one to avoid repeating mistakes and to avoid making decisions that are not well supported.[17] It includes processes that are involved in monitoring and cognitive control and it allows an individual to recognize when knowledge is lacking in a given situation or task. Metacognitive monitoring refers to those processes we engage in when monitoring our own learning, and metacognitive control refers to the ways in which we control our own cognitive processes during learning.[16] It also includes the concept of metacognitive knowledge or awareness of learning strategies such as rehearsal, mnemonics, and organizational processes.[16]

Social Cognition

An important component of cognitive functioning is social cognition or interpreting social information successfully when interacting with others. "Social cognition is the ability to correctly process information carried by socially relevant stimuli and to use it to generate adequate response in social situations."[18] Social cognition requires an understanding of verbal and nonverbal cues present in interpersonal interactions. This includes facial expressions, body language, vocal tone and rhythm, and what is referred to as "theory of mind" or the mental state of others. Social cognition refers to the "identification, perception, and interpretation of socially important information, whereas the domain of theory of mind specifically refers to the ability to infer information regarding the thoughts, intentions, and feelings of others."[19] Impairment in social cognition is recognized in several psychiatric diseases, including schizophrenia, autism, and depression.[19]

For individuals with schizophrenia, research has identified four main areas of social cognition in which impairment is probable. These areas include emotion processing, theory of mind, social perception, and attributional style. Emotion processing includes emotion perception and utilization of emotion information. Emotion perception can be further defined as understanding facial affect and vocal tone; understanding the connection between emotions and task performance; understanding emotional transitions; and regulating emotional states of self and others. Theory of mind can be succinctly defined as mind reading. Social perception is referred to as social knowledge. This includes one's knowledge of social roles, norms, and schemas regarding social situations, and one's ability to make judgments based on this knowledge. Attributional style refers to the internal or external causal explanations that one develops to understand the outcomes of situations.[20]

How do these components of cognition fit with occupational therapy practice? The focus of occupational therapy is occupational performance, which consists of purposeful activities one engages in throughout the day. All occupations require some level of cognition for the tasks associated with performance. In looking at the Occupational Therapy Practice Framework (OTPF)[21] many of the components of cognition are explicitly identified as client factors. These include sustained and divided attention; short-term, long-term, and working memory; executive function; and metacognition. Likewise, many components of social cognition are explicitly and implicitly identified as performance skills in the category of social interaction skills. Social cognition requires interpreting social information appropriately; there are 27 social interaction skills listed in the OTPF, with many including an emphasis on social appropriateness as a defining element of skill performance.

COGNITIVE DYSFUNCTION AND PSYCHIATRIC ILLNESS

Cognitive deficits are prevalent in many psychiatric disorders and have become an important area of research,

especially in schizophrenia.[22,23] Individuals diagnosed with schizophrenia have a higher probability of decreased cognitive performance.[22,23] Low IQ is a risk factor for schizophrenia, and diagnosis of the disorder is often preceded by many years of cognitive decline and intellectual underperformance. This decline may continue after diagnosis, and decreased cognitive performance is noted to be an important predictor of general functional outcome. These findings support the assertion that cognition should be recognized as the core component of schizophrenia.[24]

Many psychiatric disorders may present with deficits in cognitive regulatory functions as evidenced by neuropsychology and neuroimaging. These cognitive deficits are not established symptoms of the disorders; however, they present as regulatory problems in both traditional cognitive and emotional domains, and negatively impact daily life and occupational performance.[3] Additionally, cognitive deficits have been noted to persist in many cases after otherwise effective treatment for the disorder has been established. The reasons for the presence of cognitive deficits in many psychiatric disorders is complex, and there are multiple causes discussed in the literature. These causes include premorbid presence due to developmental vulnerability, brain injury or insult at onset of the disorder, or indirect causality resulting from effects of the disorder on cognitive systems. This may include decreased motivation or attention leading to less cognitive engagement, or it may be due to behaviors such as substance misuse or poor health habits that lead to cognitive impairment. Additionally, there are broader contributing factors such as social deprivation and decreased educational opportunities that impact cognitive functioning.[25]

Several theoretical models focused on cognitive intervention have been developed within occupational therapy and are identified in the occupational therapy literature.[1] These include the Dynamic Interactional Model,[26] Cognitive Rehabilitation Model,[27] Cognitive Disabilities Model (CDM),[28] Cognitive Orientation to Daily Occupational Performance Model (CO-OP),[29] and the Neurofunctional Approach (NFA).[30-33] Of these approaches, the CDM has been applied to individuals with severe mental illness and will be discussed in more detail in this chapter. The other approaches also can be applied to individuals with mental illness, and intervention approaches that may be considered within these models will be presented. An overview of cognitive remediation and cognitive enhancement approaches for individuals with mental illness that are documented in the psychiatric literature will be discussed. These approaches are broadly based on learning, behavioral, and neuropsychological theories. A variety of assessments and intervention approaches derived from more than one theoretical model may be used for the same client to best meet individual needs.

COGNITIVE DISABILITIES MODEL

The CDM was developed in the 1960s by occupational therapist Claudia Allen as a result of her observations of performance difficulties in routine task behaviors in adult patients with mental illness. Allen and her colleagues originally focused on the "sensorimotor actions originating in the physical or chemical structures of the brain and producing observable and assessable limitations in routine task behavior."[34] They identified cognitive abilities according to six levels of sensorimotor abilities that are hierarchal and are observable during functional activities. "Based on her observations of functional performance, Allen hypothesized that this sequence could be observed in the progression and remission of mental illness, dementia, and fatigue in adult individuals."[34]

Allen developed a screening tool, the Allen Cognitive Level Screen (ACLS), now in its fifth version, ACLS-5. The purpose of the ACLS-5 is "to obtain a quick measure of global cognitive processing capacities, learning potential, and performance abilities."[35] The construct being measured is functional cognition and the ACLS is intended to identify potential problems related to this construct. "'Functional cognition' encompasses functional performance abilities and global cognitive processing capacities. It incorporates the complex, dynamic interplay between 1) a person's information processing abilities, occupational performance skills, values and interests, 2) the increasingly complex motor, perceptual and cognitive activity demands of three graded visual-motor tasks and 3) feedback from performance of these tasks in context."[35] The screening consists of the therapist asking the client to complete three stitches: the running stitch, the whip stitch, and the single cordovan stitch. The stitches are progressively more difficult and each stitch is demonstrated to the client by the therapist. The stitches are completed on a 4-inch × 5-inch piece of leather; waxed cord is used for the whip stitch and leather lacing cord is used for the other two stitches. The test is standardized with established reliability and validity.[36] There is also an enlarged version of the ACLS-5, the Large Allen Cognitive Level Screen-5 (LACLS-5), which is intended for use with individuals with visual or fine motor coordination limitations.

When administered to an individual, the ACLS-5 provides an Allen Cognitive Level (ACL) score. There are six cognitive levels that are subdivided into 26 ordinal modes of functioning. They range from 1.0 to 6.0, and are each 0.2 points apart on the scale. The modes of performance allow therapists to observe and document improvement in functional activities. A summary of the modes of performance in the Allen Cognitive Scale is provided in Table 7.1. The actions exhibited in Level 1 are automatic actions and the actions in Level 2 are postural actions; the ACLS-5 is not designed to identify scores at these levels. The ACLS-5 detects scores at Levels 3, 4, and 5. Level 3 are manual actions, Level 4 are goal-directed actions, and Level 5 are exploratory actions.[37]

The ACLS-5 is intended to identify cognitive abilities and limitations in the range of 3.0 to 5.8 of the Allen Cognitive Scale modes of performance. Findings should be verified with other assessments within the CDM and by observations conducted by therapists experienced in the CDM.[35] The ACLS-5 is not a diagnostic tool. The findings are "used to guide occupation-based interventions at the level of activity demands, performance skills, and occupations based on the Occupational Therapy Practice Framework."[35]

Other assessments developed within the CDM include the Allen Diagnostic Module, 2nd Edition (ADM-2), the Routine Task Inventory -Expanded (RTI-E), and the Cognitive Performance Test.[38] The ADM-2 consists of 35 craft-based assessments designed to assess the functional disabilities of persons with cognitive impairments. Each assessment activity within the ADM-2 requires task procedures to complete a product that the client can keep. The 35 activities are standardized and each activity is aligned with a range of ACL modes of performance. The ACLS-5 is generally administered to the client first and then the therapist selects an ADM-2 activity that matches the client's ACLS-5 score and the client's interests. The activity is administered following the Guidelines for Use and the assessment protocol in the Allen Diagnostic Module Manual–2nd Edition.[39] The client's performance is observed and scored following the rating criteria for the activity. Results obtained from the ADM-2 assessments are one component of the overall evaluation process for each client.[40]

The Routine Task Inventory-Expanded (RTI-E)[41] is an evidence-based, semi-standardized assessment tool. It includes 25 Activities of Daily Living (ADLs) and Instrumental Activities of Daily Living (IADLs) tasks that are divided into four subscales: (1) Physical Scale-ADLs, (2) Community Scale-IADLs, (3) Communication Scale, and (4) Work Readiness Scale. It can be completed by therapist observation or by client or caregiver report using a checklist as part of an interview process with standardized questions. A mean score is calculated for each subscale and the scores are associated with the Allen Cognitive Scale. The RTI-E manual is available at no cost from the Allen Cognitive Network website.[41]

The Cognitive Performance Test (CPT) is a standardized performance-based assessment developed for the

TABLE 7.1 Cognitive Levels and Modes of Performance.

	MODES OF PERFORMANCE				
	0.0	0.2	0.4	0.6	0.8
Level	**Coma**				**0.8 Generalized reflexive actions**
Level 1 Automatic actions	1.0 Withdrawing from noxious stimuli	1.2 Responding to stimuli with one sensory system	1.4 Locating stimuli	1.6 Rolling in bed	1.8 Raising body part
Level 2 Postural actions	2.0 Overcoming gravity and sitting	2.2 Righting reactions/ standing	2.4 Aimless walking	2.6 Directed walking	2.8 Using grab bars
Level 3 Manual actions	3.0 Grasping objects	3.2 Distinguishing objects	3.4 Sustaining actions on objects	3.6 Noting effects on objects	3.8 Using all objects
Level 4 Goal-directed actions	4.0 Sequencing familiar actions	4.2 Differentiating features of objects	4.4 Completing a goal	4.6 Personalizing features of objects	4.8 Learning by rote memorization
Level 5 Exploratory actions	5.0 Comparing and changing variations in actions and objects	5.2 Discriminating among sets of actions and objects	5.4 Self-directed learning	5.6 Considering social standards	5.8 Consulting with others
Level 6 Planned actions	Typically functioning adult brain and functional cognitive capacities				

Copyright C.A. Earhart, Pasadena, CA, USA and ACLS and LACLS Committee. Camarillo, CA, USA, 2015.

assessment of older adults with cognitive deficits that can be used with a variety of diagnostic groups. It measures working memory and executive function related to occupational performance. It consists of seven tasks that include medication management, shopping for clothing, washing hands, telephone use, food preparation, dressing, and moving from one place to another. Direct observation of activity performance is used and scores range from low (1) to high (5 or 6). The test takes approximately 30 minutes to complete, and directions for standardized cues are described in the test manual. The total score represents the calculation of average task performance from the subtasks and is converted into a cognitive level based on the Allen Cognitive Scale. The CPT assists in explaining functional capabilities of the individual and can indicate the compensatory and safety requirements that are needed.[38]

In the CDM, the interventions that are used are primarily compensatory interventions. They include (1) modifying activities and environments to compensate for functional cognitive disabilities, (2) establishing and/or restoring performance skills and routines, and (3) maintenance of functional ability and prevention of cognitive decline.[42] Currently the CDM is used by occupational therapists in mental health, forensic psychiatry, rehabilitation medicine, and geriatric care. In all areas, the focus is on understanding remaining abilities to enable occupational performance in everyday life. There are other cognitive tests that can be used by occupational therapists to assess cognitive function as well, and some of these are discussed in Chapter 13.

TREATMENT APPROACHES

Treatment interventions for cognitive deficits resulting from mental illness can be classified as cognitive remediation techniques, compensatory techniques, or adaptive approaches.[43] There is a wide range of cognitive interventions for cognitive dysfunction, and mental health professionals such as occupational therapists, social workers, mental health counselors, and neuropsychologists can assess the client and determine the best approach based on the client's deficits and functional level.

In occupational therapy, functional cognition "refers to the thinking and processing skills needed to accomplish complex everyday activities such as household and financial management, medication management, volunteer activities, driving, and work."[44] Functional cognition is the interaction of cognitive skills with everyday living. AOTA identifies five approaches that occupational therapy practitioners may use when working with the client with cognitive deficits. These include Global Strategy Learning and Awareness Approaches, Domain-Specific Strategy Training, Cognitive Retraining Embedded in Functional Activity, Specific-Task Training, and Environmental Modifications and Use of Assistive Technology.[1] These approaches fall within the broad range of treatment interventions found in the literature for cognitive dysfunction in mental illness, and may be used independently or in combination based on the individual client's needs. Global strategy learning aims to increase awareness of personal cognitive processes, and therapists help clients develop compensatory techniques that are higher-order approaches they can generalize to novel situations. Domain-specific strategy training also focuses on compensatory techniques by training the individual to manage a particular deficit through use of a specific strategy. Cognitive retraining is a form of remediation in which required cognitive processes are addressed during the activity process to improve performance. Task-specific training can include adaptation of the specific task so that the client can perform it despite the cognitive deficit. Environmental modification involves adapting the environment to promote success and it may be used along with assistive technology to promote occupational performance as a component of any of the approaches.[1,44]

Cognitive Remediation

Treatment interventions described as cognitive remediation vary greatly in approach, sophistication, design, and focus. Cognitive remediation can be conducted individually or in a group, with or without a health professional facilitating the remediation. Treatment strategies may be designed with a simple approach as in paper-and-pencil exercises or puzzles, or they may involve a more complex and sophisticated approach through use of computer programs created specifically for cognitive intervention. The focus of cognitive remediation training may be neurocognition[45,46] or social cognition,[47] or a combination of both.[48] Neurocognitive remediation can be categorized as Cognitive Remediation Therapy (CRT) referring to cognitive exercises for intervention, and Compensatory Cognitive Training (CCT) referring to compensatory interventions designed to enhance cognitive functioning.[18] CRT is based on implicit learning in which the participants gain skills indirectly through repeated practice of cognitive exercises.[18] CCT involves learning strategies to compensate for impaired cognition and therefore improve daily functioning.[18]

Cognitive remediation can also be categorized as methods that provide bottom-up training and top-down training.[49,50] Bottom-up training emphasizes systematic practice with lower-level cognitive processes and builds toward higher-level processes. The low-level sensory, perceptual, and cognitive processes that are deficient are the focus of the initial tasks, and the task difficulty is gradually increased to build cognitive processes from the bottom-up. Professionals using top-down training assert that cognition can be more successfully improved via cognitive remediation that focuses initially on high-order and more complex cognitive processes. Complex executive functions are the focus of training, and some training programs include simulation of everyday activities as part of the training.

Cognitive remediation programs are also used to target social cognition. Social cognition trainings are hypothesized to be more successful than neurocognitive trainings on real-world functioning. These training programs are broad and may address decision-making in social situations, emotional processing, social perception, attribution bias, theory of mind, and other social skills.[18] Emotion perception training is a specific form of social cognition training that focuses on the impairment of emotion perception or the ability to recognize other peoples' emotions. Successful social cognition is difficult without good emotion perception, which is impaired for some individuals with mental illness.[18]

Although there is a lot of variability in cognitive remediation programs, key practice principles of these programs for individuals with schizophrenia and other mental disorders in which cognitive deficits are present, have emerged.[51] Not all programs incorporate all of these principles; however, the more effective programs do integrate them into the remediation strategies that form the program. These principles include:

- The development of mental strategies to optimize cognitive performance and task completion.
- The repetition of cognitive exercises over many sessions until performance has improved.
- The progression of targeted cognitive abilities from the basic to more complex.
- The use of external aids (usually auditory or visual) to support cognitive performance.
- The gradual removal of cues and external aids in cognitive exercises to increase difficulty.
- The adjustment of the difficulty of cognitive exercises so they remain challenging and engaging.
- The linking of cognitive exercises to "real world" behaviors and areas of functioning domains they support.
- The use of additional schizophrenia treatments and supports to maximize the benefits of cognitive remediation.[51]

Cognitive Enhancement Therapy

Cognitive enhancement therapy is a specific type of cognitive remediation. "Cognitive enhancement therapy (CET) is a performance-based, developmental intervention approach to remediation and rehabilitation in the areas of social, attention, memory, and problem-solving neuropsychological cognitive deficits."[52] CET was developed in the 1990s and originally focused on the treatment of cognitive functioning and social integration of patients with schizophrenia or schizoaffective disorder; its success has led to its use with clients with other mental health disorders who have cognitive and social deficits. CET is recognized by the Substance Abuse and Mental Health Service Administration (SAMHSA) as an evidence-based practice that helps people with mental illness that results in cognitive dysfunction to improve their processing speed, cognition, and social cognition.[53] Research[54,55] indicates that these cognitive deficits contribute to functional disability in people with mental illness. CET improves these skills and enables recovery, therefore increasing the individual's meaningful occupational engagement and quality of life in the home and community.

The main focus of CET is the emphasis on social cognition. This is distinct from cognitive remediation approaches that only target cognitive deficits such as attention, memory, and problem-solving, or approaches such as cognitive behavioral therapy that focus on changing thought processes to change beliefs. These approaches are beneficial; however, they do not address the core aspects of human relationships, including the ability to accurately perceive and understand the intentions, feelings, and behavior of another person; an understanding of how to navigate social situations; and the ability to form and maintain human relationships in an appropriate manner demonstrating empathy and meaningful interactions. Difficulty in these areas of social cognition are extremely disabling for many individuals with neurocognitive impairments.[53]

Understanding and responding to the necessity of these cognitive skills for optimal functional recovery forms the central paradigm of CET. CET addresses specific traditionally proposed areas of neuropsychological cognitive deficits along with social cognition by integrating both in the administration of training sessions and schedules. CET primarily focuses on social cognition as the primary mechanism by which all areas of cognition are effectively improved. CET recognizes that all individuals live in a social environment, consisting of specific cultural and social norms, even if that environment is limited for individuals with mental illness. It is crucial to possess the necessary social skills to negotiate social interaction for occupational performance. In CET, learning is individually self-defined through the experience of group interaction, self-reflection, and social awareness. Cognitive competencies are acquired as the individual learns to think and feel as opposed to simply learning behavioral skills. Social cognition is the central core through which the remediation of all neuropsychological cognitive impairment is addressed.[53]

A widely used CET program is the CETCleveland curriculum offered through the Center for Cognition and Recovery in Beachwood, OH. The CET curriculum consists of computer training exercises focused on attention, memory, and problem-solving skill development, along with social cognition group sessions; both are provided within a socially interactive environment. The CET computer training is conducted for 1 hour and the social cognition groups are 1.5 hours a week for 48 weeks. The structured group environment provides a socializing experience that is nonthreatening and allows the individual a way to acquire and strengthen basic abilities essential for the development of social cognition. Group activities focus on aspects of social cognition such as the use of language in a socially appropriate manner, giving and receiving constructive feedback, adjusting social interaction for a given audience and/or situation, acting empathetically and understanding other's feelings in different situations. The curriculum also includes weekly coaching and homework.[53]

Compensatory Approaches

Compensatory approaches include errorless learning, compensatory strategies, and adaptive approaches. Errorless learning assumes that some individuals with cognitive dysfunction, such as those with schizophrenia, have difficulty with the trial-and-error approach to learning. Errorless learning is structured so that errors are avoided in the process of learning new tasks.[56] A task is broken down into smaller components for training, and each component is repeated multiple times using imitative learning, thus preventing errors from occurring.[57] Training involves learning task components by use of stimulus–response connections structured from simple to more complex, with repeated and rapid succession to facilitate automation of the response.[56] Errorless learning relies on implicit memory processes or implicit learning that is often procedural and therefore unconscious, as opposed to explicit learning. For many individuals with cognitive challenges it is the explicit memory abilities that are compromised, making conscious explicit learning of new skills more difficult. By focusing on the training procedures of errorless learning and in the context where the task will be completed, intact implicit learning processes are used for learning.[56]

Compensatory strategies are largely focused on memory impairment and include low-tech and high-tech strategies and internal and external strategies.[58] Low-tech external strategies include the use of paper planners or calendars that can be posted in a commonly used area, bulletin boards or white boards for writing down important information, the use of checklists and to-do lists, and timers to remember routine tasks such as taking medication. For individuals with access to high-tech devices, smart phones and apps can be used for a variety of functions to support memory, orientation, budgeting, task completion, etc. Internal strategies include use of repetition when learning new information by reviewing the information multiple times or performing the task over and over. Strategies such as chunking information into smaller components that are easier to remember can be helpful, an example is a phone number. Chunking the information into area code, prefix, and then remaining four numbers makes it easier to remember the number. Other strategies include visualization (i.e., making up a story to remember information), use of acronyms, and listing of information into meaningful categories.

Adaptive approaches are typically used for individuals who cannot engage in cognitive remediation or make use of compensatory strategies.[59] Cognitive adaption training (CAT) focuses on environmental adaptations that support the individual's functional abilities by reducing the cognitive demands needed for task completion.[59] CAT decreases overall stress and also improves safety. The therapist works with the client to organize the home so that items are accessible and readily available in the needed context. Training involves reviewing adaptations and training the individual to recognize and use cues to access items, remember information, and complete tasks.[59]

SUMMARY

Cognitive remediation aims to improve and/or restore cognitive functioning using a variety of approaches. These approaches may be based on repeated execution of specific tasks or may involve the implementation of new strategies. They may be computerized or noncomputerized, designed for individual or group intervention, and include top-down or bottom-up approaches. They may include strategy coaching and may be individually tailored. A number of structured protocols including computer-assisted interventions have been developed and implemented in recent years, a listing of some of these protocols is provided (Box 7.1).[60]

Research supports the use of cognitive remediation for individuals with schizophrenia[61,62] and other forms of serious mental illness who demonstrate cognitive deficits.[63] A meta-analysis of 40 cognitive remediation efficacy studies (2104 participants) found positive effects on global cognition and functioning, and the effect was greater for clinically stable clients. Significantly stronger functional outcomes were found when cognitive remediation therapy was administered with psychiatric rehabilitation, such as supported employment, medication management, and/or communication skills training, and a much larger effect was present when a strategic approach to intervention was implemented.[64] A meta-analysis of 11 trials (615 participants) in early schizophrenia that examined cognitive remediation efficacy on global cognition, functioning, and symptoms showed a significant effect on functioning and symptoms. Additionally, verbal learning and memory showed a significant positive effect and five other neurocognitive domains showed borderline significant benefits. When psychiatric rehabilitation and smaller group interventions were implemented, the effect on functioning and symptoms was larger.[65] A meta-analysis of 16 studies of cognitive remediation that included diagnoses of schizoaffective disorder, affective psychosis, and unipolar and/or bipolar disorders found that cognitive remediation has at least equivalent benefits in affective and schizoaffective disorder as demonstrated in schizophrenia.[63]

Continued research is needed to determine the most effective approaches and treatment protocols for all individuals with serious mental illness who experience cognitive deficits. Functional cognition is needed for clients to engage in everyday life and maximize independence and quality of life. Early and ongoing assessment of an individual's cognitive abilities, and the impact of this on their functional abilities, is essential to providing efficient,

BOX 7.1   Selected Protocols of Structured Cognitive Remediation Interventions for Schizophrenia

Cognitive Training	Target	Duration Individual or Group
Integrated Neurocognitive Therapy	Cognitive functions and social cognition	Thirty biweekly 90-minute group sessions (6–8 per group)
Cogpack	Cognitive functions	Individual sessions, varies in duration and frequency
Cognitive Enhancement Therapy	Cognitive functions and social cognition	Biweekly group sessions for 24 months
Neuropsychological Educational Approach to Remediation	Cognitive functions and problem-solving	Individual/group 60-minute sessions twice a week, about 4 months
Neurocognitive Enhancement Therapy	Cognitive functions and social cognition	Individual/group sessions of 45 minutes at least 5 times a week for 6 months
Training of Affect Recognition	Social cognition	Twelve 45-minute sessions twice a week in pairs with a psychotherapist
Social Cognition and Interaction Training	Social cognition	Twenty-four 50-minute weekly group sessions
Social Cognitive Skills Training	Social cognition	Twelve 60-minute weekly group sessions, 60 min each one
Social Skills and Neurocognitive Individualized Training	Cognitive functions, social cognition, and social skills	Biweekly 1-hour neurocognitive training sessions (individual) and weekly 2-hour social skills training (group) for 6 months

Modified from Vita A, Barlati S, Bellani M, Brambilla P. Cognitive remediation in schizophrenia: background, techniques, evidence of efficacy and perspectives. *Epidemiol Psychiatr Sci.* 23;2014:21-25.

targeted support needs. This can be achieved through a variety of cognitive assessments as well as occupational task assessments.[66] Occupational therapy practitioners working with clients with serious mental illness are an essential part of the treatment team and can contribute significantly to the body of knowledge on cognition.

SUGGESTED LEARNING ACTIVITIES

1. Visit the Center for Cognition and Recovery website and view some of the testimonial videos highlighting the use of the CETCLEVELAND program http://cetcleveland.org/what-is-cetcleveland-2/cetcleveland-testimonials-2/.
2. Read about COGPACK software and download a free demo to try http://www.markersoftware.com/USA/frames.htm.
3. Interview an individual with serious mental illness and ask if they perceive challenges with cognitive tasks. If they do, what are the primary concerns.

REFLECTION QUESTIONS

1. What do you think is the most challenging cognitive deficit for individuals with serious mental illness? Why?
2. In your own words, articulate occupational therapy's role in addressing cognition when talking to external audiences.

REFERENCES

1. American Occupational Therapy Association. Cognition, cognitive rehabilitation, and occupational performance. *Am J Occup Ther*. 2013;67(6 suppl):S9-S31.
2. Fraser Health. Section eight: understanding cognition. In: *Dealing with Psychosis: A Toolkit for Moving Forward with your Life*. 2012. Available at: https://www.heretohelp.bc.ca/sites/default/files/dwp-understanding-cognition.pdf.
3. Etkin A, Gyurak A, O'Hara R. A neurobiological approach to the cognitive deficits of psychiatric disorders. *Dialogues Clin Neurosci*. 2013;15:419-429.
4. Kairalla ICJ, Mattos PEL, Hoexter MQ, Bressan RA, Mari JJ, Shirakawa I. Attention in schizophrenia and in epileptic psychosis. *Braz J Med Biol Res*. 2008;41:60-67.
5. Birkett P, Brindley A, Norman P, Harrison G, Baddeley A. Control of attention in schizophrenia. *J Psychiatr Res*. 2006;40:579-588.
6. Gliklich E, Guo R, Bergmark RW. Texting while driving: a study of 1211 U.S. adults with the distracted driving survey. *Prev Med Rep*. 2016;4:486-489.
7. Cowan N. What are the differences between long-term, short-term, and working memory? *Prog Brain Res*. 2008;169:323-338.
8. Cowan N. The magical number 4 in short-term memory: a reconsideration of mental storage capacity. *Behav Brain Sci*. 2001;24:87-185.
9. Squire LR, Dede AJO. Conscious and unconscious memory systems. *Cold Spring Harb Perspect Biol*. 2015;7:1-14.
10. Eriksson J, Vogel EK, Lansner A, Bergström F, Nyberg L. Neurocognitive architecture of working memory. *Neuron*. 2015;88:33-46.
11. Barak O, Tsodyks M. Working models of working memory. *Curr Opin Neurobiol*. 2014;25:20-24.
12. D'Esposito M, Postle BR. The cognitive neuroscience of working memory. *Annu Rev Psychol*. 2015;66:115-142.
13. Suchy Y. Executive functioning: overview, assessment, and research issues for non-neuropsychologists. *Ann Behav Med*. 2009;37:106-116.
14. Diamond A. Executive functions. *Annu Rev Psychol*. 2013;64:135-168.
15. Frith CD. The role of metacognition in human social interactions. *Philos Trans R Soc Lond B Biol Sci*. 2012;367:2213-2223.
16. Colbert CY, Graham L, West C, et al. Teaching metacognitive skills: helping your physician trainees in the quest to know what they don't know. *Am J Med*. 2015;128:318-324.
17. Yeung N, Summerfield C. Metacognition in human decision making: confidence and error monitoring. *Philos Trans R Soc Lond B Biol Sci*. 2012;367:1310-1321.
18. Linke M, Jarema M. Cognitive rehabilitation for people living with schizophrenia – the newest interventions. Psychiatr Pol. 2014;48:1179-1188.
19. Weightman MJ, Air TM, Baune BT. A review of the role of social cognition in major depressive disorder. *Front Psychiatry*. 2014;5:1-13.
20. McCleery A, Horan WP, Green M F. Social cognition during the early phase of schizophrenia. In: Lysaker P, Dimaggio G, Brüne M, eds. *Social Cognition and Metacognition in Schizophrenia*. 1st ed. London, UK: Elsevier; 2014.
21. American Occupational Therapy Association. Occupational therapy practice framework: domain & process, 3rd. ed. *Am J Occup Ther*. 2014;68(suppl 1):S1-S51.
22. Reichenberg A, Weiser M, Rabinowitz J, et al. A population based cohort study of premorbid intellectual, language, and behavioral functioning in patients with schizophrenia, schizoaffective disorder, and nonpsychotic bipolar disorder. *Am J Psychiatry*. 2002;15:2027-2035.
23. Zammit S, Allebeck P, David AS, et al. A longitudinal study of premorbid IQ score and risk of developing schizophrenia, bipolar disorder, severe depression and other non-affective psychoses. *Arch Gen Psychiatry*. 2004;61:354-360.
24. Kahn RS, Keefe RSE. Schizophrenia is a cognitive illness: time for a change in focus. *JAMA Psychiatry*. 2013;70:1107-1112.
25. David AS, Zammit S, Lewis G, Dalman C, Allebeck P. Impairments in cognition across the spectrum of psychiatric disorders: evidence from a Swedish conscript cohort. *Schizophr Bull*. 2008;34:1035-1041.
26. Toglia JP. The dynamic interactional model of cognition in cognitive rehabilitation. In: Katz N, ed. *Cognition, Occupation, and Participation Across the Life Span: Neuroscience, Neurorehabilitation, and Models of Intervention in Occupational Therapy*. 3rd ed. Bethesda, MD: AOTA Press; 2011:161-201.
27. Averbach S, Katz N. Cognitive rehabilitation: a retraining model for clients with neurological disabilities. In: Katz N, ed. *Cognition, Occupation, and Participation Across the Life Span: Neuroscience, Neurorehabilitation, and Models of Intervention in Occupational Therapy*. 3rd ed. Bethesda, MD: AOTA Press; 2011:277-298.
28. Allen CK, Earhart C, Blue T. *Occupational Therapy Treatment Goals for the Physically and Cognitively Disabled*. Rockville, MD: American Occupational Therapy Association; 1992.
29. Polatajko HJ, Mandich A, McEwen SE. Cognitive Orientation to Daily Occupational Performance (CO–OP): a cognitive-based intervention for children and adults. In: Katz N, ed. *Cognition, Occupation, and Participation Across the Life Span: Neuroscience, Neurorehabilitation, and Models of Intervention in Occupational Therapy*. 3rd ed. Bethesda, MD: AOTA Press; 2011:299-321.
30. Giles GM. A neurofunctional approach to rehabilitation after brain injury. In: Katz N, ed. *Cognition, Occupation, and Participation Across the Life Span: Neuroscience, Neurorehabilitation, and Models of Intervention in Occupational Therapy*. 3rd ed. Bethesda, MD: AOTA Press; 2011:351-381.
31. Giles GM, Clark-Wilson J, eds. *Brain Injury Rehabilitation: A Neurofunctional Approach*. San Diego, CA: Singular; 1993.
32. Parish L, Oddy M. Efficacy of rehabilitation for functional skills more than 10 years after extremely severe brain injury. *Neuropsychol Rehabil*. 2007;17:230-243.
33. Vanderploeg RD, Schwab K, Walker WC, et al. Rehabilitation of traumatic brain injury in active duty military personnel and veterans: defense and Veterans Brain Injury Center randomized controlled trial of two rehabilitation approaches. *Arch Phys Med Rehabil*. 2008;89:2227-2238.
34. Allen CK. *Occupational Therapy for Psychiatric Diseases: Measurement and Management of Cognitive Disabilities*. Boston, MA: Little, Brown and Company; 1985.

35. Allen Cognitive Level Screen and Large Allen Cognitive Level Screen Committee. *Allen Cognitive Level Screen-5 (ACLS-5), Large Allen Cognitive Level Screen-5 (LACLS-5), & NEW Disposable Large Allen Cognitive Level Screen (LACLS[D])* [Handout]. 2016. Allen Cognitive Group. Available at: http://allencognitive.com/wp-content/uploads/Info-2016-ACLS_5-LACLS_5-LACLS-D5-pdf.pdf.

36. McCraith DB, Riska-Williams L, Earhart CA, David SK. *ACLS-5 and LACLS-5 Test: Psychometric Properties and Use of Scores for Evidence-based Practice.* Allen Cognitive Group/ACLS & LACLS Committee. 2016. Available at: http://allencognitive.com/wp-content/uploads/Copyright ReportfPsychometricsACLS-5_3-21-2016.pdf.

37. Allen Cognitive Group. *Allen Scale/Cognitive Levels.* n.d. Available at: https://allencognitive.com/allen-scale/.

38. Douglas A, Letts L, Eva K, Richardson J. Use of the Cognitive Performance Test for identifying deficits in hospitalized older adults. *Rehabil Res Pract.* 2012;2012:638480.

39. Earhart C. *Allen Diagnostic Module Manual.* 2nd ed. Colchester, CT: S&S Worldwide; 2006.

40. Earhart CA. *Using Allen Diagnostic Module – 2nd Edition Assessments.* Colchester, CT: S&S Worldwide; 2015.

41. Katz N. *Routine Task Inventory-Expanded (RTI-E).* 2017. Available at: http://allen-cognitive-network.org/index.php/allen-cognitive-model/assessments/48-routine-task-inventory-expanded-rti-e.

42. Allen Cognitive Group. *Core Concepts.* n.d. Available at: https://allencognitive.com/core-concepts/.

43. Medalia A, Revheim N. *Dealing with Cognitive Dysfunction Associated with Psychiatric Disabilities: A Handbook for Families and Friends of Individuals with Psychiatric Disorders.* New York State Office of Mental Health. 2002. Available at: https://www.omh.ny.gov/omhweb/cogdys_manual/cogdyshndbk.pdf.

44. American Occupational Therapy Association. Occupational therapy's role in adult cognitive disorders. *AOTA Fact Sheet.* 2017. Available at: https://www.aota.org/~/media/Corporate/Files/AboutOT/Professionals/WhatIsOT/PA/Facts/Cognitive-Disorders-Fact-Sheet.pdf.

45. Fisher M, Holland C, Merzenich MM, Vinogradov S. Using neuroplasticity-based auditory training to improve verbal memory in schizophrenia. *Am J Psychiatry.* 2009;166:805-811.

46. Wykes T, Reeder C, Landau S, et al. Cognitive remediation therapy in schizophrenia: randomised controlled trial. *Br J Psychiatry.* 2007;190:421-427.

47. Horan WP, Kern RS, Tripp C, et al. Efficacy and specificity of Social Cognitive Skills Training for outpatients with psychotic disorders. *J Psychiatr Res.* 2011;45:1113-1122.

48. Hogarty GE, Flesher S, Ulrich R, et al. Cognitive enhancement therapy for schizophrenia: effects of a 2-year randomized trial on cognition and behavior. *Arch Gen Psychiatry.* 2004;61:866-876.

49. Harvey PD, Bowie CR. Cognitive remediation in severe mental illness. *Innov Clin Neurosci.* 2012;9:27-30.

50. Nuechterlein KH, Ventura J, Subotnik KL, Hayata JN, Medalia A, Bell MD. Developing a cognitive training strategy for first-episode schizophrenia: integrating bottom-up and top-down approaches. *Am J Psychiatr Rehabil.* 2014;17:225-253.

51. Eack SM. Cognitive remediation: a new generation of psychosocial interventions for people with schizophrenia. *Soc Work.* 2012;57:235-246.

52. Robinson SM. *A Brief Introduction to Cognitive Enhancement Therapy Revised.* 2018. Available at: https://www.researchgate.net/publication/323376206_A_Brief_Introduction_to_Cognitive_Enhancement_Therapy_CET_Revision.

53. Center for Cognition and Recovery. *A Foundation for Recovery Success.* 2018. Available at: http://cetcleveland.org/.

54. Eack SM, Hogarty GE, Greenwald DP, Hogarty SS, Keshavan MS. Effects of cognitive enhancement therapy on employment outcomes in early Schizophrenia: results from a 2-year randomized trial. *Res Soc Work Pract.* 2011;21:32-42.

55. Eack SM, Greenwald DP, Hogarty SS, et al. Cognitive enhancement therapy for early-course schizophrenia: effects of a two-year randomized controlled trial. *Psychiatr Serv.* 2009;60:1468-1476.

56. Kern RS, Liberman RP, Becker DR, Drake RE, Sugar CA, Green MF. Errorless learning for training individuals with schizophrenia at a community mental health setting providing work experience. *Schizophr Bull.* 2009;35:807-815.

57. Hurford I, Solomon K., Hurford M. Cognitive rehabilitation in schizophrenia. *Psychiatr Times.* 2011;8:1-9.

58. Wong K. Cognitive rehabilitation in community mental health. *BC Psychosocial Rehabilitation Advanced Practice Webinar.* March 5, 2014. Available at: https://www.psyrehab.ca/files/documents/Cog%20Rehab%20webinar%20Mar%202014-slides%20only.pdf.

59. Fredrick MM, Mintz J, Roberts DL, et al. Is cognitive adaptation training (CAT) compensatory, restorative, or both? *Schizophr Res.* 2015;166:290-296.

60. Vita A, Barlati S, Bellani M, Brambilla P. Cognitive remediation in schizophrenia: background, techniques, evidence of efficacy and perspectives. *Epidemiol Psychiatr Sci.* 2014;23:21-25.

61. Barlati S, Deste G, De Peri L, Ariu C, Vita A. Cognitive remediation in schizophrenia: current status and future perspectives. *Schizophr Res Treatment.* 2013;2013:156084.

62. Trapp W, Landgrebe M, Hoesl K, et al. Cognitive remediation improves cognition and good cognitive performance increases time to relapse – results of a 5 year catamnestic study in schizophrenia patients. *BMC Psychiatry.* 2013;13:1-9.

63. Anaya C, Aran AM, Ayuso-Mateos JL, Wykes T, Vieta E, Scott J. A systematic review of cognitive remediation for schizo-affective and affective disorders. *J Affect Disord.* 2012;142:13-21.

64. Wykes T, Huddy V, Cellard C, McGurk S, Czobar P. A meta-analysis of cognitive remediation for schizophrenia: methodology and effect sizes. *Am J Psychiatry.* 2011;168:472-485.

65. Revell ER, Neill JC, Harte M, Khan Z, Drake RJ. A systematic review and meta-analysis of cognitive remediation in early schizophrenia. *Schizophr Res.* 2015;168:213-222.

66. Clements S, Corney S, Humin Y, Karmas R, Henderson C (MHCC, edit). *Cognitive Functioning: Supporting People With Mental Health Conditions and Cognitive Impairment.* Mental Health Coordinating Council Inc.; 2015.

8

Sensory Modulation

Tina Champagne

LEARNING OBJECTIVES

1. Define and contrast the three overarching sensory integration and processing categories.
2. Identify three to five ways that occupational therapy practitioners integrate sensory modulation–related interventions as part of the occupational therapy process.
3. Recognize the interrelationship of trauma informed care and sensory modulation–related interventions.
4. Explain the significant contribution of sensory integration and processing to occupational participation across the lifespan.
5. Recognize the research evidence supporting the use of sensory modulation–related interventions as part of occupational therapy services in the mental health area of practice.

INTRODUCTION

Dr. A. Jean Ayres was an educational psychologist and occupational therapist. Ayres was the first to define the concept of sensory integration (SI) as a neurophysiologic process and to create the SI frame of reference, which is now referred to as Ayres Sensory Integration® (ASI). According to Ayres, SI refers to how people take in sensory information, from within and outside of the body, through the sensory systems, and how each person processes and perceives this information.[1,2] Ayres also promoted that SI is foundational to human development, behavior, and occupational participation.[1,2] Many other sensory-related models, assessment tools, and intervention approaches have been developed over the years, most of which have borrowed from the foundational work of Ayres. The ASI fidelity criteria and corresponding evidence-based fidelity tool are available to help distinguish between ASI and other sensory-based approaches.[3]

Sensory processing (SP) is another term that is sometimes used to describe SI; therefore, SI and SP are often used as interchangeable terms.[4-6] Throughout this chapter, *sensory integration and processing* (SIP) is the overarching term that will be used when referring to all categories of SIP, including sensory modulation, sensory discrimination, and sensory-based motor patterns and skills.[6]

For almost two decades, sensory modulation (a component of SIP) has become a significant area of focus in mental health practice across the lifespan, both within and outside of occupational therapy (OT).[7-9] Sensory modulation is known as the regulatory component of SIP and is defined as "The capacity to regulate and organize the degree, intensity, and nature of responses to sensory input in a graded and adaptive manner. This allows the individual to achieve and maintain an optimal range of performance and to adapt to challenges in daily life."[10]

Occupational therapy practitioners (OTPs) have the educational background necessary to provide services that include an emphasis on SIP as part of the OT process. OTPs engage in the OT process when working with clients, which includes occupational analysis, a skill set that is unique to OTPs (American Occupational Therapy Association [AOTA]).[11] This skill set is used to help grade activities, occupations, and environments to foster the optimal challenge and support occupational participation. In addition to the use of occupation as the primary mode of intervention whenever possible, OTPs deep understanding of neurophysiology, including SIP and the other client, cultural, contextual, and environmental factors affecting engagement in occupations, provides a unique lens from which OTPs help clients achieve positive therapeutic outcomes.[12-15] In addition to OT's distinct value, OTPs also collaborate and sometimes overlap with other professionals when working with clients who have a variety of stress, trauma, and mental health–related challenges, to promote the use of interventions that support safety, self-regulation, stress management, and occupational participation.[16-18]

Sensory modulation was introduced into general mental health care first, before SIP, because sensory modulation is directly related to self-regulation as the regulatory component of sensory processing and is more easily understood by interdisciplinary staff and clients.[7,8,17] Although sensory modulation is not separate from SIP, the addition of the concept of sensory modulation in mental health care has broadened the range of mind-body interventions supporting choice, safety, health, and the ability to participate in meaningful roles and occupations. The addition of sensory modulation–related assessment and intervention approaches have contributed to a culture change toward a more humane and nurturing way of understanding and working with people.[17,19-24] Thus, over the past two decades, there has been an increased awareness by mental health professionals and in practice settings that the OT scope of practice includes neurophysiology (of which SIP is part), trauma, and attachment informed care. This awareness has enabled OTPs to take a leadership role in supporting the expansion of the safe and responsible use of sensory modulation–related interventions in mental health. Evidence from the trauma informed care, seclusion and restraint reduction, and addiction and pain management initiatives has further emphasized the relevance of SIP-related approaches and the value of the OT in each of these areas of practice.

Research has established that there are some common SIP patterns present as part of a variety of mental health diagnoses (e.g., autism, schizophrenia),[25-28] and there are also some mental health diagnoses where there may or may not be consistent SIP patterns, such as in attention-deficit/hyperactivity disorder (ADHD).[29-31] More research is needed to understand the relationship of SIP and its correlations with mental illness better[25,32] and to gain a greater understanding of the relationships among SIP, mental health, and occupational participation.[33,34] Furthermore, it is important to note that even when a person does not have SIP or mental health challenges, sensory modulation approaches can be used to support stress management, health, and wellness.

Although there is still a long way to go in terms of the broader scale understanding and application of SIP in mental health care and in establishing a strong evidence base, there is a growing body of evidence supporting its value and promise. The bulk of the evidence in mental health related to SIP at this time is focused more on sensory modulation specifically, although a foundation of research, including the totality of SIP, is emerging. According to the AOTA,[16] OTPs, as qualified mental health practitioners, provide a broad variety of services, including those emphasizing SIP and trauma-informed care (TIC) as part of the OT process.[16] Thus, the application of the OTP's knowledge, leadership, and service provision, when adding an emphasis on SIP as part of OT services, has provided a platform from which to demonstrate the distinct value of OT in mental health care settings.

SENSORY INTEGRATION AND PROCESSING

Ayres[2] described sensation as "food for the brain" and sensory integration as "the organization of sensations for use." The work of Ayres[1,2] spearheaded the OT theory and practice of SI, which is now trademarked and known as ASI. The patterns of difficulty in occupational performance skills related to SI were first categorized by Ayres as patterns of SI dysfunction.[2,35] These patterns continue to be explored and researched, with each being directly correlated with specific sensory systems, as initially identified through neuroscience, factor analysis, and assessed using the Sensory Integration and Praxis Test.[36] An evidence-based fidelity tool has also been published to help OTPs and researchers identify when they are using ASI or some other sensory-based approach to help establish a strong evidence base.[3] The ASI fidelity tool has provided the ability to establish ASI as an evidence-based approach with children with autism.[37] Anecdotally, ASI has been used with many people with a variety of mental health needs and goals with positive results, but more research is needed to establish an evidence base.[17,21,22,38]

The taxonomy of sensory processing disorders (SPDs) is also widely used at this time and includes the following components: sensory modulation disorder, sensory discrimination disorder, and sensory-based movement disorder.[32] Box 8.1 provides a brief explanation of each of the SPDs.

The umbrella term *sensory processing disorder* (SPD) emerged out of the quest to create a uniform terminology, gain inclusion of SPD in the fifth edition of the *Diagnostic and Statistical Manual of Mental Disorders* (DSM-5),[25] and help encourage research into SIP to establish an evidence base.[10] The driving force behind the desire for SPD to be included in the DSM-5 was the hope that this initiative would also help provide more access to OT services to those in need, given that a diagnosis is required for insurance coverage in the United States. Although SPD did not achieve the level of evidence required to meet the standards and time frames necessary for inclusion in the DSM-5, a large body of research has come out of this effort and still continues, demonstrating the complexity of SIP and its relationship to mental health. A unified taxonomy that

BOX 8.1   Sensory Processing Umbrella: Sensory Processing Disorders

Sensory Modulation Disorder
- Sensory overresponsivity (SOR): hypersensitivity pattern(s)
- Sensory underresponsivity (SUR): underresponsivity pattern(s)
- Sensory seeking: behavioral response indicating an active strategy towards getting sensory needs met

Sensory Discrimination Disorder
- Difficulty distinguishing between sensory stimuli from particular sensory systems

Sensory-Based Motor Disorder
- Postural control: difficulty with the underlying sensorimotor skills that support the ability to maintain postures
- Dyspraxia: difficulty with praxis skills

Adapted from American Occupational Therapy Association. Occupational Therapy Practice Framework: Domain and Process. 3rd ed. *Am J Occup Ther.* 2014;68:S1-S48.

encompasses the work of the varied SIP theorists and research efforts within the field of OT has yet to be established. However, all of the work in this area of practice has contributed significantly to the evolution of this body of knowledge over the years. There is much debate about the future direction of the taxonomy of SIP, and much research will be needed to reach a resolution.

Sensory Modulation

Given that this chapter is primarily focused on sensory modulation, Dunn's model of sensory processing is used to describe sensory modulation in more detail due to its inclusion of a more comprehensive view of the behavioral response continuum than that represented by the model of SPD.[10] For example, in the SPD model, the behavioral response of sensory modulation identifies sensory seeking only, whereas Dunn's model includes both sensory seeking

and sensation avoiding. Table 8.1 demonstrates Dunn's representation of sensory modulation,[19,39] including terms that have been added over time, to help make the terms used to explain Dunn's four-quadrant model more understandable to the layperson.[20]

The neurologic thresholds of the Miller and Dunn models both refer to the neurologic thresholds of sensory modulation in a similar way, although the names of the thresholds differ (as shown when comparing the information provided in Box 8.1 and Box 8.2). Neurologic thresholds can also be thought of as tolerance levels for stimulation coming in from the different sensory systems, each on a continuum from low to high. Additionally, the degree of sensitivity depends on the degree of the severity within the threshold (low, moderate, or high severity) and a host of other factors (e.g., feeling well or unwell, context, environment, trauma history).

What does this look like? To have a low neurologic threshold means that sensory stimuli are very easily noticed, and the lower the threshold, the more intense and often less tolerable the stimuli become. Each of the sensory systems has its own mechanism for registering sensory input, known as the "sensory receptors," from which the stimuli are sent to the central nervous system for processing. Therefore, one or more sensory systems may have a low neurologic threshold for sensory stimuli, which results in some degree of sensory overresponsivity (hypersensitivity). The behavioral responses that correspond with having a low neurologic threshold include sensory sensitivity (sensor) and/or sensation avoiding (avoider).[19,20] For example, a person having a low threshold for tactile stimulation (touch) would tend to be more sensitive to tactile input (tactile overresponsivity), but may or may not be avoidant of it for a variety of reasons (tactile sensor or tactile avoider).

A high neurologic threshold is the opposite of a low neurologic threshold. Having a high neurologic threshold means that sensory stimuli is less noticeable than it would be to the average person in the same age range. Therefore, it takes more sensory input to be aware of it (sensory underresponsivity). The behavioral responses that correspond with having a high neurologic threshold are low

TABLE 8.1   Sensory Modulation Quadrant Model

| Neurologic Thresholds | BEHAVIORAL RESPONSE CONTINUUM | |
	Passive Strategies	Active Strategies
High threshold	Low registration (bystander)	Sensation seeking (seeker)
Low threshold	Sensory sensitivity (sensor)	Sensation avoiding (avoider)

Adapted from references 19, 20, and 41.

BOX 8.2 Self-Rating: Anxious—When I Am Anxious, I Feel

- Body: jittery, heart pounds, muscles feel tense, get a headache; gets harder to breathe
- Mind: can't focus or think straight, worry a lot, hard to know what to do, sometimes have scary thoughts, thinking gets fuzzy
- Triggers: when people are mean or rude, when I am worried, when I don't know what to do, when things get too hard
- Warning signs: I don't talk much, I stop doing what I am supposed to be doing, my body gets hyper or stops moving, sometimes I get mad or sad, or I might say "no" to what you ask me to do

registration (bystander) and/or sensory seeking (seeker). Thus, having a low threshold for tactile stimuli would mean that the individual would need more tactile input than the average person in their age range to register and notice tactile stimuli. The behavioral responses indicate whether the person would tend to seek out the tactile input needed actively (tactile seeker) or not (low registration of tactile stimuli).

Furthermore, as previously stated, it is possible to have different neurologic thresholds for different types of sensory input, which may lead to having a combination of high and low thresholds. How can this be? Because each of the sensory systems has its own "threshold" capacity, and taking into account that all the sensory systems are operating at the same time, the process is very complex. Thus, it is possible to be significantly bothered by many different types of stimulation (low neurologic threshold) such as tactile stimulation (clothing fabrics, being touched, temperatures, feeling of being wet), auditory stimulation (volume of sound, competing noises in chaotic environments), and visual stimulation (too much clutter in a classroom, fast-moving objects, or people in a space). This same person, however, may also have a high neurologic threshold for proprioceptive and vestibular input.

Let's consider what the behavioral responses of the aforementioned example might look like. Because this person is bothered by tactile input, they might avoid most types (tactile avoider), yet may or may not necessarily avoid auditory or visual stimuli (e.g., in the classroom, gym class, or cafeteria setting). This person may still feel very overwhelmed by the sensory input (sensory sensitivity [sensor]) but tolerate it to do what they need to do as part of their roles and routine. This same person also has a high threshold for proprioception and vestibular (movement) and, in this way, may be a bystander or seeker (low registration

[bystander] or sensation seeking [seeker]) of different types of movement. This is just one example of how the different neurologic thresholds and behavioral responses relate to the different sensory systems, and they may present in a very complex way.

Everyone is unique, which is why it is critical to engage in an OT assessment process that includes a focus on the entirety of SIP to help identify each individual's SIP patterns and the potential impact on participation, behavior, mental health, wellness, and quality of life.[4,40-42] Even for those with more of a neurotypical sensory profile (not too high or low in any particular sensory system), the use of sensory modulation strategies may still be helpful for stress management, participation, health, wellness, and/or quality-of-life purposes.[40] Although the focus of this chapter is primarily on sensory modulation, it is also necessary to look at all the components of SIP as part of the OT process. In mental health care, this is particularly important, because OTPs are often one of the few rehabilitation professionals involved in mental health systems of care, and if it is not identified that there are problems with SIP, these issues often go unidentified or may be considered solely as behavioral problems.

It is important also to understand that sensory modulation patterns that are not neurotypical (not similar to most people in the same age range) are not always negative or problematic. In fact, SIP patterns contribute to what makes each person different and may have a positive impact in one's daily life. For example, someone with mild auditory overresponsivity (sensitive to sound) may find that it is a strength in their role as a worker if they are a sound engineer and only bothersome when in crowds. What makes a SIP pattern become problematic is when it interferes with safety and the ability to function and participate in meaningful life roles and occupations. Thus, people may or may not want to work on strategies for coping purposes or toward changing SIP patterns if they are not perceived as problematic.

The Nervous System

The ability to understand and value the dynamic complexity of SIP requires understanding how the nervous system works and contributes to occupational performance and participation. Although is it is more obvious when someone experiences a stroke that the injury to the nervous system affects function and participation in many cases, difficulties with SIP patterns are often less obvious and not easily understood. At the same time, SIP is one of the foundational capacities that makes us human, able to function, communicate, and participate in meaningful life roles, routines, and occupations. With this knowledge, it becomes much more obvious that the nervous system supports and plays a central role in SIP and how developmental delays, trauma, or injury to the sensory systems may negatively affect occupational outcomes.

The nervous system is made up of the central nervous system (CNS—brain, brain stem, and spinal cord) and the peripheral nervous system (autonomic and somatic nervous systems). In mental health, and particularly in the literature related to trauma, there is often more of a focus on the autonomic nervous system (ANS). This heightened focus on the ANS is due to the emphasis on arousal regulation and how it corresponds with self-regulation and emotion regulation. More recently, the literature on polyvagal theory has revealed that the ANS responses that were previously understood as the sympathetic nervous system (SNS) response (fight, flight, or freeze responses) and the parasympathetic nervous system (PNS) response (rest and digest mode) also include an additional response type of the PNS known as the "freeze response."[43-45] It used to be that the freeze response was viewed as part of the SNS. We now know that the freeze response of the PNS is triggered when the sympathetic mode is not sufficient to deal with the nature of the threat.

The PNS begins to go into the freeze response (shut down) in a manner that ranges from less to more severe, depending on the person's perception of the degree of threat they are facing (e.g., dissociation, fainting, death). The freeze response mode of the PNS differs significantly from the rest and digest mode of the PNS. The rest and digest mode is the predominant PNS response when a person feels calm and relaxed. It is in the rest and digest mode of the PNS that people are able to pay attention, think most clearly, and communicate with others in the most functional manner (supports the social engagement system) and thereby engage more fully in roles, relationships, and occupations.[44,45] OTPs assist clients in becoming more aware of their ANS responses and in identifying strategies that support the ability to shift into the PNS rest and digest mode more flexibly when not threatened or in danger.

The sensory systems are part of the nervous system, and the receptors of each of the sensory systems picks up on specific information from outside and from within the body. These receptors receive the sensory input and transport that energy and information to other parts of the nervous system. Each sensory system has specific pathways from the receptor level to the level of the brain, where the information is further processed, interpreted, and ultimately perceived. How we perceive sensory input affects how we think about the world, the nature and quality of our experiences, and how we work, sleep, rest, play, and engage in roles, relationships, and other areas of occupation.

Sensory Systems

Each of the sensory systems plays a role in the ability to understand and navigate in the world. To date, we have identified that there are eight sensory systems:
1. Proprioception
2. Vestibular
3. Tactile
4. Auditory
5. Visual
6. Olfaction
7. Gustatory
8. Interoception

Each sensory system has a very specific role in helping receive and perceive our experiences over time. Table 8.2 provides a general overview of each of the sensory systems and lists examples of each system's relative contribution to self-regulation, self-awareness, and other occupational performance skills.

TABLE 8.2 **Sensory Systems**		
Sensory Systems and Receptors	**Primary Function(s)**	**Contributions**
Proprioception		
Receptors are located in the muscles, joints, ligaments, tendons, connective tissue, and fascia (e.g., muscle spindles, joint receptors, and Golgi tendon organs)	The proprioceptive system supports body awareness, the ability to assume and maintain body positions, and the grading, timing, and efficiency of movements.	Contributes to the awareness of: • Where the body and body parts are located in space and over time • Body movement • Body position
Receptors are stimulated by movements causing muscles to stretch, contract, or co-contract (particularly when movement is against resistance)	The proprioceptive system works with the tactile system to support body awareness (body-based felt sense) and the vestibular system to support efficient and fluid movements and postural control (body in space).	• Body boundaries • Body image • Proprioceptive information from the environment providing safety-related cues

TABLE 8.2   Sensory Systems—cont'd

Sensory Systems and Receptors	Primary Function(s)	Contributions
Vestibular The vestibular system structures are housed in the inner ear and include the otoliths (utricle and saccule) and semicircular canals. Receptors include tiny hair cells that bend with the movement of the fluid in the semicircular canals or by the shifting of the membrane into which the hair cells project into the otoliths. Receptors (hair cells) are activated during acceleration, deceleration, spinning, linear, angular movements, any other movements involving the head, and the pull of gravity.	The vestibular system supports the ability to be aware of the spatial orientation of the body (including equilibrium, speed, timing, and rhythmicity of positioning and movement). The vestibular system works with the proprioceptive system to support efficient and fluid movements and postural control and the visual system to support the ability to maintain a stable visual field, balance, and equilibrium. The vestibular and auditory systems are also interconnected.	Contributes to the awareness of: • Spatial awareness of where the body is in space and time • Balance • Body coordination • Muscle tone • Gravity detection • Awareness of the speed and direction of movements • Awareness of whether things around us are moving or stationary • Vestibular information from the environment providing safety-related cues
Tactile Receptors are located in the skin (most dense in the hand, mouth, and genital areas). Receptors are activated during any type of skin contact (e.g., when touching something, showering, toothbrushing, eating, drinking, grooming, dressing).	The tactile system supports the ability to detect safety, comfort, discomfort, pain sensations (protective function), and to discrimination and localize stimulation detected by the tactile receptors. The tactile system works with the proprioceptive system to support body awareness.	Contributes to the awareness of: • Tactile sensations and tactile discrimination • Pressure sensations (light, deep) • Pain coming from the pain receptors of the skin • Temperature • Vibration • Body boundaries • Tactile information from the environment providing safety-related cues
Visual Receptors are located in the retina of the eye (rods and cones) and stimulated by visual input (e.g., light, colors, contours, shades).	The visual system supports the ability to discriminate visual stimuli to see, identify, and locate—for example, objects, symbols, boundaries, people, map spatial relationships. The visual system also works with the vestibular system to support a stable visual field and supports balance and equilibrium.	Contributes to the awareness of: • Gradations of colors, light, darkness • Shapes, symbols, contours • Movement detection • Visual information from the environment providing safety-related cues
Auditory The auditory receptors are the hair cells of the cochlea located within the inner ear and stimulated by sound waves and vibrations.	The auditory system supports the ability to detect the distance, directionality, and qualities of sounds. The auditory system is interconnected with the vestibular system.	Contributes to the awareness of: • Volume of sound(s) • Tone of sound(s) • Directionality of sound(s)

Continued

TABLE 8.2 Sensory Systems—cont'd		
Sensory Systems and Receptors	**Primary Function(s)**	**Contributions**
Olfaction		
The olfactory epithelium contains the chemical receptor (chemoreceptor) of the nose and also osmoreceptors (detect osmotic pressure changes). The olfactory sense is primarily stimulated by different scents and the air through breathing.	The olfactory system supports the ability to detect and localize odors and scents, has a protective function, and has a direct connection to the limbic system (emotion center of the brain) to influence emotions. The olfactory and gustatory systems work together to enhance the sense of taste.	Contributes to the awareness of: • The nature of odors (pleasant, familiar, unpleasant) • How strong an odor is perceived to be • Olfactory information from the environment providing safety-related cues
Gustatory		
Taste buds contain the chemical receptors of the tongue and are stimulated when tasting or manipulating something in the mouth (drinking, tasting, chewing).	The gustatory system assists in the ability to discriminate between different tastes and helps gather information about stimuli entering the mouth. The gustatory and olfactory systems work together to enhance the sense of taste.	Contributes to the awareness of: • The nature of taste sensations (pleasant, familiar, unpleasant) • How strong the taste stimuli is perceived to be • Gustatory information from the environment providing safety-related cues
Interoception		
Sensory nerve endings contained within the muscles, organs, and viscera across the different systems in the body.	Interoception supports the ability to be aware of internal states, corresponding feelings, urges, and emotions.	Contributes to the awareness of: • Temperature • Pain • Hunger • Muscle tension • Sleepiness, alertness • Heart rate • Respiration rate • Digestion • Bowel and bladder functions • Itch • Tickle • Nausea • Nervousness

From Champagne T. *Sensory Modulation in Dementia Care: Assessment and Activities for Sensory-Enriched Care.* London: Jessica Kingsley; 2018.

SENSORY MODULATION AND SELF-REGULATION

Sensory modulation is the regulatory component of SIP, and for those who struggle with sensory modulation, it is critical to helping these individuals understand their sensory profile patterns whenever possible and appropriate to do so. For people who do not have problems with SIP, it may seem odd to focus on SIP patterns, and the connection between challenges with SIP and occupational participation may appear less obvious. Education is key to help people understand how SIP challenges may negatively influence safety, behavior, relationships, and occupational participation.

Once people become more aware of their SIP patterns, the information can be used to help explore interventions that support coping with and managing sensory input. Once the person is feeling more stabilized, if desired, it is also possible to help that person work on changing SIP patterns. The degree of change that may be achieved, related to one's sensory profile, depends on many variables, such as the degree of SIP pattern severity, other mental health challenges experienced, the amount and type of support(s) available, and how much the person wants to make the change. It can be difficult for a person to decide to work on changing their SIP patterns because it requires the implementation of a daily repertoire of strategies in addition to sessions with the OTP. Some of the difficulties that people face with following through with this decision are similar to those often faced when people struggle with consistent engagement in a home exercise program when in rehabilitation services. The home plan must be practical, and the supports needed to succeed must be part of the plan for optimal results.

Evaluation: Sensory Modulation

When adding the assessment of SIP patterns to the OT evaluation process, the assessment results help guide the goal setting and intervention planning.[13,46] Assessment and screening tools that look specifically at identifying sensory modulation-related patterns include some of the following (this is not an all-inclusive list):
- Adolescent/Adult Sensory Profile[19]
- Sensory Defensiveness Questionnaire[17]
- Sensory Modulation Questionnaire[17]
- Caregiver Questionnaire[17]
- Sensory Processing Caregiver Checklist[22]

There are a variety assessment tools used by OTs that look more comprehensively at different aspects of SIP, not only sensory modulation; some of these include the following:
- Adult/Adolescent Sensory History[47]
- Beery-Buktenica Test of Visual-Motor Integration (VMI)[48]
- Bruininks-Oseretsky Test of Motor Proficiency (second edition; BOT-2)[49]
- Clinical Observations of Motor Performance Skills (COMPS)[50]
- Developmental Test of Visual Perception—Adolescent and Adult[51]
- Miller Assessment for Preschoolers[52]
- Quick Neurological Screening Tool (QNST)[53]
- Sensory Integration and Praxis Test (SIPT)[36]
- Sensory Processing Measure[54]
- Sensory Profile[39]

Table 8.3 provides more detailed information about the SIP assessment tools listed above.

TABLE 8.3 Assessment Tools, Age Ranges, and Purpose

Assessment Tool	Age Range (years)	Purpose
Adult/Adolescent Sensory History[47]	13–95 years	Self-report assessment of sensory and motor behaviors of individuals with difficulties with sensory integration and processing
Beery-Buktenica Test of Visual-Motor Integration (6th ed.)[48]	2–100 years	Screens visual motor, visual perceptual, and motor coordination skills
Bruininks-Oseretsky Test of Motor Proficiency (2nd ed.) (BOT-2)[49]	4–21 years, 11 months	Comprehensive assessment of gross and fine motor skills
Clinical Observations of Motor and Postural Skills (COMPS)[50]	5–15 years	Detects a number of subtle motor control and coordination problems based on the original Ayres clinical observations.
Developmental Test of Visual Perception—Adolescent and Adult[51]	11–74 years	Assessment of different aspects of visual perception
Miller Assessment for Preschoolers[52]	2 years, 9 months–5 years, 8 months	Assessment of developmental delays and preacademic skills
Quick Neurological Screening Tool (3rd ed.) (QNST-3)[53]	4– 80 years	Assessment of neurologic soft signs related to sensory integration
Sensory Integration and Praxis Tests[36]	4–8 years, 11 months	Comprehensive assessment (17 standardized tests) of sensory integration
Sensory Processing Measure[54]	5–12 years	Caregiver questionnaire that provides the caregiver's subjective report of the child's sensory processing
Sensory Profile (Child Version)[39]	3–10 years	Caregiver questionnaire that provides the caregiver's subjective report of the child's sensory processing

Therapeutic Intervention: Sensory Modulation

After completing the OT evaluation and goal-setting processes, interventions are collaboratively identified that will help meet the individualized goals. When working on sensory modulation–related goals, given that it is the regulatory component of SIP, identification of the sensory modulation patterns (neurologic thresholds and behavioral responses) and the person's hopes and goals in this area are used to identify where to begin with interventions. Many people will begin by working with the OTP to identify strategies that will help them to feel safe and stabilized. It is also common that people want to learn more about how their nervous system responds to sensory input and identify coping skills to help them manage how they feel to support participation. When not in a crisis state and feeling more stabilized, some people may want to work on changing the way their nervous system responds to stimuli. All interventions should be directly related to the client's occupational goals. Many OTPs begin the intervention process by helping clients explore what is calming versus alerting (or the combination) and when and how these identified strategies are most helpful, ultimately having a positive impact on participation.

The Calm-Alert Continuum

When using the term *calming*, it is typically understood that what is calming is what helps a person feel relaxed, comfortable, soothed, and organized. The term *alerting* is often more complicated to understand because it can refer to what is perceived as uplifting (positive in nature) and also what is overwhelming or noxious to the person

TABLE 8.4 Continuum of Calming and Alerting Qualities	
Calming	**Alerting**
Low-stimulus intensity	High-stimulus intensity
Familiarity	Novelty
Consistency	Inconsistency
Simplicity	Complexity
Slow pace	Fast pace
Congruity	Incongruity
Neutral warmth	Cool, cold temperature

(bothersome or jarring in effect). What is calming, alerting, or the combination varies according to the individual and, therefore, OTPs help clients explore what works the best for them and consider when and how to use each strategy to gain the most therapeutic benefit. The qualities of what makes something more calming, alerting, or the combination is often thought of on a calm-alert continuum. Table 8.4 demonstrates some examples of common qualities that may foster a more calm or alert response. The information in Table 8.4 is only to be used as a guide, due to the individualized nature of each person's experience. For example, what is calming to one person may or may not be calming to another.

A general list of some sensory strategies that are often considered to be more calming versus alerting, although varying depending on the individual, is provided in Table 8.5. This table is to be used as a guide and is not a protocol.

TABLE 8.5 Calming and Alerting Strategies	
Calming Strategies	**Alerting Strategies**
Warm, hot drink	Cool or cold drink
Rocking slowly in a rocking chair	Rocking vigorously in a rocking chair
Swinging on a swing	Spinning on a swing
Swaying to music	Clapping or bouncing to music
Humming or singing quietly	Singing loudly
Deep pressure touch/massage	Light touch, tickling
Decaffeinated or herbal tea or coffee	Caffeinated tea or coffee
Soothing low-intensity scents (smelling a flower)	Intense scents (smelling eucalyptus or strong perfumes)
Slow-paced walks	Jogging or running
Slow-paced drive	Fast-paced or bumpy drive
Cooking with mild spices	Cooking with intense spices
Eating bland or mild foods	Eating spicy foods
Smooth food textures	Differing food textures

TABLE 8.5 Calming and Alerting Strategies—cont'd	
Calming Strategies	**Alerting Strategies**
Soft, low lighting	Bright, colorful lighting
Stretching	Aerobic exercise
Listening or playing slow-paced, rhythmic music	Listening or playing fast-paced music or an uneven beat
Being in a calm and quiet environment	Being in a busy, loud, or chaotic environment
Consistent routines	Inconsistent routines
Petting a cat, dog or horse (pet)	Riding a horse

Reprinted from Champagne T. The influence of posttraumatic stress disorder, depression, and sensory processing patterns on occupational engagement: a case study. Work. 2011b;38(1):67-75, with permission from IOS Press. The publication is available at IOS Press through http://dx.doi.org/10.3233/WOR-2011-1105.

INTENSITY

Part of what makes something seem more or less calming or alerting is the perception of stimulus intensity. What influences a person's perception of stimulus intensity? Although many variables may have an impact, the frequency (how often), duration (how long), degree of stimulus intensity inherent in the item or object (how much, what type), rhythm, context, and the individual's unique SIP patterns are some of the most common. The concept of intensity is important for OTPs to understand because it will guide the ability to grade activities and environmental stimuli, taking into account each of the sensory systems, the individual's SIP patterns, and the wide range of variables that are considered during the occupational analysis process. Two examples of how stimulus intensity may be graded, as it corresponds with the sensory systems, include the following:

- Taste—something sweet is often less intense than something salty, which is often less intense than something bitter.
- Vestibular—sitting upright is often less intense than linear movement, versus bending over or arching backward, which is typically less intense than spinning (rotary movement).

Grading activities, occupations, and environments, while taking into account the different types and amounts of stimulus intensity experienced, and the individual's SIP patterns is a skill set that is specific to the rehabilitation professional's scope of practice. Adding a layer of mental health and trauma-related considerations to what a person may be facing, it is easy to see how the complexity of one's experience may become significantly overwhelming. OTPs have the skill set necessary to help clients become aware of and understand how and why their nervous system responds the way it does and to consider the different types of interventions that may be helpful.

The ability to become self-aware and express one's feelings is often challenging, especially for people with more moderate to profound mental health and trauma-related challenges. The co-creation and use of self-rating tools and corresponding strategies are part of what OTPs work on with people, but take into account all the variables in addition to all the other areas that OTs assess. There are many self-rating programs (e.g., Zones of Regulation by Kuypers) and apps (e.g., Optimism, Mood Track Social Diary) available to help make the act of self-rating and increasing self-awareness more fun and engaging, including books and games. Over time, with increased self-awareness, clients are better able to create a list of triggers, warning signs, helpful strategies, and a list of things that are bothersome.

Box 8.2 and Table 8.6 summarize triggers, warning signs, and strategies that help and do not help this 9-year-old boy when he is feeling anxious. OTPs often assist clients in creating these types of tools after helping identify this information, which also serves as a concise communication tool (by parents, teachers, and residential staff). The Department of Mental Health of Massachusetts has compiled examples of practical tools used in mental health settings, known as *safety tools*, that help gather this type of information—triggers, warning signs, helpful strategies. Some of these tools include an emphasis on the sensory systems. These safety tool examples are part of a free downloadable book on trauma-informed care, *The Resources Guide: Creating Positive Cultures of Care*. It is found on this website: https://www.mass.gov/ service-details/restraintseclusion-reduction-initiative-rsri.

The ability to become aware of how other people are feeling, and how people, environments, and other stimuli influence how one feels, is an even greater skill set to master over time. Such maturation in the area of self-awareness

TABLE 8.6   Strategies

What I Can Do That Helps!	Distractions
Squeezing things	Watching baseball
Bean bag tapping	Playing with animals
Fidget with something (rubber band, stress ball, putty)	Making a snack
Pet my cat	Fishing
Mad libs, funny movies	Going out with friend
Jumping and crashing in a big bean bag or mattress	Swimming
Swinging	Legos
Ride my bike	TV
Jump on minitrampoline	Playing sports
	Playing a game
	Eating something sour
Things That Other People Can Do With Me That Might Help!	**Please Do Not:**
Sometimes, hugs	Leave me alone
Back rubs	Allow arguing or chaos near me
Massage	Tickle me
Joint compressions	Use too much deep touch pressure
Stay nearby; do not leave me alone	Put me in rooms with lots of fragile stuff
Offer me my pillow and weighted blanket	Put me in places with lots of loud noise
	Criticize me

and in the awareness of others supports occupational participation. Some clients make rating scales related to occupational participation as well. In the following study, a woman seeing an OTP in an outpatient capacity created her own 0 to 10 participation scale to help track her progress with use of the Sensory Modulation Program.[21]

The Sensory Modulation Program

There are a variety of models, frameworks, and programmatic guidelines for implementing sensory modulation–related interventions with a variety of populations across the lifespan. The Sensory Modulation Program (SMP) was developed to serve as a stand-alone therapeutic intervention approach or as an adjunct to other therapeutic approaches, when it is used in a skilled and responsible manner (e.g., Dialectical Behavior Therapy, Trauma-Focused Cognitive Behavior Therapy, Neurosequential Model of Therapeutics, 12-step programs).[17,21,22] The following is an outline of the primary components of the SMP:

- Therapeutic use of self—throughout the OT process (which is collaborative and strength-based); evaluation (include SIP), goal setting, intervention planning, outcomes monitoring, discharge planning; individual, group, and programmatic applications
- Sensory diet—a strategic routine integrating sensory-enriched preparatory and occupation-based interventions

throughout the day (for prevention, fostering participation, and crisis de-escalation purposes)
- Sensorimotor activities—any activities that will help clients reach their goals, with an emphasis on sensation that is supportive to clients' needs and goals
- Sensory-based modalities—equipment or tools that are sensory supportive of the client's SIP patterns and goals (e.g., weighted blanket, biofeedback, clinical aromatherapy, sound therapy programs, apps)
- Environmental enhancements and modifications—enhancing or modifying the physical environment(s) in a manner that is supportive of the client's SIP patterns and goals (sensory rooms, sensory stations, sensory gardens, modifications to home, school, and/or work spaces)
- Caregiver or partner education and involvement

Table 8.7 provides a brief overview of how the SMP may be implemented in an acute, inpatient, mental health setting with a 24-year-old woman named Rebecca. Although there is a growing body of evidence related to some of the different components or intervention strategies that are used as part of the SMP, the most successful outcomes have been demonstrated when using the totality of the SMP in a collaborative and individualized manner.[17,21]

A study using a sensory-based program that is similar to that of the SMP was part of a study by Pfeiffer and

TABLE 8.7 Sensory Modulation Program Components

Component	Minicase Example: Rebecca (24 years old)—Inpatient Level of Care
Therapeutic use of self	Spent time with Rebecca getting to know her strengths, areas of concern, goals, and supports
Assessment	Completed a chart review and initial assessment process, which includes sensory and trauma informed care-related questions as part of the occupational therapy process
Sensorimotor activities	Provided a variety of sensorimotor activity-based choices in group and individual sessions
Sensory modalities	Worked with Rebecca to identify the different modalities she liked: weighted blanket, aromatherapy (Bergamot), and biofeedback
Sensory diet	After working with Rebecca to complete an occupational profile, and to determine initial sensory strategies that seemed to be the most helpful to her, an individualized daily routine with sensory strategies built into her routine strategically (with prevention and crisis intervention options) was created and implemented. The sensory diet will be enhanced and modified over time. The goal of implementing a sensory diet is to support feelings of safety, comfort, and increased participation.
Physical environment	Use of the unit's sensory room to help increase feelings of safety, self-regulation, self-care and social participation
Caregiver education and involvement	Met with Rebecca's community-based outreach worker, with her permission, to educate the worker about Rebecca's sensory-based needs, goals, and helpful strategies (e.g., sensory diet) and how this is related to her recovery goals Worked with Rebecca and her outreach worker to determine a discharge plan providing the level of support needed to obtain helpful strategies and to create a plan to continue sensory diet implementation after discharge

Adapted from Champagne T. *Sensory Modulation and Environment: Essential Elements of Occupation.* 3rd rev. ed. New York: Pearson; 2011.

Kinnealey[55] that also demonstrated positive results. More research is necessary to build on the existing literature to help establish the SMP as an evidence-based practice with varied populations and age ranges and in different practice settings. As the quest continues to help mental health practices become more nurturing, healing, and recovery-oriented, the SMP has been promoted as a promising intervention. This is evident in the growing expectation that mental health services are trauma-informed and that seclusion and restraint use be significantly reduced or eliminated across mental health practice settings. Leaders of these mental health initiatives have promoted the inclusion of sensory-based approaches, such as the SMP, to help reach these goals.[8,23,56,57]

Environmental Modifications and Enhancements

When organizations are starting to begin integrating sensory modulation interventions into their programming intentionally, some choose to begin with a smaller pilot project before embarking on the totality of instituting the SMP. The creation and use of a sensory room are often more easily contained and monitored and provides a concrete example of what sensory interventions look like for the interdisciplinary staff or administrators. Training specific to the interventions therein helps organizations begin implementation in a way that is safer and decreases the probability of becoming overwhelmed with the complexity of the entirety of the SMP.[58-61] Although there are many different ways to modify and enhance the physical environment, creating a sensory modulation–style room or corner of a room in a safe and skilled manner is often a first step taken by mental health practitioners. Sensory rooms are typically conceptualized according to specific types, and the type instituted is dependent on the goals of use and skill level of the staff that will support the use of the equipment and other items in the room.[17,22]

The sensory room types that are most referred to in the literature include sensory modulation rooms, sensory integration rooms, and multisensory environments. A sensory modulation room is a room that is specifically created and used by the people that will be using them (staff and clients), preferably with the guidance and training of an OTP.

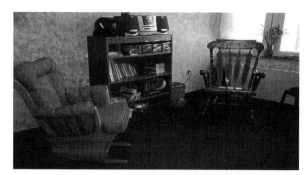

Fig. 8.1 Sensory modulation room—adult, acute, inpatient mental health unit in a hospital setting. (Courtesy Tina Champagne.)

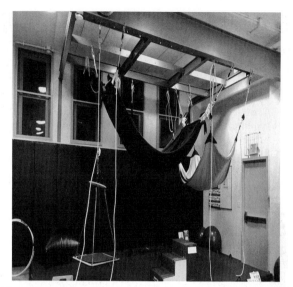

Fig. 8.2 Sensory integration room—suspended equipment and mats for safety.

A sensory modulation room is used for the purposes of supporting safety, self-regulation, self-awareness, sensory modulation–related needs and goals, and participation. They are created based on different themes and are typically named according to the theme (e.g., sensory room, comfort room, serenity room, "chillville," "explorium"). See Fig. 8.1 for an example of a sensory modulation–style room created for use in an adult, acute, inpatient mental health unit in a hospital setting.

A sensory integration style room or space is one that is created by rehabilitation professionals who are skilled in ASI and other sensory-based approaches. A sensory integration room or space is used for the purposes of evaluation and intervention. Sensory integration rooms or spaces have mats for safety and suspended, climbing, and other equipment that promotes the potential engagement of any or all of the sensory systems in a way that may be varied significantly for the grading of intensity and other therapeutic needs and goals. See Figs. 8.2 and 8.3 for examples.

A multisensory environment (MSE) is a room or space created for the purposes of fostering relaxation, socialization, and participation. Common equipment used in MSEs include a variety of lighting types, interactive switches, projectors, bubble tubes, fiberoptics, and other sensory supportive items and equipment. The MSE style of sensory room was first created for use with people with moderate to profound intellectual, developmental, and cognitive disabilities (e.g., dementia). MSEs are now being created and used for use by a large variety of populations. See Fig. 8.4 for an example.

Although these three different types of sensory rooms are the most common, rooms or spaces that combine these different room types are sometimes preferred. The use of a sensory cart is another way to bring items to the bedside or to other therapeutic spaces as needed. Sensory gardens

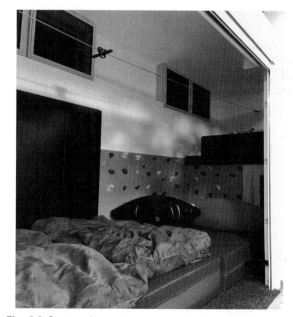

Fig. 8.3 Sensory integration space—climbing equipment and zip line.

provide sensory enrichment outdoors or even as an indoor gardening alternative. A large variety of sensory-enhanced modifications to physical environments for people with dementia are also common to decrease the probability of sensory deprivation or overstimulation and support participation and quality of life.[22]

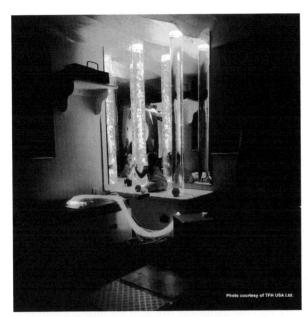

Fig. 8.4 Multisensory environment.

Sensory modulation rooms, corners, and carts are created and maintained to contain items that are safe for the clients to access, must be age- and culturally appropriate, and should be easy to clean and maintain. The following lists some common items offered in sensory modulation rooms when training, policies, and procedures are in place[17]:

- Bubble lamp or fish tank
- Rocking chair, recliner
- Desk chair that spins
- Beanbag chairs (fire-retardant)
- Hammock swing
- Bins of items for each sensory system
- Music options
- Nature and animal scene videos
- Musical instruments
- Writing, art, and coloring supplies
- Puzzles
- Zen tangles
- Self-help books
- Cards, games
- Weighted modalities (with training and proper care)
- Scented lotions
- Projectors
- Glitter wands
- Variety of tactile manipulatives
- Items offering vibration
- Soft blanket or wrap

An individualized sensory kit is a personal box or bag that contains strategies are specific to what is most helpful to the person and keeps all items organized and accessible. There are many different sensory kit themes, but the theme chosen must be one that is specific to the individual's needs and goals (e.g., mindfulness kit, sobriety kit).

The overall status of the physical environments of most mental health care settings has significantly improved due to the change in the culture of care since the introduction of the trauma-informed care initiative. Efforts to increase the safe and comfortable nature of the physical environment and that include more sensory supportive enhancements have helped contribute to this change (e.g., wall murals and decals, comfortable furnishings, sensory supportive rooms and spaces).

TRAUMA-INFORMED CARE, RESTRAINT AND SECLUSION REDUCTION, AND RECOVERY

Although SIP has been an area of emphasis in the therapeutic treatment approaches available in pediatrics, and with people with learning and developmental disabilities of all ages since its inception,[2,49] widespread application in mental health care settings and with adults with mental health diagnoses (e.g., bipolar, major depression, posttraumatic stress disorder [PTSD]) was not common until more recently.[30,62] Increasingly, the literature has been demonstrating the connection between atypical SIP patterns, trauma, and mental illness and supports the evolving understanding of the mind-body connection and the correlation with engagement in meaningful life roles, relationships, occupational participation, and quality of life.[a]

Research from many different fields of study has also contributed to the understanding of the pervasive influence of trauma on people, including the impact on SIP.[68-72] Although some people are born with SIP challenges or a genetic predisposition toward different SIP patterns, difficulty in some of the following areas may also occur as a result of traumatic experiences (this list is not all inclusive):

- Postural control
- Clumsiness
- Balance and equilibrium
- Body coordination
- Spatial awareness
- Body awareness
- Hypersensitivities (overresponsivity)
- Coordination and praxis

---

[a]References 5, 12, 21, 28, 33, 34, 38, and 63-67.

- Self-harm
- Dissociation
- Interoception
- Praxis skills
- Fine motor skills

The advent of the TIC initiative has helped spearhead a greater understanding of the value and necessity of therapeutic interventions that focus on the body, including SIP, as part of the TIC approach rather than solely on interventions that are more cognitive in nature (e.g., dialectic behavior therapy [DBT], cognitive-behavioral therapy [CBT]), talk therapy).[8,9,56] Thus, the TIC and recovery movements have helped shape how interdisciplinary professionals working with people with mental health needs and goals, within and outside of mental health settings, view mental health, mental illness, and the types of holistic, trauma-informed, and developmentally sensitive services provided, including the emphasis on SIP.

Seclusion and restraint (S/R) reduction is part of the TIC and recovery initiatives of the Substance Abuse and Mental Health Services Administration (SAMHSA).[73-76] Since these initiatives were launched in 2003 as part of the president's New Freedom Commission, a variety of international mental health organizations have joined the TIC and S/R reduction initiatives and have published guidelines to reduce S/R and other violent and restrictive interventions.[8,9,56,77,78] Many research studies have shown that the use of sensory-based approaches help reduce the use of S/R and PRN (as needed) medication use when people are distressed.[7,38,79-92]

The United States is an international leader in instituting the TIC initiative, and although there is a great deal of work still to do in terms of this national initiative and the corresponding culture change, the United States has developed national policies and evidence-based practices related to S/R reduction and trauma, including trauma and justice as part of the eight national mental health objectives.[75,76,93] In 2005, the SAMHSA created the National Center for TIC. The overall goal of these objectives, as a continued part of the current national mental health initiatives, in addition to increasing the awareness of the impact of trauma and violence, is to reduce the incidence of violence, trauma, and retraumatization in mental health systems of care for clients and staff.[8,9] These national initiatives continue to evolve on an international scale. Some countries have developed trainings, including train the trainer programs, to help institute the skilled use of sensory-based approaches as part of the S/R reduction, TIC, and recovery initiatives.[94-96] See Chapter 17 for more information on TIC.

Over time, the TIC initiative has added an emphasis on trauma-informed approaches (TIAs). This is due to the recognition that not everyone who supports people with mental illness is clinically trained (e.g., educators, police officers, prison guards). This is important because the TIC initiative has evolved to encompass the application of a TIA across other areas of practice (e.g., schools, forensic settings, rehabilitation services, skilled nursing facilities, emergency services). This is important to the OT profession in that many of the settings affected by the expansion of the TIC initiative to the TIA include an expansion into other OT practice settings.

In addition to direct care services, mental health promotion, prevention, and intervention are other areas of OT focus.[97] The Every Moment Counts (EMC) program is one example of several programs and a variety of resources created by OTPs to help teach interdisciplinary staff how to promote positive mental health and participation in academic and nonacademic activity settings.[97] The following are EMC model programs and embedded interventions:

- Refreshing recess
- Creating a comfortable cafeteria
- Embedded classroom strategies for mental health promotion
- After-school leisure coaching

SENSORY INTEGRATION AND PROCESSING AND TRAUMA-INFORMED CARE

As the understanding of SIP and the pervasive impact of trauma on early childhood development and attachment relationships evolves, the value of the use of SIP approaches that include a more comprehensive therapeutic approach addressing more than just sensory modulation is becoming increasingly evident.[38] Case Study 8.1 provides a clinical vignette demonstrating an abbreviated version of how the initial evaluation process can be used to help inform the direction of the goal-setting and intervention planning processes. It is important to note that in trauma treatment, a three-phase approach focusing on safety and stabilization, processing and grieving, and integration is the gold standard. When working with children with trauma histories, a component-based intervention approach is often used that includes fostering safety, self-regulation, relational engagement, self-reflective informational processing, positive affect enhancement, and traumatic experiences integration.[98] OTPs use these trauma therapy models in addition to traditional OT and other mental health models, given that the skilled use of sensory approaches often supports the trauma recovery process. OTPs must be skilled in trauma processing to help guide the recovery work that emerges during OT sessions. For more information on trauma and TIC, refer to Chapter 17.

CASE STUDY 8.1   Clinical Vignette: Kenny

Client Information

Child's first name: Kenny

Child's age: 5 years, 8 months

Child's year in school: Kindergarten

Parent/guardian name: Barbara (foster mother)

Reasons for referral: occupational concerns of the child and foster family

Kenny has difficulty with behavioral outbursts and head banging when frustrated or overwhelmed, poor rest and sleep, refusal to bathe and brush teeth, limited clothing (only wears soft cotton and no seams), difficulty dressing, and attachment concerns. He has difficulty leaving the house, being at school, going to stores, restaurants, and any social or community events (birthday parties, holiday events). Teachers report that he cries most of the day and will engage in head banging in the classroom, the school cafeteria, and gymnasium. He does not engage in head banging in the classroom when he is allowed to sit in the sensory corner (contains a rocker, weighted blanket, and has significantly lower stimulation than in other areas of the classroom).

Background Information

Family history: Removed from the custody of his biologic parents at birth and has been in foster care since that time (has been in numerous foster homes); biologic parents are both in prison and no longer have parental rights. Kenny has no siblings.

Medical and mental health history and diagnoses: Severe opioid withdrawal symptoms after birth, failure to thrive, fetal alcohol syndrome, and reactive attachment disorder. Problems with sensory sensitivities, fine and gross motor skills, dyspraxia, and speech and language delays. Kenny has had four psychiatric acute inpatient hospitalizations.

Developmental history: Kenny struggled to meet fine and gross motor and praxis milestones, including speech and language delays. He had and continues to have multiple and severe hypersensitivities. He received early intervention services until age 3.

Primary concerns at this time: Difficulty with very low frustration tolerance, safety (head banging), and self-regulation; severe sensory hypersensitivities and sensation avoiding, fine and gross motor delays, dyspraxia, speech and language delays, safety and impulsivity concerns; he becomes easily overwhelmed in moderate- to high-stimulus environments—all affecting home, school, play, social, and community participation.

Educational history: He was not able to attend preschool due to the severity of his behaviors. He is now in kindergarten but is rarely able to participate actively.

Evaluation of Occupational Performance
Completed Chart Review, Caregiver Interview, Structured and Unstructured Assessments
Strengths

Committed foster parents

Affectionate

Likes to sing

Enjoys children's movies

Enjoys music

Enjoys dogs

Enjoys toy cars

Enjoys swinging

Enjoys cartoons

Has some sensory tools

Structured Assessments

BOT-2 (difficulty completing)

Beery VMI (difficulty completing)

Sensory Preferences Affecting Attachment Questionnaire

Short Child Occupational Performance Evaluation (SCOPE)

Sensory Profiles (caregiver and school versions)

Unstructured Clinical Observations

Tactile, oral, and auditory sensitivities

Seeks proprioception and deep pressure touch

Easily overstimulated

Hypervigilant

Clumsiness

Poor praxis skills

Limited repertoire of interests

Primary Areas of Concern Based on the Evaluation Process

Difficulty with:

- Safety and impulse control
- Tactile, oral, and auditory sensitivities and avoiding
- Praxis skills
- Fine and gross motor control and precision
- Loud, busy or chaotic environments
- Transitions
- Poor self-awareness and self-regulation
- Speech and language delays
  Tactile, oral, and sound sensory sensitivity:
- Difficulty tolerating clothing (fabrics, seams, tags)
- Difficulty with hair brushing, face washing, nail clipping
- Very picky eater
- Difficulty with moderate and high stimulus environments (stores, restaurants, lunchroom at school)
- Startles easily

Continued

CASE STUDY 8.1   Clinical Vignette: Kenny—cont'd

Proprioceptive and deep pressure touch sensory seeking:
- Constantly seeking out movement (rocking in rocking chair)
- Seeks out self-initiated deep touch pressure (e.g., weighted blanket use; hugs)

Trauma and attachment related:
- Significant anxiety when he starts to feel close to adults (relationally)
- Hypervigilance
- Very short attention span
- Significant difficulty with rest, sleep, and nightmares
- Significant difficulty with emotion regulation
- Triggered by certain activities, places (bathing, bathroom; bed, bedroom)
- Head banging when overwhelmed, overstimulated, or frustrated

- Requires initial emphasis on safety and stabilization
- Verbal cues and hand over hand support to sequence through the steps of activities that are not overlearned (dressing, toothbrushing, school participation)
- Consistency and a slow pace to decrease feelings of overwhelm
- Sensory modulation program
  - Sensory diet for home and school (with individualized sensorimotor activities and modalities for both prevention, support of development, and de-escalation and environmental modifications and supports)
  - Caregiver education and support
- School-based consultation
- Ayres Sensory Integration (once feeling safe and more stabilized)
- Trauma-and attachment-related therapeutic supports

Other Sensory-Based Programs

With the increased focus on SIP in mental health, and the links to trauma- and attachment-informed care, a variety of other programs integrating SIP have emerged. The following lists programs not yet mentioned in this chapter, including an emphasis on SIP that have been created by OTPs or with OTP involvement:

- How Does Your Engine Run? (Williams & Shellenberger)
- Safe Place (Hughes & Koomar)
- Sensory Attachment Intervention (Bhreathnach)
- Sensory Motor Arousal Regulation Treatment (SMART Model; Warner, Cook, Westcott, & Koomar)
- Attachment Regulation and Competence (ARC) (Blaustein & Kinniburg)
- Sensory Connection (Moore)

For more information on each of these programs, refer to the resource web links at the end of the chapter.

TRAINING AND CONSULTATION

Training and consultation are part of the OT scope of practice, and those who are skilled in the application of SIP with people with trauma histories and mental illness have taken a leadership role in helping provide training and consultation to support skilled and responsible implementation. "Once a critical mass develops, it will become easier for people to model TIC, mentor others, create networks, identify TIC champions, and share ideas."[99] The same holds true for training on how to integrate SIP interventions into mental health care. There has been an increase in the literature on different ways that training is being offered by OTPs on SIP-related interventions and whether or not these specific training methods have been effective[15,59,100-102]

SUMMARY

The ability to participate in meaningful life roles, rituals, routines, and occupations is due in part to the neurophysiologic foundation that each individual possesses and the sensory input experienced when engaging in relationships and daily life occupations. There is nothing we do that is not influenced to varying degrees by the wide range of sensations experienced that come from the physical environment and from within our bodies. This input is processed at the higher levels of the central nervous system, shaping our perceptions and how we in turn engage, respond, and participate in roles, routines, and occupations. Our experiences shape our bodies, brains, perceptions, and choices over time, from birth to the end of life. Becoming aware of SIP patterns, which include sensory modulation patterns, helps us better understand why we feel and respond the way we do. Such an understanding empowers people to create ways to cope with SIP patterns that may present barriers to their mental health and participation. For some people, this knowledge also leads to a significant sense of hopefulness in realizing that it is possible to work on changing SIP patterns to support the recovery process. OTPs have the educational background and skill set necessary to support clients in skillfully exploring SIP patterns as part of the OT process and to support engagement in OT interventions that enable the individual to live life to its fullest!

SUGGESTED LEARNING ACTIVITIES

1. Explore some of the online resources and references provided; identify three things that you have learned about sensory modulation indicating that there is a growing evidence base supporting sensory modulation–related interventions as part of the OT process in mental health.

2. Take one of the sensory modulation–related questionnaires and consider whether your sensory processing patterns affect your personal roles, relationships, routines, and occupational participation.

3. Create your own sensory diet using a day of the week that tends to be the most stressful. Include in your routine sensory strategies that will help with stress management for health and wellness purposes.

4. Reflect on how different aspects of the physical environment (where you work, rest, and play) affect how you feel and participate at different times of the day.

5. Create your own personalized, sensory kit based on your sensory-based needs and occupational goals (e.g., anxiety or stress management, wellness).

6. Search the literature for articles related to sensory modulation and different mental health symptoms and diagnoses to further your understanding of the impact of sensory modulation and mental health on occupational needs and goals.

ONLINE RESOURCES

- Attachment Regulation and Competence (ARC): Available at: https://arcframework.org.
- Center for the Study of Traumatic Stress: Available at: centerforthestudyoftraumaticstress.org
- Child Trauma Academy: Available at: http://childtrauma.org.
- Child Welfare Information Gateway: Evidence-based practice for child abuse prevention. Available at: https://www.childwelfare.gov/topics/preventing/evidence.
- Every Moment Counts: Available at: http://www.everymomentcounts.org.
- How Does Your Engine Run? Available at: https://www.alertprogram.com/product/alert-program-how-does-your-engine-run/
- Massachusetts State Department of Mental Health S/R Reduction Initiative. Available at: http://www.mass.gov/eohhs/gov/departments/dmh/restraintseclusion-reduction-initiative.html
- National Center for Trauma Informed Care. Available at: https://nasmhpd.org.content/national-center-trauma-informed-care-nctic-0http://www.nasmhpd.org.content/national-center-trauma-informed-care-nctic-0
- National Center on Family Homelessness. Available at: http://www.familyhomelessness.org.
- National Child Traumatic Stress Network. Available at: www.NCTSN.org.
- OT Innovations (Sensory Modulation Program): www.ot-innovations.com.
- SAMHSA Trauma Informed Care and Alternatives to Seclusion and Restraint. Available at: http://www.samhsa.gov/nctic/trauma-interventions

- Safe Place. Available at: http://www.otawatertown.com/safe-place-2.
- Sensory Connection. Available at: http://sensoryconnectionprogram.com.
- SMART Model. Available at: http://www.traumacenter.org.clients/SMART.php
- Te Pou o te, Whakaaro Nui. Sensory modulation. Available at: https://www.tepou.co.nz/initiatives/sensorymodulation/103.
- Zones of Regulation. Available at: http://www.zonesofregulation.com/index.html.

REFERENCES

1. Ayres AJ. *Sensory Integration and Learning Disorders*. Los Angeles: Western Psychological Services; 1972.
2. Ayres AJ. *Sensory Integration and the Child*. Los Angeles: Western Psychological Services; 1979.
3. Parham LD, Roley SS, May-Benson TA, Koomar J, Brett-Green B, Burke JP, et al. Development of a fidelity measure for research on the effectiveness of the Ayres Sensory Integration intervention. *Am J Occup Ther*. 2011;65(2):133-142.
4. Dunn W. The impact of sensory processing abilities on the daily lives of young children and their families: a conceptual model. *Infants Young Child*. 1997;9(4):23-35.
5. Lane SJ, Smith Roley S, Champagne T. Sensory integration and processing: Theory and applications to occupational performance. In: Schell BAB, Gillen G, Scaffa ME, eds. *Willard & Spackman's Occupational Therapy*. 12th ed. Baltimore, MD: Lippincott Williams & Wilkins; 2014.
6. Miller LJ, Cermak S, Lane S, Anzalone M, Koomar J. Position statement on terminology related to sensory integration dysfunction. *SI Focus*. 2004:6-8.

7. Champagne T, Stromberg N. Sensory approaches in inpatient psychiatric settings: innovative alternatives to seclusion & restraint. *J Psychosoc Nurs Ment Health Serv.* 2004;42(9): 34-44.

8. National Association of State Mental Health Program Directors. *Trauma Informed Care Module.* Training Curriculum for the Reduction of Seclusion and Restraint. 1st ed. Alexandria, VA: NASMHPD; 2003.

9. National Association of State Mental Health Program Directors. *National Executive Training Institute Curriculum for the Creation of Violence-Free and Coercion-Free Treatment Settings and the Reduction of Seclusion and Restraint.* 11th ed. Alexandria, VA: NASMHPD; 2013.

10. Miller LJ, Reisman JE, McIntosh DN, Simon J. An ecological model of sensory modulation. In: Smith Roley S, Blanche E, Schaaf RC, eds. *Understanding the Nature of Sensory Integration with Diverse Populations.* San Antonio, TX: Therapy Skill Builders; 2001:57-82.

11. American Occupational Therapy Association. *Occupational Therapy Practice Framework: Domain and Process.* 3rd ed. *Am J Occup Ther.* 2014;68:S1-S48.

12. Brown C, Cromwell RL, Filion D, Dunn W, Tollefson N. Sensory processing in schizophrenia: missing and avoiding information. *Schizophr Res.* 2002;55(1-2):187-195.

13. Champagne T, Koomar J. Evaluating sensory processing in mental health occupational therapy practice. *OT Pract.* 2012; 17(5):CE1-CE8.

14. Lipskaya-Velikovsky L, Bar-Shalita T, Bart O. Sensory modulation and daily-life participation in people with schizophrenia. *Compr Psychiatry.* 2014;58:130-137.

15. Machingura T, Lloyd C. A reflection on success factors in implementing sensory modulation in an acute mental health setting. *Int J Ther Rehabil.* 2017;24:35-39.

16. American Occupational Therapy Association. Mental health promotion, prevention, and intervention in occupational therapy practice. *Am J Occup Ther.* 2014;64(suppl 2): S30-S43.

17. Champagne T. *Sensory Modulation and Environment: Essential Elements of Occupation.* 3rd rev. ed. New York: Pearson; 2011.

18. Champagne, T. AOTA Societal Statement: Stress, trauma and posttraumatic stress disorder. *Am J Occup Ther.* 2018;72: 7212410080p1-7212410080p3. doi:10.5014/ajot.2018.72S208.

19. Brown C, Dunn W. *Adolescent/Adult Sensory Profile.* Melbourne, Australia: Pearson; 2002.

20. Dunn W. *Living Sensationally: Understanding Your Senses.* Philadelphia: Jessica Kingsley; 2009.

21. Champagne T. The influence of posttraumatic stress disorder, depression, and sensory processing patterns on occupational engagement: a case study. *Work.* 2011;38(1):67-75.

22. Champagne T. *Sensory Modulation in Dementia Care: Assessment and Activities for Sensory-Enriched Care.* London: Jessica Kingsley; 2018.

23. LeBel J, Champagne T, Stromberg N, Coyle R. Integrating sensory and trauma-informed interventions: a Massachusetts state initiative, part 1. *Mental Health Spec Interest Sect Q.* 2010;33(1):1-4.

24. LeBel J, Champagne T. Integrating sensory and trauma-informed interventions: a Massachusetts state initiative, part 2. *Mental Health Spec Interest Sect Q.* 2010;33(2):1-4.

25. American Psychiatric Association. *Diagnostic and Statistical Manual of Mental Disorders.* 5th ed. Washington, DC: Author; 2013.

26. Engel-Yeger B, Palgy-Levin D, Lev-Wiesel R. The relationship between posttraumatic stress disorder and sensory processing patterns. *Occup Ther Ment Health.* 2013;29:266-278.

27. Javitt DC. Sensory processing in schizophrenia: neither simple nor intact. *Schizophr Bull.* 2009;35(6):1059-1064.

28. Javitt DC. Neurophysiological models for new treatment development in schizophrenia: early sensory approaches. *Ann N Y Acad Sci.* 2015;1344:92-104.

29. Miller LJ, Coll JR, Schoen SA. A randomized controlled pilot study of the effectiveness of occupational therapy for children with sensory modulation disorder. *Am J Occup Ther.* 2007;61:228-238.

30. Miller LJ, Nielsen DM, Schoen SA. Attention deficit hyperactivity disorder and sensory modulation disorder: a comparison of behavior and physiology. *Res Dev Disabil.* 2012;33:804-818.

31. Reynolds S, Lane S, Gennings C. The moderating role of sensory overresponsivity in HPA activity: a pilot study with children diagnosed with ADHD. *J Atten Disord.* 2009;13:468.478.

32. Miller LJ, Anzalone ME, Lane SJ, Cermak SA, Osten ET. Concept evolution in sensory integration: a proposed nosology for diagnosis. *Am J Occup Ther.* 2007;61:135-140.

33. Bailliard AL, Whigham SC. Linking neuroscience, function, and intervention: a scoping review of sensory processing and mental illness. *Am J Occup Ther.* 2017;71:7105100040p1-7105100040p18.

34. Champagne T, Frederick D. Sensory processing research advances in mental health: implications for occupational therapy. *OT Pract.* 2011;16(10):7-8.

35. Ayres AJ. *Sensory Integration and the Child: Understanding Hidden Sensory Challenges.* Rev. ed. Los Angeles: Western Psychological Services; 2005.

36. Ayres AJ. *Sensory Integration and Praxis Tests.* Los Angeles: Western Psychological Services; 1989.

37. Schaaf R, Dumont R, Arbesman M, May-Benson T. Efficacy of occupational therapy using Ayres Sensory Integration: a systematic review. *Am J Occup Ther.* 2017;72:7201190010p1-7201190010p10.

38. Champagne T. Attachment, trauma and occupational therapy practice. *OT Pract.* 2011;16:CE1-CE8.

39. Dunn W. *Sensory Profile: User's Manual.* San Antonio, TX: Psychological Corporation; 1999.

40. Bar-Shalita T, Cermak S. Sensory modulation, psychological distress, and quality of life in young adults in the general population. *Am J Occup Ther.* 2015;69(suppl 1):6911500084p1.

41. Kinnealey M, Koenig KP, Smith S. Relationships between sensory modulation and social supports and health-related quality of life. *Am J Occup Ther.* 2011;65(3):320-327.

42. Machingura T, Shum D, Molineux M, Lloyd C. Effectiveness of sensory modulation in treating sensory modulation disorders in adults with schizophrenia: a systematic literature review. *Int J Ment Health Addict.* 2018;16:764-780.

43. Porges SW. The polyvagal theory: phylogenetic substrates of a social nervous system. *Int J Psychophysiol.* 2001;42:123-146.

44. Porges SW. Social engagement and attachment: a phylogenetic perspective. Roots of mental illness in children. *Ann N Y Acad Sci.* 2003;1008:31-47.

45. Porges SW. The polyvagal perspective. *Biol Psychol.* 2007;72:116-143.

46. Dunn W, Griffith JW, Sabata D, et al. Measuring change in somatosensation across the lifespan. *Am J Occup Ther.* 2015;69:6903290020p1-9. doi:10.5014/ajot.2015.014845.

47. May-Benson T. The adult/adolescent sensory history. 2015. Available at: http://thespiralfoundation.org.ASH_home.html.

48. Beery KE, Buktenica NA, Beery NA. *Beery-Buktenica Developmental Test of Visual-Motor Integration.* 6th ed. San Antonio, TX: Pearson; 2010.

49. Bruininks RH, Bruininks BD. *Bruininks-Oseretsky Test of Motor Proficiency.* 2nd ed. Minneapolis: Pearson; 2005.

50. Wilson B, Pollock N, Kaplan B, Law M. *Clinical Observations of Motor Performance Skills.* Framingham, MA: Therapro; 2000.

51. Reynolds C, Pearson N, Voress J. *Developmental Test of Visual Perception-Adolescent and Adult.* Austin, TX: Pro-Ed; 2002.

52. Miller LJ. *Miller Assessment for Preschoolers.* San Antonio, TX: Pearson; 1988.

53. Mutti M, Martin N, Sterling H, Spalding N. *Quick Neurological Screening Test.* 3rd ed. Novato, CA: Academic Therapy; 2010.

54. Parham D, Ecker C, Miller-Kuhaneck H, Henry D, Glennon T. *Sensory Processing Measure.* Torrance, CA: Western Psychological Services; 2007.

55. Pfeiffer B, Kinnealey M. Treatment of sensory defensiveness in adults. *Occup Ther Int.* 2003;10(3):175-184.

56. Massachusetts Department of Mental Health. Resource guide: creating positive cultures of care. 2013. Available at: https://www.mass.gov/files/documents/2016/07/vq/restraint-resources.pdf.

57. National Association of State Mental Health Program Directors. *National Executive Training Institute Curriculum for the Creation of Violence-Free and Coercion-Free Treatment Settings and the Reduction of Seclusion and Restraint.* 12th ed. Alexandria, VA: NASMHPD; 2018.

58. Bobier C, Boon T, Downward M, Loomes B, Mountford H, Swadi H. Pilot investigation of the use and usefulness of a sensory modulation room in a child and adolescent psychiatric inpatient unit. *Occup Ther Ment Health.* 2015;31(4):385-401.

59. Martin B, Suane S. Effect of training on sensory room and cart usage. *Occup Ther Ment Health.* 2012;28:118.128.

60. Novak T, Scanlan J, McCaul D, MacDonald N, Clarke T. Pilot study of a sensory room in an acute inpatient psychiatric unit. *Australas Psychiatry.* 2012;20(5):401-406.

61. West M, Melvin G, McNamara F, Gordon M. An evaluation of the use and efficacy of a sensory room within an adolescent psychiatric inpatient unit. *Aust Occup Ther J.* 2017;64:253-263.

62. King LJ. A sensory-integrative approach to schizophrenia. *Am J Occup Ther.* 1974;28:529-536.

63. Bar-Shalita T, Vatine JJ, Parush S, Deutsch L, Seltzer Z. Psychophysical correlates in adults with sensory modulation disorder. *Disabil Rehabil.* 2012;34(11):943-950.

64. Engel-Yeger B, Palgy-Levin D, Lev-Wiesel R. Predicting fears of intimacy among individuals with post-traumatic stress symptoms by their sensory profile. *Br J Occup Ther.* 2015;78:51-57.

65. Kurtz MM. Neurocognitive impairment across the lifespan in schizophrenia: an update. *Schizophr Res.* 2005;74(1):15-26.

66. Olson LM. Examining schizophrenia and sensory modulation disorder: a review of the literature. *Sens Integr Spec Interest Sect Q.* 2010;33(1):1-3.

67. Olson LM. *Sensory Modulation Disorder and Schizophrenia: Linking Behavioral Measures.* Ann Arbor, MI: ProQuest, LLC; 2011.

68. Moskowitz A. Schizophrenia, trauma, dissociation, and scientific revolutions. *J Trauma Dissociation.* 2011;12:347-357.

69. Perry BD. Examining child maltreatment through a neurodevelopmental lens: clinical applications of the neurosequential model of therapeutics. *J Loss Trauma.* 2009;14:240-255.

70. Read J, Fosse R, Moskowitz A, Perry B. The traumagenic neurodevelopmental model of psychosis revisited. *Neuropsychiatry.* 2014;4:65-79.

71. van der Kolk B. Developmental trauma disorder. *Psychiatr Ann.* 2005;35(5)401-408.

72. van der Kolk, B. *The Body Keeps the Score: Brain, Mind, and Body in the Healing of Trauma.* New York: Penguin; 2014.

73. Substance Abuse and Mental Health Services Administration. Guiding principles of trauma-informed care. *SAMHSA News.* 2014;22(2):1.

74. Substance Abuse and Mental Health Services Administration. *Trauma-Informed Care in Behavioral Health Services.* Rockville, MD: Author; 2014.

75. Substance Abuse and Mental Health Services Administration. Trauma-informed care & alternatives to seclusion and restraint. 2015. Available at: http://www.samhsa.gov/ nctic/ trauma-interventions.

76. Substance Abuse and Mental Health Services Administration. Recovery and recovery support. 2017. Available at: https://www.samhsa.gov/recovery.

77. Azeem MW, Aujla A, Rammerth M, Binsfeld G, Jones RB. Effectiveness of six core strategies based on trauma informed care in reducing seclusions and restraints at a child and adolescent psychiatric hospital. *J Child Adolesc Psychiatr Nurs.* 2011;24:11-15.

78. Substance Abuse and Mental Health Services Administration. *SAMHSA's Working Concept of Trauma and Framework for a Trauma-Informed Approach, National Centre for Trauma-Informed Care (NCTIC).* Rockville, MD: SAMHSA; 2014c.

79. Björkdahl A, Perseius KI, Samuelsson M, Lindberg MH. Sensory rooms in psychiatric inpatient care: staff experiences. *Int J Ment Health Nurs.* 2016;25:472-479.

80. Chalmers A, Harrison S, Mollison K, Molloy N, Gray K. Establishing sensory-based approaches in mental health inpatient care: a multidisciplinary approach. *Australas Psychiatry.* 2012;20(1):35-39.

81. Champagne T, Mullen B, Dickson D, Krishnamurty S. Researching the safety & effectiveness of the weighted blanket with adults during an inpatient mental health hospitalization. *Occup Ther Ment Health.* 2015;31:211-233.

82. Cummings KS, Grandfield SA, Coldwell CM. Caring with comfort rooms: reducing seclusion and restraint use in

psychiatric facilities. *J Psychosoc Nurs Ment Health Serv.* 2010;48(6):26-30.

83. ForsythAS, Trevarrow R. Sensory strategies in adult mental health: a qualitative exploration of staff perspectives following the introduction of a sensory room on a male adult acute ward. *Int J Ment Health Nurs.* 2018;27: 1689-1697.

84. Gardner J. Sensory modulation treatment on a psychiatric inpatient unit: results of a pilot program. *J Psychosoc Nurs Ment Health Serv.* 2016;54:44-51.

85. Knight M, Adkison L, Kovach, JS. A comparison of multi-sensory and traditional interventions on inpatient and psychiatric and geriatric nueorpsychiatry units. *J Psychosoc Nurs & Ment Health Serv.* 2010;48(1):24-31.

86. Lee SJ, Cox A, Whitecross F, Williams P, Hollander Y. Sensory assessment and therapy to help reduce seclusion use with service users needing psychiatric intensive care. *J Psychiatr Intensive Care.* 2010;6(2):83-90.

87. Lloyd C, King R, Machingura T. An investigation into the effectiveness of sensory modulation in reducing seclusion within an acute mental health unit. *Adv Ment Health.* 2014;12(2):93-100.

88. Mullen B, Champagne T, Krishnamurty S, Dickson D, Gao R. Exploring the safety and therapeutic effects of deep pressure stimulation using a weighted blanket. *Occup Ther Ment Health.* 2008;24(1):65-89.

89. Scanlon JN, Novak T. Sensory approaches in mental health: a scoping review. *Australian Occup Ther J.* 2015;62: 277-285.

90. Smith S, Jones J. Use of a sensory room on an intensive care unit. *J Psychosoc Nurs Ment Health Serv.* 2014;52:22-30.

91. Sutton D, Wilson M, Van Kessel K, Vanderpyl J. Optimizing arousal to manage aggression: a pilot study of sensory modulation. *Int J Ment Health Nurs.* 2013; 22(6):500-511.

92. Van Pomeren V. Sensory modulation: one approach to reducing the use of seclusion and restraint at Northland District Health Board. 2009. Available at: https://www. tepou.co.nz/assets/images/content/your_stories/files/ story045.pdf.

93. US Department of Health and Human Services. *Developing trauma-informed systems of care.* 2003. Available at: https:// www.nasmhpd.org.sites/default/ files/TraumaExperts Mtgreport-final.pdf.

94. Department of Health. *Providing a Safe Environment for All: Framework for Reducing Restrictive Interventions.* Melbourne, Australia: Department of Health; 2013.

95. Scottish Government. Mental health strategy for Scotland 2012-2015. Edinburgh: Scottish Government; 2012. Available at: www.scotland.gov.uk/Resource/0039/00398762.pdf.

96. Te Pou. Sensory modulation. 2018. Available at: https:// tepou.co.nz/initiatives/sensory-modulation/103.

97. Bazyk S. *Mental Health Promotion, Prevention, and Intervention for Children and Youth: A Guiding Framework for Occupational Therapy.* Bethesda, MD: American Occupational Therapy Association; 2011.

98. Cook A, Spinazzola J, Ford J, et al. Complex trauma in children and adolescents. *Psychiatr Ann.* 2005;35(5):390-398.

99. Sweeney A, Clement S, Filson B, Kennedy A. Trauma-informed mental health care in the UK: what is it and how can we further its development? *Ment Health Rev J.* 2016; 21(3):174-192.

100. Azuela G, Robertson L. The effectiveness of a sensory modulation workshop on health professional learning. *J Ment Health Train Educ Pract.* 2016;11:317-331.

101. Blackburn J, McKenna B, Jackson B, et al. Educating mental health clinicians about sensory modulation to enhance clinical practice in a youth acute inpatient mental health unit: a feasibility study. *Issues Ment Health Nurs.* 2016;37: 517-525.

102. Meredith P, Yeates H, Greaves A, et al. Preparing mental health professionals for new directions in mental health practice: evaluating the sensory approaches e-learning training package. *Int J Ment Health Nurs.* 2018;27: 106-115.

9

Mood Disorders

Nancy Carson

LEARNING OBJECTIVES

1. Identify the types of mood disorders as defined by the DSM-5.
2. Describe the symptomology of the different mood disorders.
3. Understand the prevalence and risk factors for suicide.
4. Recognize assessment methods for mood disorders.
5. Assess the impact of mood disorders on occupational performance.
6. Discuss treatment approaches for mood disorders, including psychopharmacology and psychotherapeutic approaches.
7. Articulate occupational therapy's role in the treatment of mood disorders.

INTRODUCTION

Mood disorders include a group of psychiatric illnesses that involve a serious disturbance in mood or internal emotional state.[1] Everyone experiences changes in mood that span the continuum of extreme sadness and irritability to elevated feelings of joy and happiness. Changes in mood can generally be correlated with experiences in everyday life, interactions with others, internal thoughts and feelings, personal successes and failures, or a response to other external and internal factors. When mood or emotional state is distorted or inconsistent with everyday circumstances and interferes with daily occupational functioning, a mood disorder is indicated.

Mood disorders are divided into two categories by the American Psychiatric Association's Diagnostic and Statistical Manual of Mental Disorders, 5th edition (DSM-5).[2] The first category is depressive disorders, which includes eight types or diagnoses:
- Disruptive Mood Dysregulation Disorder
- Major Depressive Disorder, Single and Recurrent Episodes
- Persistent Depressive Disorder (Dysthymia)
- Premenstrual Dysphoric Disorder
- Substance/Medication-Induced Depressive Disorder
- Depressive Disorder Due to Another Medical Condition
- Other Specified Depressive Disorder
- Unspecified Depressive Disorder.

The second category is bipolar and related disorders and includes seven types or diagnoses:
- Bipolar I Disorder
- Bipolar II Disorder
- Cyclothymic Disorder
- Substance/Medication-Induced Bipolar and Related Disorder
- Bipolar and Related Disorder Due to Another Medical Condition
- Other Specified Bipolar and Related Disorder
- Unspecified Bipolar and Related Disorder

DEPRESSION

Depression affects 4.4% of the world's population, more than 320 million people of all ages worldwide, and it is the world's leading cause of disability.[3] It is a major contributor to the overall global burden of disease,[3] and in 2015, depressive disorders were the single largest contributor to nonfatal loss of health worldwide.[4] Between 2005 and 2015, the number of people in the world living with depression increased by 18.4% with close to half of those individuals residing in South-East Asia and Western Pacific regions.[4] In 2016, the prevalence of a major depressive episode in US adults 18 years and older was 16.2 million or 6.7% of the adult population. The prevalence of a major depressive episode was higher among adult females (8.5%) compared with males (4.8%), and it was highest among individuals aged 18–25 (10.9%).[5]

Common symptoms of depression include increased or decreased sleep, appetite, and activity level; lack of concentration, energy, and interest in activities; and feelings of sadness, hopelessness, low self-worth, guilt, and suicidality. To be diagnosed with depression, either depressed mood or a loss of interest or pleasure must be reported along with four other symptoms over a period of 2 weeks or longer.[6-8] Symptoms of depression can greatly differ from person to person, and additionally, some individuals will experience physical symptoms such as headaches, muscle aches, or digestive problems that do not have a discernible medical cause.

Persistent depressive disorder, also referred to as dysthymia, is a depressed mood that occurs for the majority of time over a period of at least 2 years. The individual experiences chronic depression that is not as severe as the depression experienced in major depressive disorder, but it is longer lasting. There may be fluctuating episodes of mild to moderate to major depression, and the symptoms interfere with relationships and daily life. Symptoms include increased or decreased appetite and/or sleep, fatigue, low self-esteem, decreased concentration, and feelings of hopelessness. At least two of these symptoms must be present.[8] Approximately 1.3% of adults in the US experience persistent depressive disorder in their lifetime.[9]

Depression does not have a single specific cause. It may occur as a result of a stressful life event or circumstance, difficult relationships, financial difficulties, a physical illness, or it may occur for no apparent reason. Research has indicated several factors that can contribute to depression. Childhood trauma can change the way an individual responds to stress, which may lead to depression. There may be a genetic predisposition to the development of a mood disorder. Conditions such as sleep disorders, chronic pain, and substance abuse are also associated with depression.[7]

Sometimes depression is clearly related to a life event, such as following childbirth. Postpartum depression is indicated by the specifier "with peripartum onset" for major depressive episode in the most recent diagnostic criteria of the American Psychiatric Association.[6] This refers to a depressive episode occurring during pregnancy as well as in the 4 weeks following delivery.[6] Regardless of the established criteria, women with a depressive episode in the first year following birth are generally classified in clinical practice as having postpartum depression. Currently, the epidemiological evidence to support the time span past 4 weeks postpartum is not substantial enough to warrant the distinction in the DSM-5; however, it is encouraging that depression during pregnancy and in the first 4 weeks postpartum are included.[10] The recognition of postpartum depression is relatively recent despite the assertion that it is a common and serious mental health problem. Estimates of prevalence range from 13% to 19%, especially in the first 6 months after delivery.[11] Postpartum depression is much more severe than the mild symptoms of depression and anxiety that many women experience in the first 2 weeks after childbirth. Postpartum depression is characterized by extreme sadness and anxiety as well as physical exhaustion that can make it difficult for a new mother to care for her newborn child.[8]

BIPOLAR DISORDER

Mood disorders classified as bipolar disorders are also referred to as manic-depressive illness. They are characterized by significant changes in mood, energy, and activity levels.[12] An estimated 2.8% of US adults have bipolar disorder with a similar prevalence for both males and females. An estimated 4.4% of US adults experience bipolar disorder at some time in their lives.[13] Manic moods or episodes involve extremely elated and energized behavior; less severe episodes are called hypomanic episodes. Depressive episodes manifest in behavior that presents as unusually sad and hopeless. There are three primary types of bipolar disorder: bipolar I disorder, bipolar II disorder, and cyclothymic disorder.[12] Bipolar I disorder is defined by manic episodes that last at least a week, or by manic symptoms that are so severe that the person requires hospitalization or immediate medical care. Depressive episodes are also present and usually last at least 2 weeks. Bipolar II disorder consists of a series of depressive episodes and hypomanic episodes without the intensity of manic episodes experienced in bipolar I disorder. Cyclothymic disorder is characterized by depressive and hypomanic symptoms that are recurrent over a 2-year period but are not of the intensity to be classified respectively as depressive or hypomanic episodes.[12]

Bipolar disorder is often underdiagnosed, as making a correct diagnosis relies strongly on the report of past hypomanic or manic episodes. Clients often have difficulty with confirming this via self-report alone, therefore interviews with family members and significant others and the use of more in-depth interviewing are suggested.[14] The mood episodes that define bipolar illness are characterized

BOX 9.1 Characteristics of Manic and Depressive Episodes

Manic Episode	Depressive Episode
• Decreased need for sleep	• Have trouble sleeping; sleep too much or not enough
• Engaged in many activities at once	• Feel very sad, down, empty, or hopeless
• Talking a lot and/or speaking loudly, quickly, or with pressured speech	• Have very little energy
• Easily distracted	• Have decreased activity levels
• Increase in risky behaviors such as spending money, gambling, or sexual promiscuity	• Do not enjoy anything
• Rapid thinking and flight of ideas	• Feel worried and empty
• Grandiose thinking	• Have trouble concentrating
• Hostility and/or increased irritability	• Forget things a lot
• Excessive religious focus	• Eat too much or too little
• Wearing bright clothing, accessories, excess makeup	• Feel tired or "slowed down"
• Impulsive behavior	• Think about death or suicide
• Difficulty finishing projects	• Feeling worthless
	• Social isolation
	• Flat affect and decreased speech

by behaviors and moods that are not representative of the person's usual behaviors and mood. The person may experience and display unusually intense emotions as well as notable changes in energy, activity level, and sleep quantity.[12] Box 9.1 outlines characteristics of manic and depressive episodes. Sometimes a mood episode has mixed features, meaning it includes symptoms of both manic and depressive symptoms. When experiencing a mixed episode, the individual can feel very sad and hopeless yet highly energized at the same time. The assessment of the depressive feature that can occur during mania is important as those individuals appear to show a more severe form of bipolar disorder.[15]

SUICIDALITY

Depression, bipolar disorder, and substance use are strongly linked to suicidal thinking and behavior.[16] Suicide is the tenth leading cause of death in the United States. Approximately 45,000 Americans die by suicide each year, and for every person that dies by suicide there are about 25 people who have attempted suicide.[17] Put in other words, approximately 123 Americans die by suicide each day, or one death by suicide occurs every 12 minutes.[18] The annual age-adjusted suicide rate is 13.42 per 100,000 individuals in the United States.[17] Worldwide, close to 800,000 people die from suicide every year; this equates to one person every 40 seconds. Globally, suicide is the second leading cause of death for individuals between 15 to 29 years old. In 2016, 79% of suicides occurred in low- and middle-income countries, and suicide accounted for 1.4% of all deaths, making it the 18th leading cause of death worldwide.[19] Approximately 90% of people who die by suicide are estimated

to have a mental health condition of which many are treatable.[16] Depression is the most common psychiatric disorder associated with suicide and nonfatal suicidal behavior; therefore it is essential for clinicians to be aware of risk factors for suicide in depression. One risk factor identified for suicide in people with depression is male gender. Men die by suicide 3.5 times more than women, and white males account for seven out of ten suicides.[17] Additional risk factors include family history of psychiatric disorder, previous attempted suicide, more severe depression, hopelessness, and comorbid disorders, including anxiety and substance abuse.[20]

The suicide rate for Americans 10 years of age and older in the United States increased 30% from 2000 to 2016, with increases occurring in almost all states. The highest increase was 57% in North Dakota. A total of 25 states experienced suicide rate increases of more than 30%. The suicide rate increased for females of all ages, with the highest increase in young girls from 10 to 14 years of age and for all men under 75 years old. As of 2018, suicide is the second leading cause of death for all Americans 10 to 34 years old.[21] There are also increases seen in specific populations such as the veteran population. According to the US Department of Veterans Affairs (2016),[22] the risk of suicide among veterans is 21% greater than among the civilian population. While the suicide rate for men 75 years of age and older has decreased, it remains the highest suicide rate (38.8/100,000 deaths) of any age group for both men and women.[21]

The significant increase in the suicide rate in recent years highlights the need for vigilance in diagnosing and treating depression to decrease the number of undiagnosed individuals. The American Foundation for Suicide Prevention asserts that depression and bipolar disorder are strongly associated with suicidal thinking and behavior, and that 90% of people who die by suicide have a potentially treatable mental health disorder. Occupational therapy professionals can help people find positive solutions when struggling with brain functions, such as decision-making and behavioral control that are related to suicidal behavior.[16] Of people who survive a suicide attempt, 85%–90% are able to participate in life successfully,[17] and occupational therapy can support productive and meaningful life activities. Assessment and treatment of vulnerable individuals is essential to reduce the suicide rate in the future.

ASSESSMENT

There are several standardized instruments that are used to screen and detect depression. One scale is the Beck Depression Inventory-II (BDI-II).[23] The BDI-II is a 21-item self-report scale that indicates the severity of depression in adolescents and adults. Each item on the BDI-II includes four statements arranged in increasing severity about a symptom of depression. The symptoms align with the DSM-IV, the version that was current in 1996. The BDI-II takes approximately 5 minutes to complete and is the most widely used instrument for detecting depression. Numerous studies support its reliability and validity across different populations.[24]

The Patient Health Questionnaire-9 (PHQ-9) is another well-validated and widely used tool for assessing severity of symptoms and tracking response to therapy over time. It has been validated for use with adults, including older adults.[25,26] The Patient Health Questionnaire-2 (PHQ-2) contains only the first two questions of the PHQ-9. These two questions ask about depressed mood and anhedonia, and the PHQ-2 is often used as an initial screen; if a person screens positive on the PHQ-2, the PHQ-9 is then administered to the individual.[27] Both the Beck Depression Inventory and the PHQ can be administered by the occupational therapist (OT).

Diagnosis of depressive disorders by the psychiatric health care provider occurs through the psychiatric interview, client observation, and history-taking with the client and significant others, as possible. The psychiatric interview and client observation provides the context for the mental status examination (MSE). The components of the MSE include appearance, general behavior, movement, posture, mood, affect, speech, language, perceptions, thought process, flow, content, cognitive status, insight, judgment, and executive function.[28] The individual experiencing a depressive episode will typically present with flat affect and may exhibit decreased speech and movement, delayed thought process, and some manifestation of impaired cognition or judgment. The individual experiencing a manic episode will typically present with an animated affect and may exhibit a euphoric or agitated mood, pressured speech, psychomotor agitation, racing and grandiose thought processes, and impulsivity. Individuals may also present somewhere in between the continuum of depressive and manic symptoms when being interviewed or participating in therapeutic sessions.

The occupational therapy interview differs from the psychiatric interview by focusing on occupation and the development of the occupational profile.[29] The Occupational Therapy Practice Framework[30] guides the evaluation process and the occupational therapy interview focuses on the person's occupational history and current occupational performance. The interview also allows for development of a therapeutic relationship with the client; therapeutic use of self is essential in facilitating the interview process. There are occupational therapy interview guidelines that can be used to provide a specific structure to the process if desired, including the Occupational Performance History Interview (OPHI-2),[31] the Canadian Occupational Performance Measure (COPM),[32] and the Occupational Self-Assessment.[33] The OT observes the client during the interview process, and while engaged in various occupational contexts, works with the client to determine appropriate therapy goals.

The OT may also choose from a wide range of specific assessments and tools to gain additional information regarding the client's occupational performance. For example, the OT may want to further evaluate the individual's quality of life, occupational satisfaction, motivation, leisure interests, time management, social interaction skills, cognition, or sensory processing abilities to fully assess the individual's strengths and deficits.

THERAPEUTIC MANAGEMENT

It is important that the individual receive a thorough evaluation to determine the best treatment approach. Psychopharmacology and psychotherapeutic approaches are often used to treat mood disorders. They may be used together or separately. Some individuals will respond very well to medication alone, and other individuals will benefit from counseling or psychotherapy without the use of medication. Most clients will reap maximum benefit from a combination of approaches. Additional methods to treat mood disorders include brain stimulation techniques and alternative and holistic approaches.

Psychopharmacology

Medications used to treat depression are referred to as antidepressants and can be very effective in treating symptoms and mood. There are different types of antidepressants, and most take several weeks to reach maximum effectiveness. Some people may need antidepressants for several months and some people may need to continue the use of antidepressants for many years. The decision to discontinue the use of antidepressants should always be made in consultation with the prescribing healthcare provider.[8]

The most commonly prescribed antidepressants are selective serotonin reuptake inhibitors (SSRIs). They work by blocking the reabsorption of the neurotransmitter serotonin so that it is more available in the brain. SSRIs tend to have fewer side effects than other classes of antidepressants. The second most commonly prescribed antidepressants are serotonin and norepinephrine reuptake inhibitors (SNRIs), which block the reabsorption of both serotonin and norepinephrine. For some people SNRIs may be more effective than SSRIs. Another type of antidepressant is norepinephrine and dopamine reuptake inhibitors (NDRIs), which block the reabsorption of norepinephrine and dopamine. Two older types of antidepressants include tricyclic antidepressants (TCAs) and monoamine oxidase inhibitors (MAOIs). Both of these antidepressants have more adverse side effects, some being very serious, so they are only used when other antidepressants are not effective. MAOIs can also interfere with the breakdown of certain foods and medications.[34]

Mood stabilizers are medications used to treat the hypomanic and manic episodes present in bipolar disorders. They are believed to affect neurotransmitters in the brain that are responsible for mood; however, the mechanism of action is not fully understood. Antidepressants and antipsychotic medications may also be used to treat bipolar disorder when mood stabilizers are not effective.[35] Lithium is the most widely used mood stabilizer for the treatment of bipolar disorder and has been the gold standard for bipolar disorder treatment for over 60 years. Lithium is effective in treating acute manic and depressive episodes and in reducing the recurrence of mood episodes.[36] Recent studies emphasize additional benefits of lithium including the enhancement of antidepressant and psychotropic medication, positive effects in depression and suicide prevention, lower incidence of dementia in old age, increased telomere length, and decreased incidence of some medical illnesses. Potential side effects include hand tremors, increased urination, mild thirst, diarrhea, vomiting, and drowsiness; however, side effects of lithium can be well managed at the usual therapeutic doses, and if needed, doses can be reduced to below the side effect threshold and still reap benefits of its usage.[37] Refer to Box 9.2 for examples of the different types of medications used to treat mood disorders.

Psychotherapy

Psychotherapeutic intervention is also used in the treatment of mood disorders and may be used along with medications or alone. Two common evidence-based approaches are cognitive-behavioral therapy (CBT) and interpersonal

BOX 9.2 Examples of Antidepressants and Mood Stabilizers

Class	Generic and Brand Names
SSRIs	citalopram (Celexa)
	escitalopram (Lexapro)
	fluoxetine (Prozac)
	paroxetine (Paxil)
	sertraline (Zoloft)
SNRIs	duloxetine (Cymbalta)
	desvenlafaxine (Pristiq)
	levomilnacipran (Fetzima)
	venlafaxine (Effexor)
TCAs	amitriptyline (Elavil)
	desipramine (Norpramin)
	doxepin (Sinequan)
	imipramine (Tofranil)
	nortriptyline (Pamelor)
	protriptyline (Vivactil)
	clomipramine (Anafranil)
	trimipramine (Surmontil)
MAOIs	isocarboxazid (Marplan)
	phenelzine (Nardil)
	selegiline (Emsam)
	tranylcypromine (Parnate)
Dopamine reuptake blocker	bupropion (Wellbutrin, Forfivo, Aplenzin)
Mood stabilizers	lithium
	valproic acid (Depakene)
	carbamazepine (Carbatrol, Epitol, Equetro, Tegretol)
	lamotrigine (Lamictal)
	divalproex sodium (Depakote)
Antipsychotics (used to treat mania)	olanzapine (Zyprexa)
	risperidone (Risperdal)
	clozapine (Clozaril)
	quetiapine (Seroquel)
	ziprasidone (Geodon)

psychotherapy (IPT).[2] CBT focuses on the identification and management of negative thoughts, beliefs, and behaviors that individuals with depression experience.[6] CBT is discussed in depth in Chapter 6. CBT is an umbrella term that includes a variety of different interventions that are empirically supported. There are also approaches that have diverged from the earlier days of CBT, such as schema-focused therapy, metacognitive therapy, and acceptance or mindfulness-based approaches. CBT approaches may vary in length of time and are considered relatively short compared with psychoanalytic approaches. There is no standard length of time for CBT; however, it is structured and time-limited. It is typically provided in 5–20 weekly sessions of 30 minutes to 1 hour but can also be provided as group therapy.[38] Occupational therapy practitioners can use techniques of CBT to assist clients in achieving occupational performance goals. For example, clients with mood disorders can benefit from CBT to address negative thoughts and beliefs that contribute to their depression.

Interpersonal Therapy (IPT) is an evidence-based therapy in which individuals learn to improve their relationships with others by accurately communicating their feelings.[2] Interpersonal stressors are categorized and understood in terms of role transitions, role disputes, loss, and social communication skills.[20] The practitioner guides the individual to develop improved communication skills and accurate expression of affect to improve current interpersonal relationships in order to build support for coping with depressive symptoms and life stressors. The therapeutic relationship can provide a platform for understanding and developing positive external relationships. IPT should be individualized to meet the specific needs of the individual and identify specific coping strategies that can promote recovery.[39] OTs are skilled at working with clients to identify goals and problem-solve potential strategies, therefore the use of IPT for addressing interpersonal stressors and relationship difficulties fits well into the realm of practice for occupational therapy practitioners. Further training and education related to specific protocols and approaches to evidence-based CBT and IPT are suggested as well.

Brain Stimulation Techniques

Additional therapies that have been successful in the treatment of depression and other neuropsychiatric conditions are brain stimulation techniques. These include transcranial magnetic stimulation (TMS), electroconvulsive therapy (ECT), deep brain stimulation, and vagus nerve stimulation.[40] TMS is a noninvasive method that stimulates the brain by applying magnetic stimulation to the scalp. A rapid succession of pulses, called repetitive TMS (rTMS), is administered during treatment with a session typically including 4 seconds of rTMS stimulation followed by 26 seconds of rest, repeated for 20–40 minutes. Treatment is provided 5 days a week for 4–6 weeks. TMS also has potential in treating Parkinson disease and chronic pain.[40]

ECT is effective for many individuals who do not respond well to antidepressants or TMS. The procedure has been refined to reduce the negative side effects previously associated with ECT, such as short-term memory loss or headaches. During ECT the individual is under anesthesia, and a muscle relaxant, succinylcholine, is administered to completely relax the muscles. A series of low-voltage currents are administered to one side of the brain for several minutes via electrode patches positioned on the face and temple. Typically, about seven treatments are administered during a 2- to 3-week period. Approximately 50% of individuals with depression report improvement.[40]

A newer technique, deep brain stimulation (DBS), is a procedure in which a very fine wire with electrodes is inserted into the brain. The electrodes are activated and create a permanent lesion. DBS is FDA-approved for the treatment of Parkinson disease, essential tremor, and dystonia, and is currently being used to treat depression in those individuals who do not respond to medication, TMS, or ECT.[40]

Another technique that is FDA-approved for the treatment of epilepsy is stimulation of the vagus nerve in the left cervical region. A vagus nerve stimulation (VNS) device is implanted and generates electrical stimulation to the vagus nerve.[40] Research is currently being conducted on the use of VNS for patients with major depression who did not respond to traditional antidepressants, and some promising results have emerged.[40]

Occupational Therapy Approaches

With individuals who have mood disorders, the OT identifies the areas of occupational performance that are of concern to the client and works with the client to set appropriate goals and treatment strategies. Challenges to functional performance are related to where symptoms and behaviors fall on the continuum from depression to mania. For clients experiencing depressive episodes, there will be concerns such as decreased self-esteem, interest, and pleasure in engaging in occupations. Activities of daily living (ADL) functioning may be impaired due to decreased motivation and concentration. The individual's routine may become unstructured and the individual may be unfocused and have difficulty participating in roles and previous occupations. Changes in sleep quality and quantity and in appetite can also impact the individual's routine and occupational performance.

The role of the occupational therapy practitioner will be individualized for each client and may include a variety of approaches. Strategies to support occupational engagement, performance, and satisfaction may include a focus on restructuring the individual's routine to identify optimal times of day for each activity to maximize energy level and social and environmental support. Assessing use of time through completion of a time-use diary and assisting the client in developing an appropriate and realistic daily schedule may be warranted. The schedule should include an emphasis on self-care, with time allotted for meaningful activities. For individuals with sleep disturbances, a focus on sleep hygiene and strategies to promote a healthy sleep routine can be addressed. For example, the use of strategies to promote sleep can be incorporated into the bedtime routine. These may include allowing time to unwind and time to engage in relaxation activities such as guided imagery, progressive muscle relaxation, or mindfulness. The importance of maintaining a consistent sleep routine should be emphasized.

For the individual diagnosed with depression, a lack of motivation or desire to engage in occupation can be a significant barrier to progress in treatment. The occupational therapy practitioner can work with the individual to identify occupations that have the most potential to enhance motivation by identifying and selecting occupations that reflect the client's values and interests. Identifying external factors in the environment that can support occupational engagement can also address a lack of internal motivation. Identifying occupations that may naturally increase serotonin, such as exercise, or identifying sensory activities that are alerting and energizing can also be beneficial in addressing amotivation in the client. Use of motivational interviewing techniques can help the client identify strategies for change.

For clients experiencing hypomania or mania, there will be difficulty concentrating and following through on tasks. The person may present as being distractible and restless. Hyperactivity may be observed, with racing speech and tangential thoughts. Mania can present as exaggerated thinking with unrealistic ideas and plans expressed either with euphoria or extreme frustration if resistance is met. Risk-taking behavior and impulsivity may be present leading to activities such as excessive spending, excessive drinking, reckless driving, and promiscuity. The individual may also experience increased productivity and creativity during manic episodes, which may serve to negate concerns from self or others; however, increased mania can result in decreased self-care or self-care that is highly exaggerated as in heavily applied makeup and flamboyant attire. Increased mania can also result in multiple projects being started but not finished due to impulsivity and difficulty concentrating on one activity at a time. Self-awareness of social cues and interactions may be affected, which can lead to social tension; for example, the individual may be overfamiliar or inappropriate with others, even strangers, leading difficulties in social relationships.

The role of the occupational therapy practitioner will also be individualized for the client experiencing hypomania and mania. Strategies to support occupational engagement, performance, and satisfaction may be difficult to implement during manic episodes due to poor awareness and difficulty focusing on self-behavior. Providing education to increase awareness of bipolar disease should be provided as tolerated. Consistent structure and limits on behavior during therapy sessions with feedback should be implemented. Medication compliance may need to be supported, as the individual may not recognize the need for medication or may be resistant to decreasing productivity and creativity. Assessing routines and working with the client to achieve occupational balance between sleep, self-care, work, and leisure to support healthy routines can be addressed.

Complementary Approaches

In addressing mood disorders, OTs may also use complementary mind-body approaches such as yoga. A review of 18 research studies on yoga and depression between 2005 and 2011 found yoga to be beneficial as a complementary therapy for depression and depressive symptoms.[41] A more recent review of 23 yoga interventions also concluded that yoga is effective in reducing depression.[42] In this review, study sizes ranged from 14 to 136 participants and there were variations in the length of the interventions, with most being at least 6 weeks. Various types of yoga were used, and there was not one type that was found to be more effective. Yoga includes a focus on physical postures, breathing regulation techniques, meditation, and relaxation. Overall benefits of yoga include improving flexibility, increasing energy level, and reducing muscle pain, respiration, heart rate, blood pressure, and stress.

Exercise can also be used as a complementary approach in the treatment of depression and as a direct intervention for some individuals with mild or moderate depression. Multiple studies have emphasized the effectiveness of exercise in the treatment of depression for various populations. Variations on intensity and length vary from 30–60 minutes 3–5 times a week for up to 12 weeks, with the most frequent form of exercise being running or walking. Exercise has many benefits and can be used for people who cannot take medications.[43]

Mindfulness is another approach that is being used to treat depression. One example is mindfulness-based cognitive therapy (MBCT), which is a group therapy program designed to address depressive relapse in recurrent depression. MBCT is based on CBT and traditional mindfulness practices such as Kabat-Zinn's mindfulness-based stress reduction (MBSR) program.[44] Mindfulness is used within MBCT to let go of repetitive negative thoughts that constitute cognitive vulnerability in individuals with depressive relapses. MBCT increases awareness of thoughts, feelings, and bodily sensations and focuses on changing the ways in which they are viewed. Instead of focusing on these negative internal events, disengagement from automatic negative cognitive patterns is emphasized.[45]

SUMMARY

Mood disorders are common across all ages and populations. Occupational therapy practitioners will work with individuals affected by mood disorders at times, regardless of practice setting and the client's primary reason for treatment. As stated earlier, depression affects approximately 16 million American adults at any time.[5] In addressing the occupational needs of recipients of occupational therapy, it is important to collaborate and employ a team approach in addressing mental illness and the psychosocial well-being of the individual. Simple strategies suggested for primary care settings have implications for health care teams in any setting.[46] These suggestions for improving depression care include:

- Create a mechanism to enable the team to identify clients with depression and track their progress.
- Refer clients to behavioral health providers when needed and consult with them for optimal care of the client.
- Use a standardized, structured rating scale, such as the PHQ-9, to identify individuals at risk for depression and to track changes over time.
- Empower and train all team members to proactively track symptoms of depression, treatment adherence, and adverse effects.
- Use evidence-based motivational interviewing techniques to improve patient engagement and adherence to supportive mechanisms for depression management.
- Communicate regularly with the team regarding the psychosocial well-being of every client.[47]

CASE STUDY 9.1   Major Depression

Susan is a 17-year-old female diagnosed with major depression. She dropped out of high school 8 months ago, halfway through her junior year. She states that she plans to eventually get her General Equivalence Diploma for high school and attend the local community college. However, she is not sure what she wants to study and has not made any plans. She was an average student in school and did not participate in any extracurricular activities. She states that she does not feel like there is anything she is good at doing or is interested in doing. She lives at home with her mom; her parents are divorced and she has a very distant relationship with her father. She has not spoken to him in over a year, and he is remarried and lives 2 hours away. Her boyfriend of 2 years recently broke up with her and she is very upset about this; she has one close friend and works part time at a retail store at the mall. Her leisure interests include watching TV and shopping. She states that she used to spend a lot of time with her boyfriend. She exhibits difficulty concentrating, decreased appetite, increased fatigue, low self-worth, flat affect, and lack of motivation. Her mother has become increasingly concerned about her and scheduled an appointment with a psychiatrist who diagnosed her with major depression. She was referred to an outpatient mental health program targeted at teenagers and young adults having difficulty transitioning into adulthood. The part-time program includes group therapy sessions led by clinical counselors three times a week, and each participant is also evaluated by an OT and vocational counselor. The program is funded by a non-profit agency, and occupational therapy sessions are limited to one individual session per week. Clients are enrolled into the program for a 12-week session. Following completion of the 12-week session, clients are seen monthly for follow-up by members of the treatment team for up to a year or longer if warranted.

Occupational Profile

The COPM is administered to structure the interview process, gather information, and assess the client's self-perception of occupational performance. Susan presents with flat affect and answers questions with short verbalizations; she requires much encouragement to expand on her answers.

Client's concerns: Susan acknowledges a lack of motivation but she has difficulty verbalizing specific concerns relative to engaging in occupations.

Successful occupations: She is unable to identify any occupations in which she feels successful. Overall, she feels her skills are limited and most of the time she doesn't feel like doing anything.

Barriers: She views her lack of motivation and lack of skills as barriers.

Supports: She states that her mother and her friend are supportive but she feels that they are tired of her being depressed.

Occupational history: She has experience in retail and she babysits occasionally.

Values and interests: She has difficulty identifying values and interests.

Daily life roles: She identifies worker and daughter as her primary roles.

Current and past routines: Her routine has become less structured as she is sleeping more and has less energy and motivation to engage in occupations.

Client's priorities and desired targeted outcomes: She states that she would like to feel better, she would like

CASE STUDY 9.1 Major Depression—cont'd

to be happier and feel more energized. She states that she misses her boyfriend and wishes they would get back together. She is not interested in dating anyone else and does not believe any other boys her age would be interested in dating her because she is not as pretty, smart, or interesting as her peers.

Analysis of Occupational Performance

Occupations: She is asked to complete the Interest Checklist, and while she initially indicates a lack of interest in any occupational activities, she does indicate a current interest in baking and expresses a desire to learn to make jewelry. She is able to complete her ADLs and instrumental activities of daily living (IADLs) but lacks motivation to complete them consistently. Her social participation and leisure activities are diminished.

Client factors: Unable to identify values and beliefs and does not consider spirituality to be of importance to her at the current time. Her body functions are intact but diminished.

Performance patterns: Susan is asked to complete a time-use diary, which she has difficulty completing. She has difficulty identifying what she is doing some of the time, and she is spending a lot of time sleeping and watching television.

Intervention

Susan is educated on the importance of establishing consistent routines, and her therapist works with her to establish some structure in her daily life. Strategies for reinforcing consistent sleep and wake time periods and consistent meal times are discussed. Susan is educated on the use of exercise to affect mood and agrees to walk with her mom or her friend for 30 minutes every day. Motivational interviewing skills are used to elicit her input into strategies that she feels she can successfully implement. Susan agrees to try to maintain a more consistent schedule, and together with her OT, a daily schedule is devised. She agrees to check off the activities she completes and bring the schedule back to discuss at her next session. A cognitive-behavioral approach of graded task assignments to engage in baking is incorporated into her daily schedule too, as she indicated a current interest in this activity. Additional cognitive-behavioral approaches including targeting dysfunctional assumptions and learning new self-statements are used to address her low self-esteem and irrational beliefs. Her desire to learn to make jewelry is incorporated into therapy and she makes a letter bead bracelet with a positive self-statement and is asked to repeat the self-statement several times during the day. Susan's affect is improved after putting on the bracelet, and she states she enjoyed making it. Future sessions will focus on establishing a healthy routine and habits and the incorporation of meaningful occupations into her daily schedule.

CASE STUDY 9.2 Bipolar II Disorder

Sharon is a 44-year-old woman diagnosed with chronic pain and bipolar II disorder. She is married and has two sons ages 10 and 14 and a daughter age 8. She worked part time as a medical technologist until being diagnosed with breast cancer (right side) 4 years ago. She underwent a mastectomy and received treatment; she has been in remission ever since. The mastectomy resulted in chronic pain and discomfort in her chest and axilla; she was not a candidate for reconstructive surgery at the time. She has experienced depression intermittently since adolescence along with periods of hypomania manifested by rapid speech and impulsivity. She reports periods of sadness along with a lack of interest/motivation that have become increasingly worse over the years. She reports that medication helps some and she is compliant with her meds. She also has chronic sinusitis, migraine headaches, asthma, respiratory allergies, and intermittent joint pain of unknown etiology. She takes prescription-strength painkillers intermittently. Her husband is supportive, although she reports they tend to fight often. Her mother and stepfather live close to her; however, she reports that her mother can be difficult and argumentative at times. Sharon has difficulty maintaining the household, often not feeling well enough to cook, clean, and transport her children to their activities. Her oldest child has a learning disability and the youngest child has ADHD. Sharon has not been receptive to participating in chronic pain management programs or in complementary pain management approaches. She presents with a flat affect and cannot identify any specific interests or activities outside of watching TV or participating in basic household tasks and childrearing activities. She reluctantly agreed to attend outpatient occupational therapy at the suggestion of her physician to address chronic pain, edema, and gradual decreased range of movement (ROM) of right upper

Continued

CASE STUDY 9.2   Bipolar II Disorder—cont'd

extremity and ADL functioning. She states that she is tired of feeling bad all of the time.

Occupational Profile

The COPM is administered to structure the interview process, gather information, and assess the client's self-perception of occupational performance. Sharon presents with flat affect, she elaborates when answering some questions but is very negative in her responses and does not feel there is anything she can do to improve her situation.

Client's concerns: Sharon states that she is tired of the chronic pain she has been experiencing and feels bad for not being more of a mother to her children. She wants to be able to resume her prior household and caretaker duties. She states she would like to be pain free and experience joy in her life again.

Successful occupations: She is unable to identify any current successful occupations.

Barriers: She states that her pain is her primary barrier to being more engaged.

Supports: She feels that her husband and mother are intermittently supportive; she feels her children are supportive but also frustrated with her.

Occupational history: She worked as a medical technologist previously; not employed for the past 4 years.

Values and interests: She values her children and wants to do more for them. She does not have any interests outside of parenting and household tasks.

Daily life roles: She identifies mother, daughter, and homemaker as her primary roles.

Current and past routines: Her routine has become less structured as she takes frequent breaks from her household tasks to rest due to pain.

Client's priorities and desired targeted outcomes: She wants to regain the strength and movement of her right arm. She wants to be pain free and able to care for her children and home again.

Analysis of Occupational Performance

Occupations: She is limited in most occupations due to her pain and decreased movement and strength in her right arm. She is observed to be independent in her self-care ADLs with increased time and some modifications. When asked to rate her pain while completing her ADLs, she reports it to be a 7 or 8 on a scale of 10.

Client factors: Her right shoulder flexion/abduction is limited to 90 degrees with pain, unable to assess strength due to pain.

Performance patterns: She is asked to complete a time-use diary and she includes an average of ten 30-minute breaks a day to rest due to pain and fatigue. She also indicates that she is up and down at night as she has difficulty staying asleep and getting comfortable. She admits to watching more TV as she gets bored. She includes time for household tasks and time with her children but it is variable from day to day due to her children's extracurricular activities and homework.

Intervention

Sharon is further evaluated on her ADLs and provided with energy conservation and work simplification techniques to incorporate into her routine to decrease pain and to increase efficiency of movement as well as ROM and strength. She values her role of mother, so she was asked to identify any activities that she could do with her children that would be fun. After much discussion and brainstorming, she said that her children were interested in making homemade pizza. She agreed to try making pizza at her next session and identify steps of the process that her children could do with her at home. She is educated on a variety of complementary approaches for pain management and at first is very resistant; however, with the use of motivational interviewing skills and the suggestion to try yoga, she decides that she could try some yoga at her next session and then show her children what she has learned and that would be a good activity to do with them. She also thinks that yoga might be good for her child with ADHD. She was also provided with information on other complementary approaches such as mindfulness and guided imagery for both pain management and to address her difficulty sleeping. She is encouraged to read the information for discussion at a future session. Her daily routine is discussed, and she agrees to start monitoring the amount of time she spends watching TV and the number and length of rest periods she takes during the day to increase her awareness of both and work toward creating more balance in her schedule. Cognitive-behavioral strategies are used throughout the session such as reframing her current situation to identify positive aspects and explore other options. Role-playing is used to improve her communication skills with her husband and mother. Future sessions will further explore these interventions with a focus on establishing a healthy routine and healthy habits that will help address her pain and movement.

CASE STUDY 9.3 Bipolar I Disorder

John is a 30-year-old male diagnosed with bipolar I disorder. He graduated from high school in the top 10% of his class and attended college on a scholarship. He majored in business but he did not graduate as he began experiencing symptoms of mania and was subsequently diagnosed with bipolar I disorder. He has had multiple jobs over the years, the majority have been in sales. He currently works as a salesman for a company that sells office equipment to large businesses. He has also worked as a waiter, cook, tour guide, and realtor. His parents are divorced and they both live about 2 hours away; he reports a good relationship with them. He has a younger brother who lives in another state and they talk occasionally. He was married at 23 and divorced a year later; he has had multiple relationships over the past 6 years with the longest relationship lasting 2 years. He feels like his relationships usually end with constant arguing and an inability to communicate. He lives in an apartment with a friend and was admitted to an acute care hospital several days ago due to an acute manic episode. His medication compliance is questionable and he admits forgetting to take his medicine at times. This is his first inpatient hospitalization; the average length of stay is 7–10 days. The treatment team includes occupational therapy services.

Occupational Profile

The COPM is administered to structure the interview process, gather information, and assess the client's self-perception of occupational performance. John presents with elevated mood and pressured speech. He is easily distracted and displays some grandiose thinking regarding his plans for getting out of the hospital and finding a more exciting and higher-paying job. He is pacing and repeatedly sits down and stands up. He keeps looking at the door expecting his roommate to arrive to visit him.

Client's concerns: John states that he is in the hospital because he forgot to take his medicine and he will be fine and out of the hospital in a day or two. He denies any additional concerns.

Successful occupations: He states that he is a very successful salesman and will be able to get a better job soon. He states he likes working in sales but needs to make more money.

Barriers: He sees this hospitalization as a barrier, as he is anxious to get his "life on track."

Supports: John states that his family and his friend are supportive.

Client's priorities and desired targeted outcomes: John has difficulty answering the questions during the initial interview, and was therefore unable to assess his values, roles, and routines. His current priorities are "getting his medication sorted out" and "finding a better paying job."

Analysis of Occupational Performance

Occupations: John has a good work history but has had multiple jobs over the years, which could be a result of impulsivity and difficulty with interpersonal relationships.

Client factors: John is exhibiting symptoms of mania, he is exhibiting rapid thinking with flight of ideas, he cannot sit still and he is slightly agitated at times.

Performance skills and patterns: Difficult to assess role performance and routines at this time.

Intervention

Since John is currently exhibiting symptoms of mania, he is scheduled for an individual occupational therapy session to observe his occupational performance in ADLs and simple tasks. Occupational therapy intervention is primarily provided in a group context in this setting, therefore John is also scheduled to participate in structured task groups for further evaluation of his skills and to monitor medication effectiveness through task abilities. He also participates in movement groups that provide an outlet for his physical energy, and he participates in life skills groups that focus on the importance of establishing healthy routines through a variety of activities and discussion. During this group he is encouraged to discuss his medication compliance, to explore how and when he takes his medications and how it fits into his routine. Each client is provided with a daily calendar template and precut activities are provided to arrange on their calendar to construct an ideal schedule. John is encouraged to identify daily activities that support healthy living and medication compliance; memory strategies are also discussed, such as setting his phone alarm and keeping his medication by his toothbrush or another object used daily to trigger him to take his medication. As he progresses and prepares for discharge, the treatment team recommends outpatient therapy for medication management and counseling. He agrees to weekly sessions through the hospital's outpatient behavioral health program and identifies a need to work on his social interaction skills and to learn more about establishing healthy habits in his routine. He is scheduled to alternate sessions between the clinical counselor and the OT.

SUGGESTED LEARNING ACTIVITIES

1. Visit the National Institute of Mental Health website and watch the following two videos on depression and reflect on your understanding of depression:
   "Baby Blues" – or Postpartum Depression? (https://www.youtube.com/watch?v=_thfjbAtTT8)
   One Woman's Experience With Depression (https://www.youtube.com/watch?v=_thfjbAtTT8)
2. Participate in an advocacy event in your community to promote suicide prevention awareness. Contact your local mental health center, local or state National Alliance on Mental Illness organization, or local or state Mental Health America affiliate to find an event in your area. September is National Suicide Awareness month.
3. If possible, interview someone who has been diagnosed with depression or bipolar illness to gain an understanding of the lived experience of depression. Identify the occupations that were impacted as a result of the disease.

REFLECTION QUESTIONS

1. What is the difference between being diagnosed with depression and experiencing occasional and situational feelings of sadness? Why do some individuals need medication and/or therapy to treat depression?
2. How would you describe yourself on the mood continuum most of the time? Do you experience more periods of depressed mood or elevated mood?
3. What strategies do you use to maintain a positive mood?
4. What complementary approaches have the most evidence-based support?

REFERENCES

1. Mental Health America. *Mood Disorders*. 2018. Available at: http://www.mentalhealthamerica.net/conditions/mood-disorders.
2. American Psychiatric Association. *Diagnostic and Statistical Manual of Mental Disorders.* 5th ed. Washington, DC: American Psychiatric Association; 2013.
3. World Health Organization. *Depression.* Fact Sheet. March 22, 2018. Available at: http://www.who.int/news-room/fact sheets/detail/depression.
4. World Health Organization. *Depression and Other Common Mental Disorders: Global Health Estimates*. Geneva, Switzerland: WHO; 2017.
5. National Institute of Mental Health. *Major Depression*. November, 2017. Available at: https://www.nimh.nih.gov/health/statistics/major-depression.shtml.
6. American Psychological Association. *Overcoming Depression*. 2018. Available at: https://www.apa.org/helpcenter/depression.aspx.
7. National Alliance on Mental Illness. *Depression*. 2018. Available at: https://www.nami.org/Learn-More/Mental-Health-Conditions/Depression.
8. National Institute of Mental Health. *Depression*. February, 2018. Available at: https://www.nimh.nih.gov/health/topics/depression/index.shtml.
9. National Institute of Mental Health. *Persistent Depressive Disorder (Dysthymic Disorder)*. November, 2017. Available at: https://www.nimh.nih.gov/health/statistics/persistent-depressive-disorder-dysthymic-disorder.shtml.
10. Segre LS, Davis WN. Postpartum depression and perinatal mood disorders in the DSM. *Postpartum Support International*. June, 2013. Available at: http://www.postpartum.net/wp-content/uploads/2014/11/DSM-5-Summary-PSI.pdf.
11. O'Hara MW, McCabe JE. Postpartum depression: current status and future directions. *Ann Rev Clin Psychol*. 2013;9:379-407.
12. National Institute of Mental Health. *Bipolar Disorder*. April, 2016. Available at: https://www.nimh.nih.gov/health/topics/bipolar-disorder/index.shtml.
13. National Institute of Mental Health. *Bipolar Disorder*. November, 2017. Available at: https://www.nimh.nih.gov/health/statistics/bipolar-disorder.shtml.
14. Regeer EJ, Kupka RW, Have MT, Vollebergh W, Nolen WA. Low self-recognition and awareness of past hypomanic and manic episodes in the general population. *Int J Bipolar Disord*. 2015;3:22.
15. Reinares M, Bonnín C del M, Hidalgo-Mazzei D, et al. Making sense of DSM-5 mania with depressive features. *Aust N Z J Psychiatry*. 2015;49:540-549.
16. American Foundation for Suicide Prevention. *Research & Suicide Prevention: Top 10 Findings*. n.d. Available at: https://chapterland.org/wp-content/uploads/sites/13/2018/01/13531_Research_Top10_Flyer_Rebrand_m2.pdf.
17. American Foundation for Suicide Prevention. *Suicide Statistics*. 2018. Available at: https://afsp.org/about-suicide/suicide-statistics/.
18. Suicide Awareness Voices of Education. *Suicide Facts*. 2018. Available at: https://save.org/about-suicide/suicide-facts/.
19. World Health Organization. *Mental Health: Suicide Data*. 2018. Available at: http://www.who.int/mental_health/prevention/suicide/suicideprevent/en/.

20. Hawton K, Comabella CC, Haw C, Saunders K. Risk factors for suicide in individuals with depression: a systematic review. *J Affect Disord*. 2013;147:17-28.

21. Centers for Disease Control and Prevention. *Suicide Rates Rising Across the U.S.* June 7, 2018. Available at: https://www.cdc.gov/media/releases/2018/p0607-suicide-prevention.html.

22. U.S. Department of Veterans Affairs. VA Conducts Nation's Largest Analysis of Veteran Suicide. July 7, 2016. Available at: https://www.va.gov/opa/pressrel/pressrelease.cfm?id=2801.

23. Beck AT, Steer RA, Brown GK. *Manual for the Beck Depression Inventory-II*. San Antonio, TX: Psychological Corporation; 1996.

24. Wang YP, Gorenstein C. Psychometric properties of the Beck Depression Inventory-II: a comprehensive review. *Braz J Psychiatr*. 2013;35:416-431.

25. Kroenke K, Spitzer RL, Williams JB. The PHQ-9: validity of a brief depression severity measure. *J Gen Intern Med*. 2001;16:606-613.

26. Kroenke K, Spitzer RL, Williams JB. The patient health questionnaire-2: validity of a two-item depression screener. *Med Care*. 2003;41:1284-1292.

27. Kroenke K, Spitzer RL, Williams JB, Löwe B. The patient health questionnaire somatic, anxiety, and depressive symptom scales: a systematic review. *Gen Hosp Psychiatry*. 2010;32(4):345-359.

28. Tesar GE, Austerman J, Pozuelo L, Isaacson JH. *Behavioral Assessment of the General Medical Patient*. Cleveland, OH: Cleveland Clinic Center for Continuing Education; 2010.

29. American Occupational Therapy Association. *AOTA Occupational Profile Template*. 2017. Available at: https://www.aota.org/,/media/Corporate/Files/Practice/Manage/Documentation/AOTA-Occupational-Profile-Template.pdf.

30. American Occupational Therapy Association. Occupational therapy practice framework: domain & process (3rd ed.). *Am J Occup Ther*. 2014;68(suppl 1):S1-S51.

31. Kielhofner G, Mallinson T, Crawford D, Nowak M, Rigby M, Henry A. *Users Manual for the OPHI-II. Version 2.1*. Model of Human Occupation Clearinghouse. Chicago, IL; University of Illinois; 2004.

32. Law MC, Baptiste S, Carswell A, McColl MA, Polatajko HJ, Pollock N. *Canadian Occupational Performance Measure (COPM)*. 4th ed. Thorofare, NJ: Slack Inc.; 2005.

33. Baron K, Kielhofner G, Iyenger A, Goldhammer V, Wolenski J. *The Occupational Self Assessment OSA; Version 2.0*. Model of Human Occupational Clearinghouse. Chicago, IL: University of Illinois; 2002.

34. Smith K. *Depression Medications*. 2018. Available at: https://www.psycom.net/depression-medications/#typeofantidepressants.

35. Smith K. *Bipolar Disorder Medications*. 2018. Available at: https://www.psycom.net/bipolar-disorder-medications.

36. Machado-Vieira R, Manji HK, Zarate Jr CA. The role of lithium in the treatment of bipolar disorder: convergent evidence for neurotrophic effects as a unifying hypothesis. *Bipolar Disorder*. 2009;11(suppl 2):92-109.

37. Post RM. The new news about lithium: an underutilized treatment in the United States. *Neuropsychopharmacology*. 2018;43:1174-1179.

38. Fenn K, Byrne M. The key principles of cognitive behavioural therapy. *InnovAiT*. 2013;6:579-585.

39. Law R. Interpersonal psychotherapy for depression. *Adv Psychiatr Treat*. 2011;17:23-31.

40. Medical University of South Carolina. *The Brain Stimulation Lab at MUSC*. n.d. Available at: http://academicdepartments.musc.edu/psychiatry/divisions-and-programs/bsl/index.htm.

41. Mehta P, Sharma M. Yoga and complementary therapy for clinical depression. *Complement Health Pract Rev*. 2010;15:156-170.

42. Bridges L, Sharma M. The efficacy of yoga as a form of treatment for depression. *J Evid-Based Complementary Altern Med*. 2017;22:1017-1028.

43. Tasci G, Baykara S, Gurok MG, Atmaca M. Effect of exercise on therapeutic response in depression treatment. *Psychiatry Clin Psychopharmacol*. 2018. doi:10.1080/24750573.2018.1426159.

44. Kabat-Zinn J. Mindfulness-based interventions in context: past, present, and future. *Clinical Psychol: Sci Pract*. 2003;10:144-156.

45. MacKenzie MB, Kocovski NL. Mindfulness-based cognitive therapy for depression: trends and developments. *Psychol Res Behav Manag*. 2016;16:125-132.

46. Cozine EW, Wilkinson JM. Depression screening, diagnosis, and treatment across the lifespan. *Prim Care*. 2016;43:229-243.

47. Unützer J, Park M. (2012). Strategies to improve the management of depression in primary care. *Prim Care*. 2012;39:415-431.

10

Anxiety Disorders

Nancy Carson

LEARNING OBJECTIVES

1. Identify the anxiety disorders, obsessive-compulsive disorders, and trauma- and stressor-related disorders defined by the DSM-5.
2. Describe the symptomology of the different disorders.
3. Understand the prevalence and risk factors of the different disorders.
4. Recognize assessment methods for the different disorders.
5. Discuss treatment approaches including psychopharmacology, psychotherapeutic, and complementary approaches.
6. Articulate the role of occupational therapy in the treatment of these disorders.

INTRODUCTION

Anxiety is a normal part of everyday life. It is typical to feel some level of anxiety or stress when engaging in new activities, meeting new people, or learning new skills. The experience of taking a test or being evaluated on competency skills can create high levels of anxiety. Public speaking can create enormous anxiety, and many people work hard to learn how to control the anxiety they experience when required to engage in public speaking or similar anxiety-provoking activities. Driving in heavy traffic or unfamiliar places can result in anxiety, but it also promotes the hypervigilance needed to be observant, alert, and cautious, thereby preventing an accident. Many self-help books and articles are available to offer suggestions on how to deal with daily stress and combat anxiety. The healthy aspect of anxiety is the motivation it creates to learn skills that enable one to engage in occupations while dealing effectively with any resulting anxiety.

When anxiety becomes extreme and disrupts the individual's ability to function, it indicates the presence of an anxiety disorder. Anxiety disorders are different from stress-induced transient anxiety or otherwise developmentally normal types of stress in that it is out of proportion to the source of the anxiety, it is persistent, and it interferes with the individual's daily occupational functioning.[1] Anxiety disorders often co-occur with other mental disorders such as major depression, substance use disorders, and personality disorders, and if untreated, it tends to recur chronically. Women experience anxiety disorders almost twice as often as men.[1]

More than 260 million people globally, 3.6% of the world's population, are affected by anxiety disorders, including generalized anxiety disorder, panic disorder, posttraumatic stress disorder, and obsessive-compulsive disorder. The prevalence of anxiety disorders increased by 14.9% globally between 2005 and 2015, and anxiety disorders are now the sixth largest cause of disability worldwide.[2] Approximately 40 million adults in the United States (18%) and 8% of children and teenagers have an anxiety disorder, making it the most common mental health concern in the United States.[3] The DSM-5 lists three categories of disorders that were previously combined into one category of anxiety disorders in the Diagnostic and Statistical Manual of Mental Disorders, 4th ed. (DSM-IV). These three categories are anxiety disorders, obsessive-compulsive disorders, and trauma- and stressor-related disorders.[4]

ANXIETY DISORDERS

This category includes generalized anxiety disorder, separation anxiety disorder, selective mutism, specific phobia, social anxiety disorder, panic disorder, and agoraphobia.

Anxiety disorders are a group of related conditions that are defined by persistent excessive fear or worry in situations that do not warrant it. Each disorder has additional unique symptoms.[3] Separation anxiety and selective mutism were formerly classified as childhood disorders, but now both children and adults can be diagnosed with either disorder.[4]

General Anxiety Disorder

Generalized anxiety disorder (GAD) produces chronic, exaggerated worrying about everyday life that occurs most of the time for at least 6 months. In addition, at least three physical or emotional symptoms are present such as restlessness, increased fatigue, impaired concentration, irritability, increased muscle aches, or difficulty sleeping.[5] GAD impacts an individual's quality of life as the person with GAD does not know how to stop worrying; it is a constant theme and the person cannot stop it even though the awareness that it is unwarranted for the situation is apparent. Some people believe that worrying about something will somehow prevent it from occurring so there is hesitancy to try to stop worrying.

Separation Anxiety Disorder

Separation anxiety disorder is an inappropriate and excessive anxiety regarding separation, actual or imagined, from home or major attachment figures, causing significant distress or impairment in functioning. Symptoms may include recurrent excessive stress when anticipating or experiencing separation from home or major attachment figures, or symptoms may focus on potential harm to or loss of them. Symptoms are present for at least 4 weeks or more in children and adolescents and at least 6 months in adults.[6]

Selective Mutism

Selective mutism is consistent failure to speak in specific social situations in which there is an expectation for speaking. An example is a child who does not speak at school but speaks without difficulty at home. Symptoms must be present for at least 1 month. Selective mutism may occur along with social phobia, separation anxiety disorder, or specific phobia.[7]

Specific Phobia

An irrational and fearful reaction to a place, situation, event, or object is referred to as a phobia. The reaction can be very powerful, causing the individual to go to great lengths to avoid whatever it is that is causing the fear, and there may be multiple triggers that elicit a fear response to a phobia. Phobias affect approximately 19 million adults, with women being two times more likely than men to have a specific phobia.[3] Some people experience multiple specific phobias simultaneously. When multiple phobias or types of triggers are present or are frequent, the person may go to great lengths to avoid the triggers, and these actions can take over the person's life, disrupting healthy occupational functioning.[8]

Phobias can be divided into four categories depending on the source of the phobia: natural, mutilation, animal, and situational. An example of a natural phobia is astraphobia (fear of thunder and lightning). An example of a mutilation phobia is iatrophobia (fear of the doctor). A common situational phobia is claustrophobia (fear of enclosed spaces). Cynophobia, the fear of dogs, is an example of an animal phobia. It can be particularly debilitating in communities where there is a high prevalence of dogs.[8]

A phobia is different from a fear or dislike of an object, place, or situation. A phobia elicits unreasonable, excessive, persistent, and intense fear that is markedly greater than the actual danger or threat posed by the object or situation. The individual may use extreme methods to avoid exposure to the source of the phobia and this negatively impacts daily life.[8]

Social Anxiety Disorder

This anxiety disorder is characterized by intense fear or anxiety about social interaction in one or more social settings. Social anxiety disorder is different from shyness or disliking social events or settings. The individual experiences irrational fears of humiliation related to not knowing what to say or saying something that others reject. The person may avoid participating in social conversations or avoid school or work discussions. Panic attacks may occur if the person is forced into social interaction, or may result in anticipation of social interaction.[3]

The person with social anxiety disorder may experience racing thoughts, increased heart rate, flushing, and sweating at the thought of going to a social event or conversing with someone they do not know. This may lead the person to avoid social situations, therefore becoming isolated and feeling very much alone. Excessive fear of potential humiliation and possible rejection from others can interfere with daily roles and activities, and can negatively impact work, school, and relationships. Social anxiety disorder affects approximately 15 million, or 7%, of American adults and those affected are at a greater risk for substance use disorder and major depressive disorder.[9]

Panic Disorder

This disorder is characterized by episodic, unexpected panic attacks, and sudden feelings of terror, sometimes striking repeatedly and without warning or without an evident trigger. A panic attack may be mistaken for a heart attack, as it may result in chest pain, heart palpitations, dizziness, shortness of breath, and stomach upset. A panic attack is described as a rapid onset of intense fear that usually peaks within 10 minutes. There are at least four symptoms present, such as accelerated heart rate, sweating, shortness of breath, nausea, dizziness, fear of losing control, or fear of dying. Many people will go to desperate measures to avoid an attack, including social isolation.[5] A panic attack specifier can be applied to any diagnostic category such as depression with panic attack.[10]

Agoraphobia

In the DSM-5, agoraphobia is identified as a separate disorder. Agoraphobia is defined as intense fear or anxiety in at least two situations or places such as using public transportation and being in public places such as stores. It can also include being outside the home alone or being in open spaces. The individual exhibits avoidance behaviors that may increase over time. If a person experiences intense fear in one specific situation or place, similar places may be avoided for fear of having the same experience. Over time these limits impair the person's relationships with others and ability to work or engage in other satisfying occupational roles and activities. Quality of life and overall functioning is negatively impacted as a result of the avoidance behaviors.[4]

OBSESSIVE-COMPULSIVE DISORDERS AND RELATED DISORDERS

This is a new category that includes obsessive-compulsive disorder, body dysmorphic disorder, hoarding disorder, trichotillomania (hair-pulling), and excoriation (skin-picking) disorder. Hoarding disorder and excoriation disorder are both newly defined disorders in the DSM-5. Obsessive-compulsive disorders were previously categorized as anxiety disorders in the DSM-IV; however, researchers determined there to be unique differences justifying a separate category for DSM-5.[4]

Obsessive-Compulsive Disorder

Obsessive-compulsive-disorder (OCD) is defined by a cycle of obsessions and compulsions that are extreme, time consuming, and that interfere with valued occupations on a regular basis. Obsessions are thoughts, images, or impulses that the individual does not want and that trigger intensely distressing feelings. The obsessions occur repeatedly and are disturbing to the person. They usually do not make sense and may be accompanied by personal despair and disgust, as well as the need to do something in a specific way. Because of the obsessions,

the person engages in behaviors called compulsions that are perceived to decrease the distress and alleviate the obsessions. Common obsessions may be related to germ exposure, perfectionism, harming others accidently or acting on unwanted impulses to harm someone, unwanted sexual thoughts, religious obsessions, physical illness, or superstitions.

Compulsions are repetitive behaviors or thoughts that a person uses to alleviate the distress created by the obsession. They are usually recognized as a temporary solution, but the person does not feel there is any other option for dealing with the distress. They are time consuming and usually occur at the expense of valued activities. Compulsions may include avoiding situations that trigger obsessions.[11] It is important to discern between repetitive activity and OCD. There are times when an individual may appear obsessed or engage in repetitive behavior that is positive and does not interfere with daily life or cause distress. Some examples include strict bedtime routines or religious practices. These may serve as important components of the individual's daily life. Learning a new skill or completing a desired project may require short-term repetition or focus at the temporary expense of other valued activity. The context and level of distress to the individual must be considered. Usually, individuals with OCD feel driven to engage in the compulsive behavior even when they do not want to. Common compulsions include excessive washing of hands or showering, checking that one did not make a mistake, arranging items in a specific order, repeating routine activities, body movements, or activities and mental compulsions such as counting, reviewing events, or praying.[11]

Body Dysmorphic Disorder

Excessive and persistent preoccupation with perceived defects or flaws in personal appearance is referred to as body dysmorphic disorder (BDD). These flaws are relatively unnoticed by others but are a source of great distress to the individual. The most common concerns are facial features and hair, and the individual engages in repetitive behaviors such as excessive grooming or checking their appearance in the mirror repeatedly. Left untreated, BDD typically follows a chronic course and results in functional impairment both socially and occupationally. There is high comorbidity with major depressive disorder, social anxiety disorder, and obsessive-compulsive disorder. There are also increased rates of suicidality in untreated BDD.[12]

Hoarding Disorder

In 1996, the behavior of hoarding was defined as acquiring objects without being able to discard those objects when warranted.[13] In the DSM-5, hoarding disorder (HD) was added as a disorder within the OCD category. The criteria include persistent difficulty discarding items, the desire to save items to avoid negative feelings associated with discarding them, significant accumulation of possessions that clutter active living areas, and significant distress or impairment in areas of functioning.[14] Hoarding is typically explained by the individual to be necessary due to the objects having a current or future purpose or there is an emotional attachment to the object. Severe hoarding can create major clutter that may be a public health or safety concern. HD does not include the intrusive or repetitive thoughts associated with OCD. Compulsive hoarding affects about 2%–5% of the population. Stressful or traumatic events may be associated with the onset of hoarding symptoms, and there is a comorbidity of major depression approximately half of the time.[15]

Trichotillomania

Chronic hair-pulling is a disorder that primarily affects women and can cause significant psychosocial impairment. Trichotillomania (TTM) is characterized by the repeated pulling of hair that results in significant hair loss. TTM most commonly manifests at approximately 13 years of age, and 0.6%–3.6% of adults are affected. Those individuals who experience TTM feel shame about the behavior and struggle with low self-esteem. Individuals with TTM are mostly able to suppress the behavior in public and wait to engage in the behavior while alone or while engaged in sedentary activities. Negative affective experiences such as stress and anxiety often exacerbate pulling, which in turn alleviates the negative feelings. Research indicates that persons with TTM suffer mild to moderate life impairment in many functional domains.[16]

Excoriation Disorder

Excoriation disorder (ED) or skin-picking is characterized by recurrent picking of skin. The prevalence is estimated to be between 1.4% and 5.4%, with the majority being women. Skin-picking triggers include emotions such as stress, anger, anxiety, boredom, and sedentary activities. Skin-picking most commonly occurs on the face, followed by the hands, fingers, arms, and legs. An inability to stop picking despite repeated efforts to do so is typical and may lead to shame, anxiety, and depression. Individuals with ED often spend a significant amount of time on repetitive picking and then on concealing the resulting skin lesions or scars to avoid social embarrassment. Severe cases may result in infections, lesions, scarring, and even serious physical disfigurement. ED is also associated with comorbidities such as TTM, OCD, BDD, and depression. Individuals with ED may not commonly seek treatment for their condition due to social embarrassment or a belief that it is just a bad habit and not treatable.[17]

TRAUMA- AND STRESSOR-RELATED DISORDERS

Trauma- and stressor-related disorders include disorders in which exposure to a traumatic or stressful event is listed explicitly as a diagnostic criterion. These include reactive attachment disorder, disinhibited social engagement disorder, posttraumatic stress disorder, acute stress disorder, and adjustment disorders.[4]

Reactive Attachment Disorder

Reactive attachment disorder is caused by social neglect or a lack of attachment to a caregiver at an early age. It results in an inability for the child to form normal relationships with others. The child presents with withdrawn behavior and depressive symptoms, does not seek comfort when distressed, and presents with persistent social and emotional disturbances even when a nurturing caregiver is provided. Reactive attachment disorder is diagnosed in children at least 1 year old and develops within the first 5 years of life.[18]

Disinhibited Social Engagement Disorder

Disinhibited social engagement disorder is an emotional disorder that results from social neglect during childhood. It is similar to reactive attachment disorder but presents with externalizing behavior and disinhibition rather than internalizing and withdrawn behavior with depressive symptoms. A criterion for diagnosis is a pattern of behavior in which the child actively approaches and interacts with unfamiliar adults. The behavior may include overly familiar verbal or physical behavior, diminished checking back with the adult caregiver in social settings, and a willingness to go off with an unfamiliar adult with minimal or no hesitation.[19]

Posttraumatic Stress Disorder

Posttraumatic stress disorder (PTSD) is a common mental health disorder that affects 8.7% of people during their lifetime.[20] There are four core PTSD symptoms: (1) reexperiencing the trauma psychologically, (2) avoiding reminders of the trauma, (3) hyperarousal or hypervigilance, and (4) cognition and mood symptoms referred to as emotional numbing.[20,21] To be diagnosed with PTSD, an adult must have at least one of each of the four core symptoms for at least 1 month. Reexperiencing symptoms include flashbacks in which the person relives the trauma over and over, and the experience is usually accompanied by physiological symptoms such as a racing heart. Reexperiencing symptoms also include bad dreams and frightening thoughts. Avoidance symptoms include avoiding situations, places, events, or anything else that serves as a reminder of the traumatic experience, and avoiding thoughts or feelings related to the traumatic event. An individual may go to great lengths to stay away from people or places or avoid situations that could trigger the reexperiencing symptoms. This can create disruptions to the individual's routine and role responsibilities and negatively impact occupational functioning and satisfaction. For example, a person who was the victim of a violent crime in the parking lot of a store in the early evening may avoid parking lots, stores, and being in the car at night. Anything related to the traumatic experience can be a trigger. The person's routine may be restructured and the person may avoid attending certain events. The person may not be able to fulfill prior role responsibilities and may even change jobs or forego participation in certain activities.

Another core PTSD symptom is arousal and reactivity, which include being easily startled or angered, feeling tense, and/or having difficulty sleeping. Arousal symptoms do not require triggers to occur; they are usually constant and can interfere with concentration and the ability to successfully engage in activities of daily living and meaningful occupations. Cognition and mood symptoms also interfere with daily activities. They include difficulty remembering the trauma, negative thoughts, feeling guilt or blame, and loss of interest in satisfying occupations. These symptoms create a sense of emotional numbing that makes the person appear and feel detached from others.[21]

Acute Stress Disorder

Acute stress disorder (ASD) can develop after exposure to one or more traumatic events. It usually occurs within 1 month and lasts from 3 days to 1 month. The symptoms are similar to those experienced with PTSD, and individuals with ASD are at a greater risk of developing PTSD. It is natural for people to exhibit some of the core symptoms of PTSD following a traumatic event. People experiencing ASD may find that occupational functioning, roles, and routines may be severely limited for a few hours, days, or weeks. If the symptoms continue for longer than 1 month, the person may be diagnosed with PTSD. For some individuals, symptoms of PTSD do no emerge until weeks or months following the trauma.[21]

Adjustment Disorder

An adjustment disorder is the experience of greater stress than would normally occur following a stressful or unexpected situation. As a result, the individual experiences significant problems in occupational activities or relationships. There is difficulty recovering from the stressful event that results in behaviors such as feeling hopeless, frequent crying, worrying, decreased activities of daily living (ADL)

functioning and participation, and potential for suicidal thoughts or behaviors. Symptoms usually begin within 3 and 6 months but can last longer and result in chronic or persistent adjustment disorder. Stressful events may include divorce, relationship problems, unemployment, chronic illness, and losing a loved one.[22]

ASSESSMENT

There are many instruments that are used to screen and detect anxiety disorders, obsessive compulsive disorders, and trauma- and stressor-related disorders. A few of the instruments that can be used and may be of interest to the occupational therapist (OT) are discussed here.

State-Trait Anxiety Inventory

The State-Trait Anxiety Inventory (STAI) is a commonly used measure of trait and state anxiety[23] that is used to diagnose anxiety and to distinguish it from depressive syndromes. There are 20 items for assessing state anxiety and 20 for trait anxiety. State anxiety is a psychophysiological state of reactions that occur during adverse situations in a specific moment. Trait anxiety is a personality trait and indicates individual differences related to how state anxiety manifests over time.[24] Examples of state anxiety inventory items include: "I am tense," "I am worried," "I feel calm," and "I feel secure." Examples of trait anxiety inventory items include: "I worry too much over something that really doesn't matter" and "I am content." All items are self-reported rated on a four-point scale. Evidence supports the construct and concurrent validity of the scale.[25]

Holmes and Rahe Stress Scale

The Holmes and Rahe Stress Scale[26] is a self-report scale that asks the individual to select life events, from a list of 43 life events, that have been experienced in the previous year. Each event is called a Life Change Unit (LCU) and has a different value that reflects the level of stress of the event. The point value of all selected LCUs are added together to obtain a score. Scores higher that 150 points indicate a 50% change of a major health concern in the next 2 years, and scores higher than 300 points increase it to 80%. The scale is well researched and consistent across cross-cultural differences. It is free to use and available to download or use online from several different websites.[27]

Generalized Anxiety Disorder Screening Tool

The Generalized Anxiety Disorder-7 (GAD-7)[28] has been validated as a diagnostic tool and a severity assessment scale. There are seven items that are rated on a scale of 0–3 from "not at all" to "nearly every day." Examples of items include "Not being able to stop or control worrying" and

"Being so restless that it is hard to sit still." A higher score on the GAD-7 correlated with increased functional impairment.[28]

Current Anxiety Level Measure

The Current Anxiety Level Measure (CALM)[29] was developed by OTs with the purpose of developing a fast, free, valid, and reliable current or state anxiety assessment. The CALM consists of 16 self-report statements. Each statement is scored on a scale of 0–3 from "not at all" to "extremely." The maximum score is 64 and the minimum score is 0. Higher scores indicate higher levels of anxiety. The CALM demonstrates strong concurrent validity and strong reliability.[29] OTs can benefit from using this tool to determine the effectiveness of short-term occupational therapy intervention, as it is fast and easy to administer and score.

Yale–Brown Obsessive-Compulsive Scale

The Yale–Brown Obsessive-Compulsive Scale (Y-BOCS) is considered the gold-standard assessment tool for OCD symptom severity. It consists of a symptom checklist and severity scale to consecutively rate 54 common obsessions and compulsions that are grouped according to thematic content (e.g., contamination) or behavioral expression (e.g., checking behaviors). Symptom severity is rated according to frequency, interference, distress, resistance, and degree of control. The Y-BOCS total severity score shows good internal consistency, excellent inter rater reliability, and good test–retest reliability. There is also a self-report version of the Y-BOCS in which individuals are asked to identify the presence/absence of obsessions and compulsions and rate their severity. This self-rate scale, the Y-BOCS-SR, shows fair to good internal consistency and good short-term test–retest reliability in nonclinical samples, and it does appear to have utility as a diagnostic screening measure.[30]

Obsessive-Compulsive Inventory–Revised

The Obsessive-Compulsive Inventory–Revised (OCI-R) is a brief self-report measure consisting of 18 items rated on a five-point scale. Brief self-reports are ideal for identifying symptoms and severity quickly, are cost effective, and require minimal training to administer and interpret. The OCI-R tool possesses reliability, validity, and diagnostic sensitivity, with a total score of 21 corresponding to an OCD diagnosis.[30]

Dimensional Obsessive-Compulsive Scale

The Dimensional Obsessive-Compulsive Scale (DOCS) is a 20-item self-report scale designed to look at four dimensional factors: (1) germs and contamination; (2) responsibility for harm, injury, or bad luck; (3) unacceptable obsessional thoughts; and (4) symmetry, completeness, and exactness. Each factor is measured across five items related to time, avoidance, distress, impairment, and resistance. Psychometric properties of the DOCS support its use as a clinically informative assessment tool; however, it is limited in a treatment-planning context.[30]

Trauma Assessments

Heath care providers should assess patients for a history of trauma exposure because trauma and trauma-related problems are common, PTSD affects physical health, individuals who experience trauma have high medical utilization rates, and PTSD is under recognized by practitioners. Many patients receiving services for other conditions have been exposed to trauma and have posttraumatic stress symptoms but have not received appropriate mental health care such as education, counseling, or referrals for mental health evaluation. This is due in part to the individual's avoidance of trauma reminders, and it leads to a lack of individuals who spontaneously report their trauma experiences or related symptoms.[31]

Health care providers can screen individuals for trauma-related symptoms by asking questions or using a self-report screening tool during an evaluation or treatment session. The Primary Care PTSD Screen (PC-PTSD)[32,33] is a brief symptom-driven tool developed for use in primary care and other medical settings. There are four questions asking about the presence of behaviors in the past month that include nightmares or bad thoughts, avoidance of situations, hypervigilance, and emotional numbing in response to a past experience that was frightening or extremely upsetting. If a patient answers "yes" to three items, it is indicative that a patient may have PTSD or trauma-related problems, and further investigation of trauma symptoms by a mental health professional is warranted.

The National Center for PTSD[34] provides a listing of the measures authored by the National Center and measures that assess trauma and PTSD provided by other organizations. A list of some of the measures authored by the National Center for PTSD and measures provided by other organizations can be found in Box 10.1. They are available either to download or by request as indicated by the National Center for PTSD at https://www.ptsd.va.gov/professional/assessment/list_measures.asp#list2. Measures developed by other organizations can be requested via contact information on the page for the specific measure.

Occupational Therapy Assessment

In evaluating individuals with anxiety, obsessive-compulsive, and trauma- and stressor-related disorders, the OT will

BOX 10.1   PTSD and Trauma Measures

Interview
Clinician-Administered PTSD Scale for DSM-5 (CAPS-5)
National Center for PTSD

Structured Interview (PSS-I)
Davidson JRT, Kudler HS, Smith RD. Assessment and pharmacotherapy of posttraumatic stress disorder. In: JEL Giller, ed. *Biological Assessment and Teatment of Posttraumatic Stress Disorder.* Washington, DC: American Psychiatric Press; 1990:205-221.

Self-Report
Dissociative Subtype of PTSD Scale (DSPS)
National Center for PTSD

Mississippi Scale for Combat-Related PTSD (M-PTSD)
National Center for PTSD

PTSD Checklist for DSM-5 (PCL-5)
National Center for PTSD

Posttraumatic Diagnostic Scale
Foa E, Cashman L, Jaycox L, Perry K. The validation of a self-report measure of PTSD: the Posttraumatic Diagnostic Scale. *Psychol Assess.* 1997;9:445-451.
Foa E. *Posttraumatic Diagnostic Scale Manual.* Minneapolis, MN: National Computer Systems; 1996.

Trauma Symptom Checklist-40 (TSC-40)
Elliot DM, Briere, J. Sexual abuse trauma among professional women: validating the Trauma Symptom Checklist-40 (TSC-40). *Child Abuse Negl.* 1992;16:391-398.
Briere JN, Runtz MG. The Trauma Symptom Checklist (TSC-33): early data on a new scale. *J Interpers. Violence.* 1989;4:151-163.

PTSD Screens
SPAN
Davidson J. *SPAN Addendum to DTS Manual.* New York: Multi-Health Systems Inc.; 2002.
Short Post-Traumatic Stress Disorder Rating Interview (SPRINT)
Connor K Davidson J. SPRINT: a brief global assessment of post-traumatic stress disorder. *Int Clin Psychopharmacol.* 2001;16:279-284.
Davidson JRT, Colket, JT. The eight-item treatment-outcome post-traumatic stress disorder scale: a brief measure to assess treatment outcome in post-traumatic stress disorder. *Int Clin Psychopharmacol.* 1997;12:41-45.

Trauma Screening Questionnaire (TSQ)
Brewin CR, Rose S, Andrews B, et al. Brief screening instrument for post-traumatic stress disorder. *Br J Psychiatry.* 2002;181:158-162.

Trauma Exposure
Brief Trauma Questionnaire (BTQ)
National Center for PTSD

Combat Exposure Scale (CES)
National Center for PTSD

Life Events Checklist for DSM-5 (LEC-5)
National Center for PTSD

Life Stressor Checklist-Revised (LSC-R)
National Center for PTSD

BOX 10.1 PTSD and Trauma Measures—cont'd

Trauma History Screen (THS)
National Center for PTSD

Stressful Life Events Screening Questionnaire (SLESQ)
Goodman L, Corcoran C, Turner K, Yuan N, Green B. Assessing traumatic event exposure: general issues and preliminary findings for the Stressful Life Events Screening Questionnaire. *J Trauma Stress*. 1998;11:521-542.
Green B, Chung J, Daroowalla A, Kaltman S, DeBenedictis C. Evaluating the cultural validity of the Stressful Life Events Screening Questionnaire. *Violence Against Women*, 2006;12(12):191-213.

Trauma Assessment for Adults (TAA)
Resnick HS, Falsetti SA, Kilpatrick DG, Freedy JR. Assessment of rape and other civilian trauma-related post-traumatic stress disorder: emphasis on assessment of potentially traumatic events. In: TW Miller ed. *Stressful Life Events*. Madison: International Universities Press; 1996:231-266.

Trauma History Questionnaire (THQ)
Hooper L, Stockton P, Krupnick J, Green B. Development, use, and psychometric properties of the Trauma History Questionnaire. *J Loss Trauma*. 2011;16:258-283.

BOX 10.2 Examples of Medications to Treat Anxiety

Class	Generic and Brand Names
SSRIs	citalopram (Celexa)
	escitalopram (Lexapro)
	fluoxetine (Prozac)
	paroxetine (Paxil)
	sertraline (Zoloft)
SNRIs	duloxetine (Cymbalta)
	desvenlafaxine (Pristiq)
	venlafaxine (Effexor)
Benzodiazepines	alprazolam (Xanax)
	clonazepam (Klonopin)
	chlordiazepoxide (Librium)
	diazepam (Valium)
	lorazepam (Ativan)
	oxazepam (Serax)
Beta-blockers	propranolol (Inderal)
	atenolol (Tenormin)
Other anxiolytic (antianxiety)	buspirone (BuSpar)
	hydroxyzine (Vistaril, Atarax)

SNRIs, Serotonin-norepinephrine reuptake inhibitors; SSRIs, Selective serotonin reuptake inhibitors.

use the Occupational Therapy Practice Framework[35] to guide the evaluation process and determine how the individual's occupations, roles, and routines are impacted by the disorder. The Canadian Occupational Performance Measure[36] or the Occupational Performance History Interview (OPHI-2)[37] may be used to guide the interview process, and skilled observation of the client's behaviors during the interview and while engaged in occupations will provide additional information. Depending on the client, the OT may also choose specific assessments to gain additional information regarding the client's occupational performance. For example, the OT may want to evaluate sensory modulation because the ability to respond appropriately to sensory stimuli may be impacted by stress and trauma. This is discussed in detail in Chapter 8, with examples of assessments that may be used. Evaluation of leisure interests and wellness approaches can also provide useful information to understand what occupations the individual may be using or not using to effectively manage stress and anxiety.

THERAPEUTIC MANAGEMENT

The various disorders discussed in this chapter each have unique symptoms, and the response to treatment approaches can vary depending on the specific diagnosis. There are also many similarities among the anxiety, obsessive-compulsive, and trauma- and stressor-related disorders that result in common types of treatment that are used. A thorough evaluation by a mental health professional is essential for determining effective treatment for those individuals diagnosed with one of these disorders. Most individuals will respond best to a combination of psychopharmacology and psychotherapeutic approaches, whereas some individuals will respond well to medication alone, and other individuals will benefit from counseling or psychotherapy without the use of medication. Additional methods to treat anxiety, obsessive-compulsive, trauma- and stressor-related disorders include a variety of complementary approaches and wellness approaches, such as exercise.

Psychopharmacology

There are several different categories of medications that may be prescribed to treat anxiety depending on the symptoms experienced. They include selective serotonin reuptake inhibitors (SSRIs), serotonin-norepinephrine reuptake inhibitors (SNRIs), benzodiazepines, beta-blockers, and some medications that do not fit into these categories, such as buspirone and hydroxyzine.[38] As with depression, the most commonly used medications for anxiety are SSRIs, which work by blocking the reabsorption of the neurotransmitter serotonin in the brain.[38,39] They are commonly used to treat anxiety disorders including OCD. They can cause side effects such as sleep problems, weight gain, and sexual issues, but these are usually less intense than with other medications and are more manageable by the prescribing provider. They are not habit-forming, but may take several weeks to achieve their maximum effectiveness. SNRIs are similar to SSRIs, but they block the reabsorption of both serotonin and norepinephrine in the brain. These medications promote neuroplasticity in the brain and can take several weeks to be effective. Higher levels of norepinephrine and serotonin are thought to stimulate neurons and create changes in neural circuitry, which promotes flexibility and allows the brain to adapt to higher levels of serotonin and norepinephrine.[40]

Benzodiazepines are sometimes prescribed because they act quickly to reduce anxiety; however, individuals can develop a tolerance to the medication with the potential to become addicted, and therefore they are not used for the long-term treatment of anxiety. They may be prescribed along with SSRIs or SNRIs until that medication reaches it full effect, but they are not usually considered the first course of treatment for anxiety.[38]

Beta-blockers are sometimes used for performance or situation-specific anxiety. Beta-blockers work by blocking physical symptoms of anxiety including rapid heart rate and sweating.

For example, an actor may use a beta-blocker to deal with stage fright or a person may take a beta-blocker before engaging in public speaking. A person with social anxiety disorder may use a beta-blocker prior to situations requiring interaction with other people. They may be used with specific phobias too, with the premise that with the absence of the physical symptoms associated with the phobia, eventually the fear may diminish or even subside completely. The use of beta-blockers with cognitive behavioral therapy (CBT) can also be very beneficial for some people. Situations that cause intense anxiety but are necessary for role performance may be addressed with the use of beta-blockers.[41]

There are other medications that do not fit into the above categories that are sometimes prescribed to treat anxiety disorders. One example is buspirone (brand name Buspar), which has fewer of the sexual side effects associated with SSRIs. It is typically used to treat generalized anxiety disorder. Buspirone is an anxiolytic medication but is not related to other antianxiety medications, such as benzodiazepines, barbiturates, or other sedative/ anxiolytic drugs.[42] Hydroxyzine (Atarax, Vistaril) is another anxiolytic medication prescribed for anxiety. It works quickly and is not addictive. Hydroxyzine is an antihistamine that is used to treat allergic reactions and also has an effect on the processing of serotonin.[43] The occupational therapy practitioner can support the client by asking about medication compliance, providing education regarding how the medications work, and providing strategies within the client's routine to help the client remember to take medications as prescribed.

Psychotherapy

CBT is the most validated nonpharmacologic approach for anxiety disorders overall. The CBT approach or technique that is most effective will depend on the specific diagnosis. CBT is a treatment approach that focuses on changing maladaptive emotional responses by changing the individual's thoughts and/or behaviors. Two of the most commonly used CBT treatment approaches for anxiety disorders are exposure therapy and cognitive therapy.[44]

Exposure therapy modifies thought processes by activating the fear or anxiety and then providing new information that disputes the unrealistic associations currently believed. The desired outcome is that successful confrontation decreases the fear or anxiety. Exposure may be imaginal, in vivo (in real life), or interoceptive. Imaginal exposure is vivid imagination of the feared situation without avoiding the resulting anxiety. In vivo exposure involves gradual exposure to the actual source of the fear or anxiety. Interoceptive exposure, which is mostly used in treating panic disorder, involves deliberately inducing the physical sensations of a panic attack. In general, exposure therapy is typically completed in about 10 sessions.[44]

Cognitive therapy targets distorted thinking such as all-or-nothing thinking, jumping to conclusions, disqualifying the positive, overgeneralization, catastrophizing, etc. Therapy may include approaches such as challenging and changing maladaptive thoughts, recognizing inaccurate thinking, discussing the evidence for and against automatic thoughts, and adapting or changing problematic behaviors. Cognitive therapy is typically problem-focused and completed in about 20 sessions or less.[44]

One specific CBT approach for GAD is self-monitoring of anxiety, in which patients are requested to think about anxiety-provoking situations and become aware of the physical and mental reactions. The patient is taught to recognize these cues early and implement coping mechanisms before the anxiety escalates and becomes overwhelming. Other CBT approaches for GAD includes cognitive therapy techniques specific to anxiety-provoking thoughts and beliefs, imagery rehearsal of coping skills, and relaxation training.

Exposure therapy is well validated for the treatment of social anxiety disorder. Exposure therapy involves repeated exposure to the social situation with the expectation that the symptoms will diminish over time and allow the patient to engage socially without the overwhelming anxiety. Exposure and response prevention is effective for the treatment of OCD. Individuals are exposed to situations that provoke anxiety or fear and in which compulsory behavior subsequently occurs. These behaviors are suppressed with the expectation that the individual can learn to control the behavior and suppress the obsessive thoughts or desires. An example is exposing a person to a cluttered or disorganized closet and suppressing the desire to organize it.

An important distinction can be made in the types of dysfunctional beliefs that occur in the different obsessive-compulsive and related disorders. OCD generally involves irrational beliefs that cannot be factually supported, whereas HD and BDD generally involve distorted beliefs that often have a rational basis. For example, when considering BDD, it is understandable that one values personal appearance; however, it is a distortion of that belief if one believes one's entire worth is determined by something trivial that is judged to be a flaw. Individuals with HD do not believe in throwing away items that may be useful or have value; however, it is a distortion of that value to believe that nothing should ever be discarded. This distinction is important, as irrational beliefs are somewhat simpler to treat than distorted beliefs. It is generally easier to refute irrational beliefs than distorted beliefs as distorted beliefs are grounded in an extreme of acceptable beliefs or practices. Without recognition of distorted beliefs, motivation for treatment is poor because there is no reason to change the belief. This can create difficulty in the treatment of HD and BDD.[4]

Examples of some specific therapies used in PTSD include prolonged exposure, in vivo exposure by directly confronting the trigger, cognitive restructuring and processing, and relaxation techniques. Although CBT is found to be as effective, if not more so, than medication in the treatment of some anxiety disorders, the evidence is not as strong for PTSD treatment to suggest psychotherapy is more effective than pharmacotherapy. Another approach in treating PTSD is eye movement desensitization and reprocessing (EMDR),[45] which is the use of a patient's eye movements to decrease the power of emotionally charged memories of past traumatic events. The therapist directs eye movements of the patient while the patient recalls a disturbing event. Gradually, the therapist guides the patient to alter thinking to pleasant thoughts. A growing body of research indicates that trauma experiences negatively impact the individual leading to a variety of psychologic and physiologic symptoms. EMDR therapy research has shown that processing memories of such experiences can significantly decrease negative emotions, beliefs, and physical sensations related to the memory. Evidence indicates the potential for wider application for patients with stress-related disorders.

Occupational Therapy Approaches

In working with individuals with anxiety, obsessive-compulsive, and trauma- and stressor-related disorders, the OT identifies the areas of occupational performance that are of concern to the client and works with the client to set appropriate goals and treatment strategies. The occupational performance of these patients may be affected by difficulty with cognitive and physiologic hypersensitivity to threat, thereby negatively affecting occupational participation. Evaluating the sensory profile of individuals with posttraumatic stress (PTS) symptoms can be useful, and there is some evidence of hypersensitivity and low registration with PTS symptoms.[46] Sensory modulation intervention using calming sensory input can effectively manage the hypersensitivity and physiologic arousal associated with anxiety. There is evidence for sensory modulation approaches in community mental health service provision when strategies are used during task performance. Sensory modulation can support occupational engagement and participation in everyday life.[47] Sensory modulation strategies can also be implemented successfully in day programs by offering sensory tools and schemes to target debilitating hypervigilance and hyperarousal while engaging in community-living experiences.[48]

For individuals with OCD who describe a constant uncomfortable feeling of imperfection toward sensory stimuli referred to as "not just right experiences," addressing sensory over-responsivity to manage the sensory-cognitive experiences that lead to obsessive-compulsive symptoms may be warranted. This is rarely addressed in conventional approaches to OCD, and occupational therapy is well suited to provide appropriate intervention.[49] There is growing evidence for targeted sensory strategies including proprioceptive input,[50] deep pressure touch,[51-53] auditory input,[54-56] and olfactory input.[57] There is also evidence for the use of sensory rooms to manage acute anxiety.[58] Chapter 8 provides a more in-depth description of sensory modulation and approaches for occupational therapy practice, and Chapter 17 provides an in-depth discussion of trauma-informed care.

The role of the OT practitioner will be individualized for each client and may include a variety of approaches. Evaluation of the individual's daily routine can provide information related to stressors and potential triggers. Lack of a consistent routine or structure for daily activities and sleep can be stressful. Long commutes and noisy overstimulating environments can add unwanted stressors. Strategies to support occupational engagement, performance, and satisfaction for individuals with anxiety and stress-related disorders may vary depending on the population and the setting. For example, the value of occupational therapy in addressing combat and operational stress is presented in the literature.[59,60] Occupational therapy providers within the combat and operational stress control unit can provide targeted use of activity to maximize performance. OTs in this setting provide distinct services through focusing on functional performance skills that affect overall mission readiness and ability to handle stress.[59] The Kawa Model is used to address and implement culturally relevant occupation-based interventions that address the specific needs of this military population.[60] The Redesigning Daily Occupations (ReDO)-Program is targeted to assist women who have stress-related disorders and it supports return to work. The focus is on lifestyle changes through organizing and analyzing daily occupations. Strategies for change are implemented to support occupational performance.[61]

Complementary Approaches

There is growing evidence suggesting that complementary therapies may be beneficial as adjunctive treatments for anxiety.[62] Examples of complementary approaches include yoga, massage therapy, aromatherapy, pet therapy, Qigong, Reiki touch therapy, auricular acupressure, acupuncture, music therapy, and relaxation techniques.[62,63] A review of aquatic therapy found that it may be an effective modality in reducing symptoms of PTSD.[64] Therapeutic horseback riding as an intervention for combat veterans found a clinically significant decrease in PTSD symptoms, improved social functioning, improved vitality, less interference of emotions on daily activities, and increased participation. Exercise as a complementary approach has been researched and a review of the evidence from multiple randomized control trials indicates that exercise training can improve anxiety symptoms among healthy adults, patients with a chronic illness, and patients with panic disorder and GAD; these results are comparable to other treatments.[65,66] Mindfulness meditation approaches are increasingly promoted to address anxiety and stress. The first randomized control trials comparing the manualized Mindfulness-Based Stress Reduction program to a group intervention with active control for GAD suggest that mindfulness meditation training can reduce anxiety symptoms in patients with GAD.[67] Additionally, using nature to creating therapeutic outdoor environments for correctional staff at risk for high levels of stress was explored with favorable results and presented as a new role for occupational therapy.[68]

SUMMARY

Anxiety and trauma-related problems are common among the general population, and such problems affect physical and psychological functioning as well as occupational performance. Occupational therapy practitioners will work with clients with anxiety, obsessive-compulsive, and trauma- and stressor-related disorders in all practice settings. The client may be referred to occupational therapy for treatment of a physical diagnosis, yet present with anxiety or stress-related symptoms and behaviors impeding progress. There may be a mental health diagnosis, although oftentimes disorders such as PTSD are under recognized by medical practitioners. Occupational therapy's holistic approach and evaluation of occupational performance provides opportunity to recognize and address anxiety and stress and provide management approaches to maximize quality of life.

CASE STUDY 10.1   **Panic Disorder**

Steve is a 40-year-old divorced male diagnosed with panic attacks that have become gradually more severe for the past 4 months. He feels like he "may be dying" when these attacks occur, and his physician convinced him to attend an outpatient program for anxiety management offered two evenings a week at a behavioral health clinic. He is a chain smoker who started smoking at age 13. He admits to drinking "more alcohol than he should" several times a month but does not see that as a problem. He reports frequent restlessness and impaired concentration. He has always worked for himself in areas such as landscaping, printing, and real estate. He is currently working in real estate and he bartends one night a week. He sees himself as intelligent and has attended college off and on. He was briefly married at age 20 but the marriage only lasted 1 year. His wife left him; they did not have any children. Since then he has had several long-term relationships but has never remarried. After his

CASE STUDY 10.1 Panic Disorder—cont'd

divorce, he returned to his parents' home and lived there until 6 months ago when he moved into his current girlfriend's home. He states that he has no hobbies and he is not sure about participating in the program; he believes there is a physical reason for the anxiety attacks, and he will be getting a complete physical in the next 2 weeks. The outpatient program provides education on anxiety management, and sessions are co-led by clinical counselors and an OT. Each client participates in a 30-minute evaluation session with either the counselor or the OT prior to participating in the sessions.

Occupational Profile

Participants complete a questionnaire that includes questions about home life, work, relationships, current stressors, and goals. A semi-structured interview is conducted and participants are asked to identify their primary concerns, sources of anxiety/stress, and history of coping skills and strategies. The participant is asked to describe a typical weekday and weekend. The OT completes the interview with Steve. He presents as restless and distracted during the interview; he is constantly looking around, tapping his fingers, and fidgeting. He participates willingly in the interview but appears anxious. When asked how he is feeling, he denies anxiety and says he is just trying to get used to the environment. He states he would like a cigarette before the group starts.

Client's concerns: The panic attacks are very concerning and he does not understand why they are occurring.

Successful occupations: He denies any problems with ADLs or instrumental activities of daily living (IADLs). He states that he does not like to cook or clean, he does admit to being "messy" but has been trying harder to participate in chores and help his girlfriend keep the home they share clean. He keeps up with the news and socializes some with friends. He does not have any other leisure interests or hobbies.

Barriers: He states that his only barrier are the panic attacks he is experiencing.

Supports: His parents and girlfriend are supportive.

Occupational history: He prefers to work for himself and set his own hours; he has had several different jobs in the past. He states he is not very good at managing his money.

Daily life roles: He identifies with the roles of boyfriend, friend, son, and worker.

Current and past routines: He states his routine varies a lot depending on when he needs to work.

Client's priorities and desired targeted outcomes: Steve is focused on finding the physical reason for his anxiety attacks.

Analysis of Occupational Performance

There is not additional time for evaluation outside of the initial 30-minute session. Steve did complete the initial questionnaire, and when asked to describe his daily routine he states that his routine is never the same as he does not have structured job hours. He does not have consistent meal time or sleep/wake times, as it depends on what he needs to accomplish for the day. He states he is concerned about the quality of his work and social occupations due to increased restlessness, distraction, and increased worry about having a panic attack.

Intervention/Rationale

Group intervention is the only type of intervention provided in this program. The group sessions are educational and use a CBT approach that is problem-focused and incorporates skill-building. Steve participates in the following group sessions with the following outcomes:

- Self-monitoring of anxiety is introduced and participants begin to work on identifying physical and mental reactions to stress.
  - After the first two sessions, Steve starts to talk more about his ability to sense when a panic attack is beginning and identifies some potential triggers.
- Awareness of cues and strategies for implementing coping mechanisms prior to the panic attack are discussed.
  - Steve gradually begins to verbalize potential strategies and he is instructed to try using them.
- Negative coping mechanisms are discussed and Steve identifies tobacco use and alcohol use as negative coping mechanisms.
  - He states he can choose not to drink but he feels he cannot give up smoking at this time, as he has tried many times before without success. He admits that he likes smoking and has difficulty believing he can stop.
- Positive coping mechanisms are discussed and practiced, including deep breathing, guided imagery, progressive muscle relaxation, and mindfulness meditation.
  - Participants are given homework to practice one technique at home. Steve tries deep breathing and focusing on his breathing patterns and body awareness when he is in potentially stressful situations. He struggles with doing this and feels uncomfortable initially.

Continued

CASE STUDY 10.1 **Panic Disorder—cont'd**

- Sensory modulation is defined and sensory strategies for self-regulation are introduced.
  - Participants are given homework to incorporate one sensory strategy into daily routine. Steve is focusing on music for both calming and grounding. He states that he has always enjoyed music and can see how music can help with mood. He is motivated to build a personalized playlist of songs to incorporate into his routine.

Steve starts off apprehensive about attending the group session and later admits that he only started coming at the persistence of his girlfriend. He is eventually able to identify some potential triggers, and with encouragement he begins to experiment with different strategies. After 4 weeks he states that he feels much more aware of how his body reacts to stress and he is beginning to realize that he can use positive coping strategies to deal with stress and anxiety. He has difficulty with establishing a more consistent routine and addressing his smoking and use of alcohol as a coping mechanism. He agrees to continue attending the program.

CASE STUDY 10.2 **Generalized Anxiety Disorder**

MaryAnn is a 29-year-old female recently diagnosed with rheumatoid arthritis (RA). She was also diagnosed with generalized anxiety disorder in her early 20s. She is married and has one child, aged 8 months. She had experienced problems prior to her pregnancy, but it was not until after her son was born that she was diagnosed. She is experiencing a very severe flare-up, primarily in the small joints of bilateral hands, but affecting other joints as well. She was taking an SSRI prior to becoming pregnant and has not resumed taking it. She has received counseling for the anxiety disorder intermittently. MaryAnn was married at age 24. She has a college degree and is an elementary school teacher. She worked prior to the birth of her son but has not returned to work and is not sure if she will. She enjoys reading, cooking, scrapbooking, socializing, and shopping. She has a happy, stable marriage and her husband is supportive. She is very concerned about being able to take care of her son and about the prognosis of her illness. She would like to have one more child but she is concerned about her ability to care for another child. She is also concerned about finances—she had planned on resuming work when her child or children were in preschool; however, she is not sure that will be feasible. She is also concerned about the financial burden of a chronic illness on her family. Her weight is also of concern to her: she weighs 25 pounds more than she did before she was pregnant and she is having difficulty losing weight since the birth of her child. She has always struggled with her weight, finding it difficult to maintain her desired weight; she does not like to exercise and has always preferred more sedentary activities. She feels that her anxiety disorder is becoming worse now; however, she is reluctant to take medication for it since she is now taking medication for her RA. She was referred to outpatient occupational therapy to provide treatment for her RA through exercise, education, pain management, and ADLs.

Occupational Profile

The Canadian Occupational Performance Measure (COPM) is administered to structure the interview process, gather information, and assess the client's self-perception of occupational performance. MaryAnn presents as anxious and very focused on her physical concerns. She catastrophizes regarding the future and believes she will not be able to take care of her son and her home if her RA is not managed. She is willing to participate in OT sessions but presents with skepticism as to its efficacy.

Client's concerns: She believes she will get progressively worse and she is worried about her health, her ability to care for her family, and the financial implications of her illness.

Barriers: She feels her RA is a barrier to her future well-being.

Supports: Her husband and her parents are supportive.

Occupational history: She previously taught school and enjoyed it. She has several leisure interests.

Values and interests: She values being a good mother and taking care of her family. She valued teaching and helping others.

Daily life roles: Mother, wife, homemaker, daughter, friend, former teacher.

Current and past routines: She maintains a consistent routine taking care of her son and her home; however, she no longer works outside of the home and her ADLs and IADLs sometimes take longer to complete depending on how she is feeling physically.

Client's priorities and desired targeted outcomes: She wants to be able to take care of her son and her home without difficulty and she would like to have another child.

CASE STUDY 10.2 Generalized Anxiety Disorder—cont'd

Analysis of Occupational Performance

Occupations: Currently MaryAnn can complete all ADLs and IADLs most of the time with some modifications. When she has acute exacerbations, or is experiencing increased pain, she requires more assistance and has difficulty with tasks requiring increased fine motor co-ordination and hand strength.

Client factors: She presents with distorted beliefs, stating she will continue to get worse and have increased difficulty with her occupations. She also presents with irrational beliefs such as "If I cannot continue to take care of my family and home in the same way, I will not be a good wife and mother."

Intervention/Rationale

MaryAnn is provided with an exercise program, customized joint protection and work simplification techniques, appropriate adaptive devices, and strategies for organizing her home and routine. Her anxiety is a barrier as she is consumed with worry about the future and spends excessive time focusing on these concerns. She expresses concern about her ability to continue doing what she is currently able to do and often stops during therapy and perseverates her concerns. She continues to be resistant to medication. The OT uses CBT techniques to target her dysfunctional assumptions and to keep her focused on the present and what she is currently able to do. She is encouraged to reframe her thinking to accept that doing something differently is good enough if she can continue doing it; for example, there may be some tasks that she cannot do at times and she can plan to approach the task differently or plan to have assistance to complete the task. She is asked to rate the importance of different activities, and therapy is focused on the most important tasks initially to build her confidence through success. She is also encouraged to create new self-statements such as "I am a good mother because I spend time reading to my son." She makes a list of meaningful activities she can engage in with her family that do not increase physical stress on her joints. She is also encouraged to incorporate different relaxation techniques into her routine and she expresses interest in learning new techniques. Future sessions will explore techniques that can enhance her occupational functioning.

CASE STUDY 10.3 Obsessive-Compulsive Disorder

Dawn is a 31-year-old female participating in a mental health program at the community mental health department. Dawn reports elaborate cleaning and washing rituals. She is concerned with exposure to germs and anything considered dirty. She is specifically fearful of contracting the flu or a respiratory infection that will require hospitalization, and she is fearful of being hospitalized and exposed to other patients. Her rituals include elaborate handwashing routines, excessive showering, and lengthy wiping and cleaning rituals of certain items such as doorknobs. She spends many hours a day obsessing about exposure to germs and ways to avoid germs. Her behaviors developed in her 20s and have become increasingly worse. She is not married; she worked as a bookkeeper but was let go due to her decreased productivity at work; and she lives at home with her parents who are greatly concerned about her mental health. She is attending weekly occupational therapy group sessions focused on coping skills.

Occupational Profile

COPM is administered to structure the interview process, gather information, and assess the client's self-perception of occupational performance. Dawn presents as anxious and is fixated on the need to avoid exposure to germs.

Client's concerns: Dawn can verbalize awareness that her compulsive handwashing and other rituals are irrational, but she is not able to stop her behaviors.

Successful occupations: Dawn is not able to identify successful occupations.

Barriers: She states that her obsessive thoughts and behaviors are a barrier to her ability to engage in meaningful occupations.

Supports: Her parents are supportive.

Occupational history: She previously worked as a bookkeeper and states she was good at her job and enjoyed it.

Values and interests: She is not able to identify any values or interests.

Daily life roles: It takes her a long time to complete her ADLs each day due to her compulsions; she also spends time watching TV or browsing the internet.

Client's priorities and desired targeted outcomes: She states she wants to be normal again; she recognizes that she cannot continue to engage in her compulsory behaviors but does not know how to stop.

Continued

CASE STUDY 10.3   Obsessive-Compulsive Disorder—cont'd

Analysis of Occupational Performance

Dawn presents with obsessions and compulsory behaviors that greatly impact her occupational performance. She spends excessive time on her rituals and expresses irrational beliefs associated with cleanliness. She is no longer able to maintain her job or social relationships, and she does not have any significant meaningful occupations.

Intervention/Rationale

Dawn is being seen by the mental health center physician and is being treated with an SSRI. Her physician refers her for individual counseling with a clinical counselor for CBT, specifically exposure and response-prevention therapy. She is also referred to attend weekly occupational therapy groups at the mental health center to learn coping skills. Group sessions use a CBT approach and focus on identification of stressors, skill-building, and wellness. Group participants include individuals with anxiety, obsessive-compulsive, and trauma- and stressor-related disorders. For the first 4 weeks, Dawn participates very little in the group sessions but she does comply with her medication. She slowly becomes more engaged as she feels more in control of her compulsory behaviors.

Dawn participates in the following group sessions with the following outcomes:

- Educational session with a discussion on defining and discussing irrational thoughts and distorted thinking; potential neurobiological and psychosocial causes are discussed.
  - Dawn is very interested in understanding OCD and feels supported by the group members.
- Positive coping mechanisms including deep breathing and mindfulness meditation for dealing with stress are discussed and practiced.
  - Dawn is interested in mindfulness as she has read about it previously, but she has never been motivated to try it. She agrees to try mindfulness at least once a day when she has obsessive thoughts.
- Importance of structure and balance in daily routines is discussed and participants complete a daily schedule identifying different wellness activities that are included or not included.
  - Dawn recognizes the amount of time her compulsory behaviors require and the lack of balance she has in her daily life. She creates her ideal schedule and makes a goal to incorporate one new meaningful occupation into her schedule. She wants to reengage in social relationships but is fearful of meeting people in public. She also wants to return to work so she decides to enroll in an online accounting course to maintain her skills and develop advanced skills.

Dawn continues to experience obsessive thoughts and the urge to engage in previous compulsory behaviors; however, she is gradually learning how to deal with them. She understands that she needs to continue taking her medication and incorporate coping strategies into her daily life. She continues to participate in the group sessions with her primary goal of adding more meaningful occupations into her routine, returning to work, and developing meaningful relationships.

SUGGESTED LEARNING ACTIVITIES

1. Make a list of the things you do to manage stress and anxiety on a daily/weekly basis. What works best for you and why?
2. Try a stress management or relaxation technique you have not tried before such as mindfulness, music, or yoga. Evaluate its effectiveness for you.
3. Explore apps designed for relaxation, meditation, and managing anxiety and stress. Use each one for a week at a time and compare how well each works for you.

REFLECTION QUESTIONS

1. If possible, interview someone who has been diagnosed with one of the obsessive-compulsive or related disorders or a trauma- and stressor-related disorder. What occupations were most affected by the disorder? What, if anything, has worked best to alleviate symptomology for this person?
2. Reflect on a time when you were extremely anxious, fearful, or experienced a panic attack. If possible,

identify the source of the stress or fear and how you felt at the time. What behaviors did you exhibit? How long did the episode or feelings persist and how did you resolve the situation? What occupations were most affected?

3. What complementary approaches for managing anxiety and stress do you believe has the most evidence-based support? Should more emphasis be placed on the use of complementary approaches instead of medication? Why or why not?

REFERENCES

1. Craske MG, Stein MB. Anxiety. *Lancet.* 2016;388:3048-3059.
2. World Health Organization. *Depression and Other Common Mental Disorders: Global Health Estimates.* Geneva, Switzerland: WHO; 2017. Document Production Services. License: CC BY-NC-SA 3.0 IGO.
3. National Alliance on Mental Illness. *Anxiety Disorders.* December, 2017. Available at: https://www.nami.org/Learn-More/Mental-Health-Conditions/Anxiety-Disorders.
4. Zupanick CE. *The New DSM-5: Anxiety Disorders and Obsessive-Compulsive Disorders.* 2018. Available at: https://www.mentalhelp.net/articles/the-new-dsm-5-anxiety-disorders-and-obsessive-compulsive-disorders/.
5. Locke AB, Kirst N, Shultz CG. Diagnosis and management of Generalized Anxiety Disorder and Panic Disorder in adults. *Am Fam Physician.* 2015;91:617-624.
6. Carmassi C, Gesi1 C, Massimetti E, Shear MK, Dell'Osso L. Separation anxiety disorder in the DSM-5 era. *J Psychopathol.* 2015;21:365-371.
7. Selective Mutism Foundation. *Selective mutism in the DSM.* 2018. Available at: https://www.selectivemutismfoundation.org/knowledge-center/articles/view-selective-mutism-in-the-dsm.
8. Fritscher L. *DSM-5 Diagnostic Criteria for a Specific Phobia.* 2018. Available at: https://www.verywellmind.com/diagnosing-a-specific-phobia-2671981.
9. Mental Health America. *Social Anxiety Disorder.* 2018. Available at: http://www.mentalhealthamerica.net/conditions/social-anxiety-disorder.
10. Star K. *New Diagnostic Criteria for Panic Disorder, Agoraphobia.* Available at: https://www.verywellmind.com/new-diagnostic-criteria-for-panic-disorders-2583933.
11. International OCD Foundation. *About OCD: What is OCD?* 2018. Available at: https://iocdf.org/about-ocd/
12. Krebs G, Fernández de la Cruz L, Mataix-Cols D. Recent advances in understanding and managing body dysmorphic disorder. *Evid Based Ment Health.* 2017;20:71-75.
13. Frost RO, Hartl TL. A cognitive-behavioral model of compulsive hoarding. *Behav Res Ther.* 1996;34:341-350.
14. American Psychiatric Association. *Diagnostic and Statistical Manual of Mental Disorders.* 5th ed. Washington, DC: American Psychiatric Association; 2013.
15. Vilaverde D, Gonçalves J, Morgado P. Hoarding disorder: a case report. *Front Psychiatry.* 2017;8:1-5.
16. Woods DW, Houghton DC. Diagnosis, evaluation, and management of trichotillomania. *Psychiatr Clin North Am.* 2014;37:301-317.
17. Lochner C, Roos A, Stein DJ. Excoriation (skin-picking) disorder: a systematic review of treatment options. *Neuropsychiatr Dis Treat.* 2017;13:1867-1872.
18. Traumadissociation.com. *Reactive Attachment Disorder.* September 25, 2018. Available at: http://traumadissociation.com/rad.html.
19. Traumadissociation.com. *Disinhibited Social Engagement Disorder.* September 25, 2018 Available at: http://traumadissociation.com/disinhibited.html.
20. Traumadissociation.com. *Posttraumatic Stress Disorder.* November 25, 2018. Available at: http://traumadissociation.com/ptsd.html.
21. US Department of Health and Human Services, National Institutes of Health, National Institute of Mental Health. *Post-Traumatic Stress Disorder.* (NIH Publication No. QF 16-6388). Sept 15, 2018. Available at: https://www.nimh.nih.gov/health/publications/post-traumatic-stress-disorder-ptsd/ptsd-508-05172017_38054.pdf.
22. Mayo Clinic. *Adjustment Disorders.* 2018. Available at: https://www.mayoclinic.org/diseases-conditions/adjustment-disorders/symptoms-causes/syc-20355224.
23. Spielberger CD, Gorsuch RL, Lushene R, Vagg PR, Jacobs GA. *Manual for the State-Trait Anxiety.* Palo Alto, CA: Consulting Psychologists Press; 1983
24. Leal PC, Goes TC, da Silva LCF, Teixeira-Silva F. Trait vs. state anxiety in different threatening situations. *Trends Psychiatry Psychother.* 2017;39:147-157.
25. Spielberger CD. *State-Trait Anxiety Inventory: Bibliography.* 2nd ed. Palo Alto, CA: Consulting Psychologists Press; 1989.
26. Holmes TH, Rahe RH. The Social Readjustment Rating Scale. *J Psychosom Res.* 1967;11:213-218.
27. Noone PA. *The Holmes-Rahe Stress Inventory. Occup Med.* 2017;67:581-582.
28. Spitzer RL, Kroenke K, Williams JB, Löwe B. A brief measure for assessing generalized anxiety disorder: the GAD-7. *Arch Intern Med.* 2006;166:1092-1097.
29. Marris M, Sladyk K, St Pierre B, Dey EC. Reliability and validity of the Current Anxiety Level Measure. *Occup Ther Ment Health.* 2017;33:386-393.
30. Rapp AM, Bergman RL, Piacentini J, McGuire JF. Evidence-based assessment of obsessive–compulsive disorder. *J Cent Nerv Syst Dis.* 2016;8:13-29.
31. US Department of Veterans Affairs. *PTSD: National Center for PTSD. PTSD Screening and Referral: For Health Care Providers.* 2018. Available at: https://www.ptsd.va.gov/professional/treat/care/screening_referral.asp.
32. Prins A, Ouimette P, Kimerling R, et al. The primary care PTSD screen (PC-PTSD): development and operating characteristics. *Prim Care Psychiatry.* 2003;9:9-14.
33. Prins A, Ouimette P, Kimerling R, et al. The primary care PTSD screen (PC-PTSD): corrigendum. *Prim Care Psychiatry.* 2004;9:151.

34. U. S. Department of Veterans Affairs. *PTSD: National Center for PTSD. List of All Measures.* 2018. Available at: https://www.ptsd.va.gov/professional/assessment/list_measures.asp#list2.

35. American Occupational Therapy Association. Occupational therapy practice framework: domain & process (3rd ed.). *Am J Occup Ther.* 2014;68(suppl 1):S1-S51.

36. Law MC, Baptiste S, Carswell A, Mccoll MA, Polatajko H, Pollock N. *Canadian Occupational Performance Measure Manual (COPM).* 4th ed. Thorofare, NJ: Slack Inc.; 2005.

37. Kielhofner G, Mallinson T, Crawford D, Nowak M, Rigby M, Henry A. *Users Manual for the OPHI-II. Version 2.1.* Model of Human Occupation Clearinghouse. Chicago, IL: University of Illinois; 2004.

38. Smith K. *Anxiety Medications.* February, 2018. Available at: https://www.psycom.net/anxiety-medications/.

39. Pittman C. *What You Need to Know About SSRIs.* 2016. Available at: https://www.anxiety.org/selective-serotonin-reuptake-inhibitor-ssri.

40. Pittman C. *What You Need to Know About Your SNRI.* 2017. Available at: https://www.anxiety.org/serotonin-norepinephrine-reuptake-inhibitor-snri.

41. National Institute of Mental Health. *Anxiety Disorders.* 2018. Available at: https://www.nimh.nih.gov/health/topics/anxiety-disorders/index.shtml.

42. National Alliance on Mental Illness. *Buspirone (Buspar).* October, 2016. Available at: https://www.nami.org/Learn-More/Treatment/Mental-Health-Medications/Types-of-Medication/Buspirone-(BuSpar).

43. National Alliance on Mental Illness. *Hydroxyzine (Vistaril, Atarax).* October, 2016. Available at: https://www.nami.org/Learn-More/Treatment/Mental-Health-Medications/Types-of-Medication/Hydroxyzine-(Vistaril%C2%AE-Atarax%C2%AE).

44. Kaczkurkin AN, Foa EB. Cognitive-behavioral therapy for anxiety disorders: an update on the empirical evidence. *Dialogues Clin Neurosci,* 2015;17(3):337-346.

45. Shapiro F. The role of Eye Movement Desensitization and Reprocessing (EMDR) therapy in medicine: addressing the psychological and physical symptoms stemming from adverse life experiences. *Perm J.* 2014;18:71-77.

46. Engel-Yeger B, Palgy-Levin D, Lev-Wiesel, R. The sensory profile of people with post-traumatic stress symptoms. *Occup Ther Ment Health.* 2013;29:266-278.

47. Wallis K, Sutton D, Bassett S. Sensory modulation for people with anxiety in a community mental health setting. *Occup Ther Ment Health.* 2018;34:122-137.

48. Holland J, Begin D, Orris D, Meyer A. A descriptive analysis of the theory and processes of an innovative day program for young women with trauma-related symptoms. *Occup Ther Ment Health.* 2018;34:228-241.

49. Ben-Sasson A, Dickstein N, Lazarovich L, Ayalon N. Not just right experiences: association with obsessive compulsive symptoms and sensory over-responsivity. *Occup Ther Ment Health.* 2017;33:217-234.

50. Mollo K, Schaaf RC, Benevides TB. The use of kripalu yoga to decrease sensory overresponsivity: a pilot study. *Sens Integr Spec Interest Sect Q.* 2008;31:1-8.

51. Heard CP, Tetzlaff A, Fryer P, et al. Mechanical chair massage and stress reduction in the seriously mentally ill consumer: a preliminary investigation. *Occup Ther Ment Health.* 2012; 28:111-117.

52. Kimball JG, Cao L, Draleau KS. Efficacy of the Wilbarger Therapressure Program™ to modulate arousal in women with post-traumatic stress disorder: a pilot study using salivary cortisol and behavioral measures. *Occup Ther Ment Health.* 2018;34:86-101.

53. Mullen B, Champagne T, Krishnamurty S, Dickson D, Gao RX. Exploring the safety and therapeutic effects of deep pressure stimulation using a weighted blanket. *Occup Ther Ment Health.* 2008;24:65-89.

54. Canbeyli R. Sensorimotor modulation of mood and depression: an integrative review. *Behav Brain Res.* 2010;207:249-264.

55. Champagne T, Koomar J. Expanding the focus: addressing sensory discrimination concerns in mental health. *Ment Health Spec Interest Sect Q/Am Occup Ther Assoc.* 2011;34(1):1-4.

56. Paula D, Luis P, Pereira OR, Joao SM. Aromatherapy in the control of stress and anxiety. *Altern Integr Med.* 2017;6(4):1-5.

57. Maddocks-Jennings W, Wilkinson JM. Aromatherapy practice in nursing: literature review. *J Adv Nurs.* 2004;48:93-103.

58. Champagne T, Stromberg N. Sensory approaches in inpatient psychiatric settings: innovative alternatives to seclusion and restraint. *J Psychosoc Nurs Ment Health Serv.* 2004;42:34-44.

59. Baumann ML, Brown AN, Quick CD, Breuer ST, Smith-Forbes EV. (2018). Translating occupational therapy's current role within U.S. Army combat and operational stress control operations. *Occup Ther Ment Health.* 2018;34: 258-271. doi:10.1080/0164212X.2018.1425952.

60. Gregg BT, Howell DH, Quick CD, Iwama MK. The Kawa River Model: applying theory to develop interventions for combat and operational stress control. *Occup Ther Ment Health.* 2015;31:366-384.

61. Erlandsson, L. The Redesigning Daily Occupations (ReDO)-Program: supporting women with stress-related disorders to return to work—knowledge base, structure, and content. *Occup Ther Ment Health.* 2013;29:85-101.

62. Sagarwala R, Nasrallah HA. Complementary treatments for anxiety: beyond pharmacotherapy and psychotherapy. *Curr Psychiatry.* 2018;17:29-36.

63. Lanning BA, Wilson AL, Krenek N, Beaujean AA. Using therapeutic riding as an intervention for combat veterans: an international classification of functioning, disability, and health (ICF) approach. *Occup Ther Ment Health.* 2017;33:259-278.

64. Herold B, Stanley A, Oltrogge K, et al. post-traumatic stress disorder, sensory integration, and aquatic therapy: a scoping review. *Occup Ther Ment Health.* 2016;32:392-399.

65. Herring MP, Lindheimer JB, O'Connor PJ. The effects of exercise training on anxiety. *Am J Lifestyle Med.* 2014;8:388-403.

66. Jayakody K, Gunadasa S, Hosker C. Exercise for anxiety disorders: systematic review. *Br J Sports Med.* 2014;48:187-196.

67. Hoge EA, Bui E, Marques L, et al. Randomized controlled trial of mindfulness meditation for generalized anxiety disorder: effects on anxiety and stress reactivity. *J Clin Psychiatry.* 2013; 74:786-792.

68. Wagenfeld A, Stevens J, Toews B, et al. Addressing correctional staff stress through interaction with nature: a new role for occupational therapy. *Occup Ther Ment Health.* 2018;34:285-304.

11

Schizophrenia

Nancy Carson

LEARNING OBJECTIVES

1. Identify the criteria for schizophrenia spectrum disorders as defined by the DSM-5.
2. Describe the symptomology of the different schizophrenia spectrum disorders.
3. Recognize assessment methods for schizophrenia spectrum disorders.
4. Discuss treatment approaches for schizophrenia spectrum disorders, including psychopharmacology and psychotherapeutic approaches.
5. Articulate the role of occupational therapy in the treatment of schizophrenia spectrum disorders.
6. Discuss the concept of functional recovery for individuals diagnosed with schizophrenia.

INTRODUCTION

Schizophrenia is a serious psychiatric disorder that has a lifetime risk of approximately 1%.[1] It remains a mysterious, frightening, and devastating illness to many. Reports of behaviors similar to the current-day understanding of schizophrenia can be found in ancient writings. The modern concept of schizophrenia was first presented as a distinct mental disorder by the German psychiatrist Emil Kraepelin in 1887. He named the disorder *dementia praecox* and identified it as a form of early dementia, to be distinguished from other forms of dementia (such as Alzheimer disease) that typically occur late in life.[1] The word *schizophrenia* was coined by Eugen Bleuler, a Swiss psychiatrist, in 1911, and it replaced the term *dementia praecox*. The former name was misleading, as the illness did not always lead to mental deterioration. Bleuler also made distinctions of the symptoms, as he was the first to describe the positive and negative symptoms that occur in the illness.[1]

Modern-day understanding of schizophrenia is still limited. For many people, the 2001 Academy Award winning film, *A Beautiful Mind*, based on the life of John Nash, is the best representation of understanding the tormented mind of someone with schizophrenia. The movie is based on Sylvia Nasar's Pulitzer Prize–nominated 1998 book[2] of the same name. John Nash was a Nobel Laureate in Economics. Although his intelligence was undeniable, his mind was consumed with delusions and hallucinations. However, for most people with the diagnosis, there are also significant cognitive deficits that impede functional performance and daily life. The cognitive deficits have received more attention in recent years.[3] Recovery of functional skills and symptom remission remains difficult for many individuals with the disease, despite the progress in therapeutic approaches.[4,5]

SCHIZOPHRENIA SPECTRUM AND OTHER PSYCHOTIC DISORDERS

The word *schizophrenia* comes from the Greek roots of *schizo* meaning "split" and *phrene* meaning "mind" and is meant to describe fragmented thinking as opposed to the idea of split or multiple personalities, which is a common misunderstanding by many lay people. Bleuler defined it as "a mind that is torn asunder."[1] The Diagnostic and Statistical Manual of Mental Disorders, 5th Ed. (DSM-5),[6] lists schizophrenia in the category of Schizophrenia Spectrum and Other Psychotic Disorders. This category also includes the following diagnoses:

- Delusional Disorder
- Brief Psychotic Disorder
- Schizophreniform Disorder
- Schizoaffective Disorder
- Substance/Medication-Induced Psychotic Disorder
- Psychotic Disorder Due to Another Medical Condition
  Schizotypal (Personality) Disorder is listed under this category as well as the category of Personality Disorders in the DSM-5 and is discussed in Chapter 14. Previously, a catatonic subtype was also included in this category but it has been eliminated in DSM-5; instead, a catatonic specifier has been added and may be used with various mental and medical disorders or may be unspecified catatonia.[6]

Symptoms of Psychotic Disorders

There are five key symptoms of psychotic disorders; they include delusions, hallucinations, disorganized speech, disorganized or catatonic behavior, and negative symptoms.[7] They can be categorized as positive, negative, and cognitive symptoms.[3] Positive symptoms are those that are easily identified or observed in the person. They include delusions, hallucinations, and abnormal motor behavior.[3] Negative symptoms are harder to observe and diagnose, as they reflect a loss or absence of something. It is usually the positive symptoms that result in hospitalization or treatment, whereas negative symptoms are more easily overlooked. Negative symptoms include blunted affect, alogia, asociality, anhedonia, and avolition.[8,9] Cognitive symptoms include disorganized speech, thought, and/or attention.[3] Difficulty with executive function and working memory may be present.[10] Cognition as related to emotional regulation and social cognition have been studied, including theory of mind processes. Perception of emotion is impaired in some individuals, and emotion regulation may be diminished due to reduced cognitive control of emotion.[11]

Positive Symptoms

A delusion is a belief that an individual has that is not real. It is not explained by the person's cultural or religious background or level of intelligence. The person firmly clings to the belief regardless of evidence that indicates it is not true. It is different from an overvalued or unreasonable idea in which the person has at least some level of doubt as to its truthfulness. A person with a delusion is absolutely convinced that the delusion is real.[12]

Delusions can be categorized as bizarre or non-bizarre delusions. Bizarre delusions are strong beliefs that are obviously not true, as they are not logical or plausible. An example might be believing that a radio transmitter has been implanted in one's brain by an alien who is listening to the person's every thought. Non-bizarre delusions are strong beliefs that could be true but are not true. It is verifiable that the belief is not true, yet the person still believes it to be true. An example is believing a close friend or family member is terminally ill despite denial and lack of evidence to support the belief.

There are different types or themes of delusions that may develop with psychosis. Persecutory delusions are those in which the person believes that they or someone close to them is being mistreated or they believe that someone is planning to harm them. Persecutory delusions may lead the individual to contact legal authorities multiple times to request intervention or to file a complaint or concern. Grandiose delusions are evident as an overinflated sense of self-worth, power, knowledge, or identity. The belief that one possesses extraordinary talent or has made a significant contribution may be evident. A somatic delusion is the belief that one has a physical defect or medical problem. The belief may focus on an abnormal body function, sensation, or belief that one's physical appearance is abnormal. The belief that one's spouse or partner is unfaithful is another type of delusion, categorized as jealous. There is no evidence of the behavior, and denial may be voiced, but the individual continues to believe the behavior has occurred.[13]

Hallucinations are sensory perceptions that occur without the presence of the corresponding external or somatic stimuli. A person may or may not be aware that a hallucination is occurring. Lack of awareness of a hallucination indicates a psychotic symptom. This is distinguished from a hallucination in which the individual is conscious of the experience not being grounded in reality, e.g., the visual hallucinations of migraine aura and sleep transition–related hallucinations. Hallucinations can be experienced in any of the sensory domains. The most frequent type of hallucination is an auditory hallucination. This type may involve hearing voices conversing with one another, or providing a running commentary on one's actions, or there may be an experience of hearing one's own thoughts spoken out loud. The second most frequent hallucination is visual, followed by tactile, olfactory, and gustatory.[14]

Visual hallucinations occur in 50% of people who have auditory hallucinations. Visual hallucinations in the absence of auditory hallucinations occur less frequently. Those individuals who experience auditory hallucinations are also more likely to experience olfactory and tactile hallucinations. Gustatory hallucinations are rarely reported.[15] Visual hallucinations are generally reported to be projected into the external world and are often life-sized, fullyformed, and dynamic, although they can be static.

They may include images of people, faces, animals, objects, or events. They may be frightening and associated with distress, or they may be non-frightening visions. They may be seen as black and white or in color. They are perceived to be real, and the person may respond behaviorally as in moving away for safety from a frightening hallucination. There is a lack of control over the content and appearance of hallucinations, and they may be rare or frequent, lasting several seconds to several minutes.[16]

Abnormal motor behavior refers to a range of reduced and involuntary movements. Abnormal motor behavior may include bradykinesia, parakinesia, or dyskinesia; spontaneous and tardive dyskinesias include abnormal, involuntary, and repetitive movements of the face, limb, and trunk muscles; abnormal involuntary face movements, grimacing, tics, or mannerisms; rigidity or catatonia; or parkinsonism.[17] Catatonia is a syndrome of abnormal motor behavior including posturing, mannerisms, immobility, rigor, catalepsy, grimacing, and waxy flexibility.[17] Muscle rigidity and bradykinesia are the most frequently reported parkinsonian signs in schizophrenia.[18] At least one abnormal motor symptom has been reported to be prevalent in 66% of first-episode, never-medicated patients,[19] and in 59% of patients upon hospital admission.[20]

Negative Symptoms

Negative symptoms are characterized by significant reductions in goal-directed behavior that results in reduced initiative and social withdrawal. They involve an absence of or deficits in experiences that are usually present in those individuals without illness. Negative symptoms tend to last longer than positive symptoms and are more difficult to treat.[21] Blunted affect, or affective flattening, refers to decreased emotional expression. There is a lack of, or minimal, facial and vocal expression. Alogia, or poverty of speech, is decreased speech resulting in little or no verbal expression or decreased verbal speed in communication. Asociality is a decreased interest in spending time with others including friends or family members. There is no apparent motivation to build or sustain meaningful relationships, resulting in social isolation. Anhedonia is a decreased ability to experience pleasure in activities that one would usually enjoy. Anticipatory pleasure may be affected more than in-the-moment pleasure, depending on the activity. A person may find pleasure in an activity that provides physical needs such as eating while engaged in the act of eating, but may not be able to think ahead with pleasure about the experience of eating. Avolition is the inability to initiate an activity and follow through to complete the task. The negative symptoms fall into two overarching domains: blunted affect and alogia can be conceptualized as diminished expression, and avolition,

anhedonia, and asociality can be conceptualized as diminished motivation and pleasure.[8]

Cognitive Symptoms

Impairments in a broad range of cognitive abilities have been consistently reported in people diagnosed with schizophrenia.[22] Cognition and cognitive deficits are discussed in Chapter 7. Cognitive and intellectual underperformance are considered risk factors for schizophrenia, and research indicates that a decline in cognitive functioning precedes the onset of psychosis by almost a decade. Cognitive decline may continue after diagnosis and is related to functional outcome.[23] An initiative of the National Institute of Mental Health (NIMH) focused on identifying the cognitive domains that are impaired in patients with schizophrenia. This initiative, the Measurement and Treatment Research to Improve Cognition in Schizophrenia (MATRICS) project, identified seven distinct cognitive domains that are impaired: speed of processing, attention/vigilance, working memory, verbal and visual learning, reasoning and problem solving, and social cognition.[24]

Social cognition includes impairments in facial affect recognition, in perceiving and interpreting social cues, theory of mind, and understanding causality.[25] Both social cognitive and neurocognitive impairments are believed to contribute to the severe functional disabilities associated with schizophrenia.[26-28] The influence of cognition on functional outcomes impacts the ability to perform critical everyday living skills,[29] therefore improvement in cognitive functions has become an increasingly significant goal in the treatment of schizophrenia.[30]

Schizophrenia

Schizophrenia is a severe and chronic mental disorder that can be difficult to diagnose, as it involves a range of cognitive, behavioral, and emotional symptoms that negatively impact social or occupational functioning and self-care. Symptoms usually present between the mid-teens and mid-30s. The peak age of onset of the first psychotic episode for males is generally in the early to mid-20s and for females it is in the late 20s. The cognitive impairments resulting from the disorder may continue to be recognized even when other symptoms are in remission.[31]

For a diagnosis of schizophrenia, two of the five key symptoms of psychotic disorders must be present and at least one symptom must be either delusions, hallucinations, or disorganized speech.[6] This varies from previous diagnostic criteria that only required one of the five symptoms if there were bizarre delusions present, or if hallucinations involved a persistent dialogue about the person's thoughts or behavior, and/or if there were two or more voices conversing. This was not included in DSM-5 due to poor reliability. It was determined to be too difficult to ascertain what is bizarre in nature, and it could also be culturally biased.[7] Impairment in either work, interpersonal relations, or self-care must also be present, and some signs of the disorder must extend for 6 months to be diagnosed.[31]

Another difference present in the DSM-5 is the elimination of types of schizophrenia. The previous version of the DSM[6] included five types of schizophrenia: disorganized, catatonic, paranoid, residual, and undifferentiated. These types were eliminated, as they were not helpful in predicting outcome and were not reliably diagnosed.[7]

Schizoaffective Disorder

Schizoaffective disorder can be described as a disorder with both mood and psychotic features. Schizoaffective disorder includes a mood episode that is present the majority of the time.[7] The disorder can be differentiated into a depressive type and a manic type. A depressive episode is present in the depressive type and a manic or mixed episode is present in the manic type.[32] Schizoaffective disorder can be difficult to diagnose because of the presence of symptoms from two different diagnoses occurring at the same time. This also makes it difficult to determine the number of people affected. It is believed to be less common than both schizophrenia and affective disorder alone. The lifetime prevalence of schizoaffective disorder is estimated to be 0.32%. The depressive type is seen more in older individuals and the bipolar type is more common in younger adults.[32]

The symptoms of schizoaffective disorder are a combination of the symptoms of schizophrenia and either depression or bipolar disorder. This makes it difficult to determine the diagnosis, and it takes time to distinguish between schizoaffective disorder, schizophrenia, and mood disorders. Symptoms of a mood disorder (severe mood changes) and schizophrenia (psychotic symptoms such as hallucinations, delusions, and disorganized thinking) need to be present simultaneously for a minimum of 2 weeks to be diagnosed with schizoaffective disorder. Symptoms of schizoaffective disorder can vary greatly from person to person and can range from mild to severe, making it more difficult to diagnose.[32]

Delusional Disorder

Delusional disorder is a mental illness in which bizarre or non-bizarre delusions are present as the primary symptom for at least one month. Delusional disorder was previously called paranoid disorder. As compared to schizophrenia it is relatively rare. The prevalence of delusional disorder in the United States is estimated to be around 0.02%.[6] It usually occurs in middle or late adulthood, and overall psychosocial functioning is not markedly impaired; however, problems arise that are directly related to the delusional belief. The delusions may appear at first to be a misinterpretation of perceptions or experiences, but upon closer examination it is evident that the situations are either extremely exaggerated or simply false. The individual may continue to function in a normal fashion with no evidence of odd or bizarre behavior except for direct references to the delusional belief. This varies from behavior in other disorders when delusions are a symptom of the disorder. It is also possible for the individual to experience more in-depth impairment of daily functioning if there is increased preoccupation with the subject of the delusion.[13]

Brief Psychotic Disorder

Brief psychotic disorder is an episode that may be as brief as 1 day and no more than 1 month in which one or more of the following symptoms are present: delusions, hallucinations, disorganized speech, or grossly disorganized or catatonic behavior. After the brief episode the person returns to their previous functional level. It is more typical to occur in an individual's late 20s or early 30s. It may occur as a result of extreme stress but cannot be diagnosed as the result of consumption of a substance or drug that results in a physiological reaction of this nature. If a brief psychotic disorder is suspected and the symptoms persist for longer than 1 month, a diagnosis of schizophrenia is considered.[33]

ASSESSMENT

There are no physical diagnostic tests that are used to diagnose schizophrenia spectrum disorders. A physician will determine the diagnosis based on the presence of clinical symptoms after ruling out other conditions that could be contributing to the symptomology, such as seizure disorders, a brain tumor, illicit drug use, or metabolic disorders. There are tools available for rating the presence and degree of intensity of clinical symptoms and tools for assessing occupational functioning.

Brief Psychiatric Rating Scale (BPRS)[34,35]

The BPRS is one of the oldest, most widely used scales to measure psychotic symptoms. It was developed in 1962 and includes 18 items to assess the following psychiatric constructs: somatic concern, anxiety, emotional withdrawal, conceptual disorganization, guilt feelings, tension, mannerisms and posturing, grandiosity, depressive mood, hostility, suspiciousness, hallucinatory behavior, motor retardation, uncooperativeness, unusual thought content, blunted affect, excitement, and disorientation. Each item is rated on a scale from 1 (not present) to 7 (extremely severe). Ratings are based on the clinician's interview with the client and observations of the client's behavior over the previous 2–3 days. It is useful in gauging the efficacy of treatment in individuals with serious psychopathology. The BPRS can be administered and scored in 20–30 minutes.

Positive and Negative Syndrome Scale (PANSS)[36,37]

The PANSS was developed in 1987 and consists of 30 items divided into three subscales (positive, negative, and general psychopathology) with scoring that ranges from 30 to 210 points.[38] The negative symptoms subscale evaluates presence of blunted affect, emotional withdrawal, poor rapport, passive/apathetic social withdrawal, difficulty in abstract thinking, lack of spontaneity and flow of conversation, and stereotyped thinking. The positive subscale evaluates presence of delusions, conceptual disorganization, hallucinatory behavior, excitement, grandiosity, suspiciousness, and hostility. The general psychopathology subscale evaluates for presence of somatic concern, anxiety, feelings of guilt, tension, mannerisms and posturing, depression, motor retardation, uncooperativeness, unusual thought content, disorientation, poor attention, lack of judgment and insight, disturbance of volition, poor impulse control, preoccupation, and active social avoidance. The PANSS is a reliable measure providing an objective gauge of clinical response to pharmacologic treatments. It is often used in clinical research and is considered by some researchers to be the gold standard measure of treatment efficacy of assessing patients chronologically throughout the course of their illness. There is some concern over the PANSS due to its length and complexity in scoring. It requires converting the PANSS into a ratio scale to interpret correct scores.[39] In comparison with the BPRS, it demonstrated better outcomes and was superior in clinical predictive power.[39]

Scale for the Assessment of Negative Symptoms (SANS)[40]

The SANS was developed in the early 1980s to specifically measure the severity of negative symptoms. The SANS consists of 25 items on a six-point scale. The items are categorized into the five domains of affective blunting, alogia, avolition/apathy, anhedonia/asociality, and attention. The SANS was the first standardized scale used to measure negative symptoms. At the time of its development, negative symptoms were often overlooked.[37,40]

Scale for the Assessment of Positive Symptoms (SAPS)[41]

The SAPS was developed after the SANS to specifically measure the severity of positive symptoms. The SAPS consists of 34 items on a six-point scale. The items are categorized into the four domains of hallucinations, delusions, bizarre behavior, and positive formal thought disorder.

The SAPS was the first standardized scale measuring positive symptoms and allowed the clinician to evaluate positive symptoms in a similar manner as the SANS for negative symptoms.[37,41]

Clinical Global Impression Schizophrenia (CGI-SCH)[42]

The CGI-SCH scale is a brief instrument that assesses the positive, negative, depressive, and cognitive symptoms and overall severity of schizophrenia. Research has found it to be a valid, reliable instrument to evaluate severity and treatment response in schizophrenia.

The scale consists of two categories: severity of illness and degree of change. The severity of illness category is based on behavior the week previous to the assessment, whereas the degree of change category assesses the change from the previous evaluation. Each category contains five different ratings (positive, negative, depressive, cognitive, and global) that are evaluated using a seven-point ordinal scale. Administering the instrument is simple, making it user friendly in routine clinical practice.[37,42]

Next-Generation Negative Symptom Scales

The Clinical Assessment Interview for Negative Symptoms (CAINS)[43] and the Brief Negative Symptoms Scale (BNSS)[44] were developed following a 2005 NIMH conference on negative symptoms. They both consist of 13 items that address the five currently recognized domains of negative symptoms, as well as aspects of anhedonia and the desire for social relationships. Older tools do not incorporate the more recent research and understanding on negative symptoms, therefore these tools are referred to as the next-generation scales. Good psychometric properties for both instruments has been reported and they are becoming more widely used.[37]

Occupational Therapy Assessment

In evaluating individuals with schizophrenia spectrum disorders, the occupational therapist (OT) will use the Occupational Therapy Practice Framework[45] to guide the evaluation process and determine how the individual's occupations, roles, and routines are impacted by the disorder. The Canadian Occupational Performance Measure (COPM)[46] may be used to guide the interview process, and skilled observation of the client's behaviors during the interview and while engaged in occupations will provide additional information.

As stated previously, cognitive deficits are a common feature of schizophrenia. A discussion of cognitive deficits is found in Chapter 7 and the Cognitive Disability Model

(CDM)[47] is one approach for the evaluation and treatment of cognitive deficits. The Allen Cognitive Level Screen (ACLS)[48] can be used to assess the cognitive level of the individual and provide insight into occupational functioning abilities. The Cognitive Performance Test (CPT)[49] is a standardized performance-based assessment that measures working memory and executive function related to occupational performance. The CPT assists in explaining functional capabilities of the individual and can indicate the compensatory and safety requirements that are needed. The Routine Task Inventory-Expanded (RTI-E)[50] assesses activities of daily living (ADL) and instrumental activities of daily living (IADL) functioning, and the scores are associated with the Allen Cognitive Scale.

Depending on the client, the OT may also choose specific assessments to gain additional information regarding the client's occupational performance. Three assessments described in Chapter 6, the Kohlman Evaluation of Living Skills (KELS), The Bay Area Functional Performance Evaluation (BaFPE), and the Performance Assessment of Self-Care Skills, Version 4.0 (PASS) may be used to assess ADL functioning. Additional tools may be used to explore concepts such as use of time, satisfaction, quality of life, and leisure interests. Evaluation that is individualized to best explore the client's needs should be implemented.

THERAPEUTIC MANAGEMENT

Psychopharmacology

Most individuals diagnosed with schizophrenia benefit from antipsychotic medication. It may be administered initially because of an acute psychotic episode. The goal is symptom management and the patient's response to the medication is closely monitored. Maintenance medication is generally necessary to help prevent relapse. The incidence of relapse among patients who do not receive maintenance therapy is 60%–80%, whereas those on maintenance therapy have a relapse incidence of 18%–32%.[3] People with schizophrenia are also sometimes prescribed antidepressants or mood stabilizers to manage mood symptoms.

There are two main categories of antipsychotic medications, typical, or first-generation medications, and atypical, or second-generation medications (Box 11.1). The second-generation (atypical) antipsychotics (SGAs) are the

---

BOX 11.1 Examples of Medications to Treat Psychosis

Class	Generic and Brand Names	Adverse Side Effects
Atypical or second generation	aripiprazole (Abilify)	Dry mouth
	iloperidone (Fanapt)	Blurred vision
	ziprasidone (Geodon)	Constipation
	paliperidone (Invega)	Dizziness
	lurasidone (Latuda)	Sleepiness
	risperidone (Risperdal)	Sexual dysfunction
	brexpiprazole (Rexulti)	Weight gain
	asenapine (Saphris)	Increased risk of diabetes
	quetiapine (Seroquel)	Tardive dyskinesia
	cariprazine (Vraylar)	Long-term use carries a risk of this condition
	olanzapine (Zyprexa)	involving repetitive, involuntary movements often of the mouth, tongue, facial muscles and upper limbs
	clozapine (Clozaril)	Increased risk for lowered white blood cell count (agranulocytosis)
	Can be prescribed if other antipsychotics do not work	
	Used if person has suicidal ideation	
Typical or first generation	haloperidol (Haldol)	Tardive dyskinesia
	loxapine (Loxitane)	Akathisia (feeling of restlessness)
	thiothixene (Navane)	Parkinsonism (tremor, slower thought processes and movements, rigid muscles, difficulty speaking and facial stiffness)
	fluphenazine (Prolixin)	
	chlorpromazine (Thorazine)	
	perphenazine (Trilafon)	Dystonia (involuntary and often painful muscle contraction and movements)
	trifluoperazine (Stelazine)	

preferred choice for first-line treatment of schizophrenia, except for clozapine.[3] Clozapine carries a risk of agranulocytosis (loss of white blood cells). It is prescribed only when other medications do not work or when a person with schizophrenia suffers from suicidal ideation, as clozapine is the only atypical medication that is indicated to help reduce suicidal thoughts. Taking the medication requires monitoring one's white blood cell count.[51]

First-generation antipsychotics (FGAs) were the first antipsychotics developed, beginning in the 1950s. Although effective in managing symptoms, they can cause serious side effects such as development of tardive dyskinesia, which is an involuntary movement disorder in which the individual may experience random movements in the muscles, eyes, tongue, jaw, and lips. It is a potentially permanent condition. FGAs are also more likely to cause extrapyramidal side effects. Extrapyramidal function refers to motor control and coordination. Some of the side effects include akathisia (feeling of restlessness), parkinsonism (tremor, slower movements and thought processes, rigid muscles, difficulty speaking, and facial stiffness), and dystonia (involuntary and often painful muscle contraction and movements). FGAs are usually prescribed when atypical antipsychotics have not been effective.[3,51]

Atypical antipsychotics or SGAs are generally the first course of medication because they have a lower risk of serious side effects and fewer extrapyramidal symptoms are associated with their use. However, SGAs tend to have metabolic side effects, such as weight gain, which can be a significant issue resulting in hyperlipidemia and diabetes mellitus. Most people taking an atypical antipsychotic can expect to gain weight, and this can contribute to the increased risk of cardiovascular mortality observed in patients with schizophrenia.[3] Of great concern is the standardized mortality rate in schizophrenia, which is about 2.5, corresponding to a 10–25-year reduction in life expectancy.[52,53] A major contributor of the increased mortality is due to cardiovascular disease (CVD), with CVD mortality ranging from 40% to 50% in most studies.[53] Adverse side effects of antipsychotic medication and suboptimal lifestyles include unhealthy diets, excessive smoking and alcohol use, and lack of exercise, and contribute to CVD in individuals with schizophrenia.[52]

There is a significant concern regarding medication nonadherence in individuals with schizophrenia. A systematic review of 39 studies found a 41% mean rate of medication nonadherence. Of the five most methodologically rigorous studies, which included defining adherence as taking medication at least 75% of the time, the nonadherence rate increased to 50%.[54] Long-acting injectable antipsychotic medications can offer an alternative option for individuals who are nonadherent to the oral medication. They can be given every 2–4 weeks or at even longer intervals, depending on the medication.[3]

Psychotherapy

Pharmacological therapy is considered essential to schizophrenia management, but nonpharmacological treatment such as psychotherapy is necessary to treat residual symptoms that persist and can support medication compliance. Psychotherapeutic approaches may include supportive counseling, psychoeducation, cognitive remediation, and cognitive behavioral therapy (CBT) including cognitive therapy and social skills therapy. A focus on life skills and wellness is beneficial, and some individuals may warrant vocational rehabilitation. Therapy may be individual or group based and should include family and caregivers to support the individual.

Cognitive deficits are a major determinant of functional disability affecting approximately 80% of individuals diagnosed with schizophrenia. Impairment is variable and may affect attention, memory, executive function, social cognition, or metacognition. Cognitive remediation can limit the impact of cognitive impairment on occupational functioning.[4] Cognitive remediation, including cognitive enhancement therapy and compensatory approaches are discussed in Chapter 7.

Psychoeducation provides information on the illness and its treatment, and includes integrating coping mechanisms that support patients or family to deal with the illness. It is led by health professionals using a collaborative relationship between the health professionals and the patients or their families. Psychoeducation programs include information about the signs and symptoms of schizophrenia, relapse prevention, and treatment of psychosis. Psychoeducation enables patients to take action and engage in disease management problem-solving and coping skills. Information on how to access community mental health care services can also be provided. Family intervention is similar to patient psychoeducation and serves to support the patient and the family by focusing on improving both patient and family outcomes, thereby reducing the burden of the disease.[4]

CBT includes social skills training and cognitive therapy. Social skills training is based on behavioral therapy principles and techniques. Programs may vary in implementation setting, duration and content, but all use similar approaches for teaching skills. These can include goal setting, role modeling, behavioral rehearsal, positive reinforcement, corrective feedback, problem-solving techniques, and home assignments to practice skills and promote generalization. Training provided in a group format provides an opportunity for peer support and enables participants to learn from each other's real-life experiences.

Social skills training targets social, independent living skills, and thus probably has an impact on factors such as social cognition, functional capacity, or symptoms. Cognitive therapy for psychosis aims to modify dysfunctional beliefs by helping people to understand the links between perceptions, beliefs, and emotional and behavioral reactions.[55] Patients learn to cope with symptoms by using structured techniques. Greater attention is now focused on negative symptoms, whereas previously, the positive symptoms were most targeted. CBT including cognitive techniques and behavioral techniques are discussed in Chapter 6.

Occupational Therapy Approaches

In working with individuals with schizophrenia spectrum disorders, the OT identifies the areas of occupational performance that are of concern to the client and works with the client to set appropriate goals and treatment strategies. Challenges to functional performance are related to the presence and severity of positive and negative symptoms and cognitive deficits, as well as the presence of environmental and social barriers. Occupational therapy practitioners are skilled in evaluating occupational performance, role function, routines, and the environment.

Occupational therapy may include psychoeducation, cognitive remediation, and CBT to support occupational performance. Additional strategies to support occupational engagement and satisfaction may include ADL training, restructuring routines to maximize independence, and social and environmental support. An example of an individualized occupational therapy program for recently hospitalized patients with schizophrenia is described in the literature.[56] The program included self-monitoring, motivational interviewing, individualized visits, handicraft activities, individualized psychoeducation, and discharge planning. Improvements in neurocognition, psychotic symptoms, and social functioning were achieved. Occupational therapy must be individualized for each client with appreciation for the client perspective. A first-person account of recovering from schizophrenia[57] describes recovery as a self-directed transformative process, as opposed to just symptom remission. Suggestions on how professionals can support recovery are included as well as an overview of recovery strategies. The OT's role in teaching sensory strategies for coping with sensory defensiveness, and the creation of a sensory diet to help modulate sensory input and affective arousal is highlighted.

Another study explored how people with schizophrenia experienced an occupational therapy intervention supporting meaningful occupational engagement in the early phases of recovery. The intervention lasted 8 weeks and provided each individual 60–90 minute weekly sessions targeting identified goals. Clients were part of the mental health center and were seen either at the facility or in the home. Goals were client-centered; examples included "working out at a fitness center," "attending a party with a friend," and "taking a bath every day." Qualitative analysis revealed that participants valued engaging in real-life meaningful occupations with support and strategies provided, and they felt that the intervention assisted in their recovery.[58]

Assessing use of time through completion of a time-use diary, and assisting the client in developing occupational balance may be warranted. One study exploring the time use of 10 individuals with schizophrenia found stagnation in the participants' occupational patterns and time use. Occupational engagement resulted primarily from the person responding to their own basic needs, whereas the environment was not recognized as being conducive to stimulating engagement. Occupational therapy was indicated to modify the environment to support satisfying role performance.[59] Another study assessed occupational balance using the Profiles of Occupational Engagement in people with Schizophrenia (POES), an assessment that includes a time-use diary and supplementary interview to rate items associated with occupational engagement. Construct validity has been established for this instrument, and it has clinical value in understanding the individual's well-being and health in real-life context.[60] Participants assessed as having occupational balance were more engaged in occupations, had better quality of life and sense of coherence, and had fewer negative symptoms than those individuals assessed as being under-occupied. This supports previous research, indicating that negative symptoms are better determinants than positive symptoms of occupational engagement for individuals with schizophrenia.[61] In the treatment of individuals with schizophrenia, occupational therapy services will depend on the individual's current level of occupational functioning, living environment, and setting in which services are provided, but most importantly it will depend on what is meaningful to the client.

FUNCTIONAL RECOVERY

Approximately 25% of individuals with schizophrenia do not respond well to first-line treatments and have poor outcomes long term.[5] In the remaining 75% of cases, the course of schizophrenia is characterized by a remission phase that alternates with relapses. Depending on how recovery is defined, research reports that the percentage of people with schizophrenia achieving recovery varies from 13.5% to 50%.[4,62] Longitudinal follow-up studies of patients diagnosed as having schizophrenia have consistently found that about 40% achieve social or functional recovery.[63]

Some researchers have suggested that recovery should be based on both clinical remission and social functioning. When using these criteria, a meta-analysis found the proportion of individuals with schizophrenia who met the criteria for recovery and appeared stable over time was only 13.5% (or about one out of seven patients) noted to recover after a first episode of psychosis despite psychiatric care.[4,5]

Recovery from mental illness is defined by psychiatric consumers as the attainment of a meaningful life, and by psychiatrists as the elimination of symptoms leading to a return to normal functioning.[4] Considering the culture-specific nature of recovery outcomes and dimensions, defining a common set of criteria to assess recovery in schizophrenia is needed. Functional outcome should be a priority target for therapeutic interventions.[62] Some of the factors affecting these functional outcomes include neurocognition, believed to account for approximately 25%–50% of the variance in real-world functional outcomes. Other variables such as intrinsic motivation and metacognition are also indicated. Social cognition is a multidimensional construct that comprises emotional processing, social perception and knowledge, theory of mind, and attributional biases. A meta-analysis showed that social cognition may have a stronger impact on variance in community outcome than neurocognition. It appears that symptoms such as amotivation and avolition have the greatest impact.[4]

The management of schizophrenia is evolving toward a more comprehensive model based on functional recovery; however, the concept of recovery is multidimensional and can be difficult to define. A panel of experts in schizophrenia identified common factors associated with functional recovery and provided recommendations to address functional recovery in research and practice. Some of the recommendations[64] for clinical practice include:

- focus on quality of life, cognition, and clinical remission when considering functional recovery in routine practice;
- focus on functional recovery as a goal in the management of patients with schizophrenia;
- gather information for appraising functional recovery from patients, their relatives (and/or caregivers), and the health care team;
- consider sociocultural background when assessing functional recovery;
- consider the combined influence of stressful life events, substance abuse, socioeconomic conditions, and family relationships when assessing successful functional recovery;
- do not focus exclusively on symptom remission when considering functional recovery; and
- include a variety of psychosocial interventions (including social skills training, family therapy, cognitive rehabilitation, social cognitive training, and occupational programs) to achieve functional recovery.

SUMMARY

Schizophrenia can be a very disabling illness that causes many of those affected to suffer a substantial decline in their functioning and in their ability to realize their full potential.[63] Despite many advances in the treatment of schizophrenia over the years, the outcomes for many patients with schizophrenia remain poor.[5] There are multiple factors that may account for these outcomes. They include those listed in Box 11.2.

BOX 11.2 Factors Affecting Outcomes in Schizophrenia[5]	
Involvement and engagement in treatment	Only 25%–40% receive stable ongoing treatment Reflects lack of adequate services and challenges in engaging patients in ongoing services
Poor treatment response	20%–30% of individuals with schizophrenia do not respond well to first-line treatments
Poor adherence	Estimated 50% rate of nonadherence to medications
Cognitive deficits	80% of individuals with schizophrenia experience cognitive deficits that impact functional abilities
Substance use disorders	Individuals with schizophrenia are at comparable risk as general population for alcohol use disorders and greater risk for cannabis use
Concurrent mental illness	Prevalence is believed to be high for other common mental disorders
Preexisting developmental problems	Significant deficits in intellectual and social functioning occur in premorbid phase of illness

Continued

BOX 11.2   Factors Affecting Outcomes in Schizophrenia—cont'd

Loss of functioning prior to diagnosis	Occurs on average 5 years before first emergence of psychotic symptoms; upon remission it is harder to return to previous functional level
Medication effects	Adverse side effects can create additional problems and may lead to nonadherence
Social determinants of health	Poverty, lack of adequate housing, health care, and education affects many individuals with schizophrenia and negatively impacts treatment
Accommodation to disability and shifting expectations	Disconnect between goals or expectations of client and those of health care provider may not align (rehab versus medical model)

More work is needed to address these concerns. Occupational therapy aligns well with the principles of functional recovery and employs strategies that address some of these factors. OTs possess the knowledge and skills to address the complex physical, mental, cognitive, emotional, and psychosocial needs of the individual. Knowledge and awareness of roles, routines, environment, and social support systems enable OTs to work with individuals to establish goals for engagement in meaningful occupations. Recovery is a unique journey for each individual, and the strengths and resources of each person must be explored on the road to recovery.

CASE STUDY 11.1

Jim is a 34-year-old man diagnosed with schizophrenia. He lives independently in an apartment complex subsidized for individuals with serious mental illness. He receives services through the state Department of Mental Health (DMH) and receives disability benefits. He has been living alone in his apartment for the past 4 years. Prior to that he lived with his mom and his younger brother and sister. He graduated from high school, and he has attended technical school in the past but has not graduated. He has worked part time in the past stocking shelves in a grocery store. He smokes 1–2 packs of cigarettes a day, does not exercise, eats a limited diet, and is within his recommended weight range. He spends some time with other residents in the apartment complex and occasionally with his family. He spends most of his time alone in his apartment.

He vividly recalls his first hospitalization and states he was taken to the hospital because the people on TV were talking to him and coming out of the TV to "get him." He remembers bright beams emanating from the TV and being blinded and scared. His father called 911 for help and he was hospitalized for 5–6 weeks. He was 19 at the time and prior to that he does not remember having problems. He went back home to live with his parents and his father died of a heart attack about a year later. His mom and siblings are supportive, but he found it difficult to live at home with them. He is on atypical antipsychotic medication and has had episodes of noncompliance in the past. His DMH caseworker checks on him periodically, and 1 month ago she noted that he was exhibiting delusional thinking and his grooming and self-care skills were diminished. He was hospitalized for 10 days and his medication was adjusted. He was discharged to the care of his family. His caseworker requested an OT evaluation and follow-up services and support for his return to independent living. You are contracted by the DMH and have been requested to evaluate and treat Jim.

Occupational Profile
The COPM is administered to structure the interview process, gather information, and to assess the client's self-perception of occupational performance. Jim presents with a blunted affect; he responds to questions adequately and without prompting.
Client's concerns: Jim states he is worried about his apartment and his stuff and he wants to be able to return to

CASE STUDY 11.1—cont'd

his apartment as soon as possible. He loves his family but is not happy living with them.

Successful occupations: He has been successful with ADLs and home management occupations in the past. He is not able to identify additional occupations other than watching TV and playing video games.

Barriers: At times he has been noncompliant with medication; more recently this resulted in emergence of delusions. Negative symptoms of blunted affect and asociality appear to be consistent; avolition and anhedonia may also be affecting his occupational engagement.

Supports: Family and case worker are supportive.

Occupational history: He worked as a stocker in the past, he states he liked doing it but would get tired after several months and would quit; on one occasion he said his boss told him it was not working out.

Values and interests: He is not able to identify any values or interests.

Daily life roles: He states he spends most of his time alone watching TV and playing video games.

Client's priorities and desired targeted outcomes: He states that he wants to return to his apartment and he wants to go back to school to become a physical therapist assistant.

Analysis of Occupational Performance

Jim is evaluated for his ability to return to his apartment. He exhibits mild problems with working memory and attention. The ACLS is administered and Jim is scored at a 4.6 cognitive level, indicating the need to live with someone for safety and problem-solving at this time. Additionally, the PASS is administered. The PASS includes four main types of ADL/IADL items: functional mobility, basic ADLs, IADLs with cognitive emphasis, and IADLs with physical emphasis. For Jim, items such as home maintenance, oven and stove-top use, taking out the garbage, and money management, are essential tasks when living independently. The PASS includes several other fundamental tasks that must be addressed for the client to live at home safely and effectively.

The Modified Interest Checklist is also administered to evaluate potential for activities that would increase his socialization. He lacks friends outside of the apartment complex and lacks social outlets. He does not date but states he would like to have a girlfriend. Jim primarily spends the majority of his time isolated in his apartment and when faced with new situations, he has difficulty with social cues and adjustment. Identifying potential interests and activities may help motivate Jim to increase his social participation. While ADL/IADLs are very important to address and must improve in order for Jim to continue to live alone, incorporating socialization and meaningful activities will increase his quality of life. Getting Jim socially engaged will be a significant building block to his recovery.

Additional concerns include medication adherence and his overall wellness. He states he sometimes forgets his medication, and he is not interested in exercise or smoking cessation. He states he does not cook much, he does not eat fruits or vegetables, and is a picky eater. He has participated in day treatment programs and groups sporadically in the past, and his goal is to return to his apartment.

Intervention/Rationale

Cognitive remediation is recommended for Jim, and he agrees to participate in a program offered at the community mental health department by the social worker and OT. The program includes computer training exercises focused on attention, memory, and problem-solving skill development, along with social cognition group sessions. The computer training is conducted for 60 minutes and the social cognition groups are 90 minutes a week. Jim will also be seen individually by the OT for 2 hours a week for the first month to further evaluate his ability to move back to his apartment. These sessions will be provided at his apartment with a family member to determine if he can move back with additional support from his family. CBT focused on problem-solving strategies is used with Jim to address ADL and IADL abilities.

Psychoeducation is provided to address medication compliance and strategies are provided to reinforce his medication schedule. Motivational interviewing is employed to discuss wellness behaviors, but Jim is very resistant to change and does not indicate a desire to quit smoking or change his eating habits. He does agree to consider increasing his activity level and states he would like to get outside and walk for exercise. Strategies for including walks into his daily routine are discussed. He agrees to walking with family or neighbors, which will also increase his social interaction. He agrees to allow the OT to assist with organizing a walking club at the apartment complex.

His functional abilities will be assessed each week to determine if he has resumed prior level of functioning to live independently, as this is his goal.

CASE STUDY 11.2

Ann is a 25-year-old woman diagnosed with schizophrenia with a predominance of negative symptoms. You are seeing her in a community mental health program designed to promote recovery. Ann has been stabilized on medication for several years. She lives with her mother and has a high school diploma. She would like to go to community college and has enrolled in courses several times over the past 2 years but keeps dropping out. She is not consistently well groomed, sometimes presenting with a disheveled appearance. She has moderate difficulty with social skills; primarily with poor eye contact and difficulty interpreting social cues for interaction. She has been assigned tasks at the community center such as filing paperwork and organizing files to evaluate her ability to follow through on tasks. She sometimes does well and sometimes presents with lots of reasons for not completing tasks. You are part of the treatment team working with her, and the team agrees that she has potential to achieve a higher level of functioning.

Occupational Profile

The COPM is administered to structure the interview process, gather information, and to assess the client's self-perception of occupational performance. Ann presents primarily with blunted affect and avolition. She answers questions cooperatively but responses are superficial.

Client's concerns: Overall, she is negative in her responses and is focused on the burden she feels from being diagnosed with schizophrenia.

Successful occupations: She is unable to identify any occupations in which she feels successful.

Barriers: Presence of negative symptoms; lack of insight and awareness of deficits.

Supports: Mother is supportive.

Occupational history: No additional work history to report. She does not demonstrate insight or problem-solving abilities related to her work skills.

Values and interests: She states she values the time she spends at the community center.

Daily life roles: She identifies her roles as daughter and friend.

Current and past routines: She is inconsistent in her self-care routine and is sometimes disheveled. She is also inconsistent with her attendance and her duties at the community center.

Client's priorities and desired targeted outcomes: She states that she wants to go back to school but she is not sure what she wants to study.

Analysis of Occupational Performance

To gather additional insight into her values and priorities, several assessments are administered to gather more information and to engage Ann in a deeper conversation about her occupational performance. The Engagement in Meaningful Activities Survey is administered to gather information on how meaningful Ann perceives her daily activities to be. The Satisfaction with Daily Occupations Instrument is administered to assess her overall satisfaction with what she is currently doing and what she would like to do. The Role Checklist is administered to increase discussion regarding past, current, and future roles. Finally, the Modified Interest Checklist is administered to learn more about Ann's interests.

Intervention/Rationale

After completing the assessments, Ann states that she finds work meaningful and she wants to establish a social network of friends her age. Since Ann has been attending the mental health center for some time and the team feels she has more potential, she will be directed to establish her own Wellness Recovery Action Plan (WRAP) to address her goals. The WRAP will increase her insight and provide empowerment. She will be asked to identify uncomfortable and distressing behaviors and situations and identify strategies for coping. She will be encouraged to complete her plan and reinforced to use it to enable her to achieve her goals.

Psychoeducation, CBT, and social skills training will be provided to support her WRAP and to empower her recovery. Psychoeducation will provide her with information and understanding regarding schizophrenia to address her feelings of being burdened by the diagnosis. CBT will address her negative thoughts through techniques such as reframing and challenging her thoughts. Social skills training will include role-playing and feedback on her skills. She will also be taught to self-monitor behaviors such as hygiene and eye contact. She will need to ask herself questions each day such as:

- Have I showered, put on clean clothes, brushed my teeth, and combed my hair?
- Have I completed my chores (at home) or job duties (at work)?

Through an individualized targeted plan, Ann will be supported to address her deficits, and as she makes progress she will be engaged in vocational rehabilitation to explore returning to school.

SUGGESTED LEARNING ACTIVITIES

1. Participate in an auditory hallucination simulation. Search online for an audio clip of distressing voices experienced by someone diagnosed with schizophrenia. Using ear buds or headphones, listen to the voices while engaging in a self-care activity or while preparing a meal or taking a walk. Write down your thoughts after the simulation.
2. Watch a movie you have not seen before about someone with schizophrenia, such as *A Beautiful Mind* or *The*

Soloist. With a fellow student, discuss the impact of the illness on the individual's occupational functioning.
3. Read the following article by Pat Deegan, a clinical psychologist diagnosed with schizophrenia, and consider how she was able to succeed in her recovery process.

Deegan PE. Recovery as a self-directed process of healing and transformation. *Occup Ther Ment Health.* 2002;17(3-4):5-21.

REFLECTION QUESTIONS

1. Reflect on the negative symptoms of schizophrenia. How do you think other people react to individuals exhibiting negative symptoms? How does this reinforce the symptoms and perpetuate dysfunctional behavior?
2. What strategies do you think work best to treat negative symptoms?

3. Why do you think there is a high rate of medication noncompliance for individuals with schizophrenia?
4. What does functional recovery mean for someone with schizophrenia?

REFERENCES

1. Lavretsky H. History of schizophrenia as a psychiatric disorder. In: Mueser KT, Jeste DV, eds. *Clinical Handbook of Schizophrenia.* New York, NY: Guilford Press; 2008.
2. Nasar S. *A Beautiful Mind.* New York, NY: Simon & Schuster; 1998.
3. Patel KR, Cherian J, Gohil K, Atkinson D. Schizophrenia: overview and treatment options. *P T.* 2014;39:638-645.
4. Morin L, Franck N. Rehabilitation interventions to promote recovery from schizophrenia: a systematic review. *Front Psychiatry.* 2017;8:100.
5. Zipursky RB. Why are the outcomes in patients with schizophrenia so poor? *J Clin Psychiatry.* 2014;75(suppl 2):20-24.
6. American Psychiatric Association. *Diagnostic and Statistical Manual of Mental Disorders.* 5th ed. Washington, DC: American Psychiatric Association; 2013.
7. Zupanick CE. *The New DSM-5: Schizophrenia Spectrum and Other Psychotic Disorders.* 2018. Available at: https://www.mentalhelp.net/articles/the-new-dsm-5-schizophrenia-spectrum-and-other-psychotic-disorders/.
8. Elis O, Caponigro JM, Kring AM. Psychosocial treatments for negative symptoms in schizophrenia: current practices and future directions. *Clin Psychol Rev.* 2013;33:914-928.
9. Remington G, Foussias G, Fervaha G, et al. Treating negative symptoms in schizophrenia: an update. *Curr Treat Options Psychiatry.* 2016;3:133-150.
10. National Institute of Mental Health. *Schizophrenia.* 2018. Available at: https://www.nimh.nih.gov/health/topics/schizophrenia/index.shtml.

11. Aleman A. Neurocognitive basis of schizophrenia: information processing abnormalities and clues for treatment. *Adv Neurosci.* 2014;2014:104920. Available at: http://dx.doi.org/10.1155/2014/104920.
12. Kiran C, Chaudhury S. Understanding delusions. *Ind Psychiatry J.* 2009;18:3-18.
13. Bressert S. Delusional disorder symptoms. *Psych Central.* 2018. Available at: https://psychcentral.com/disorders/delusional-disorder-symptoms/.
14. Arciniegas DB. Psychosis. *Continuum (Minneap Minn).* 2015;21(3 Behavioral Neurology and Neuropsychiatry):715-736. doi:10.1212/01.CON.0000466662.89908.e7.
15. Ford JM. Current approaches to studying hallucinations: overcoming barriers to progress. *Schizophr Bull.* 2017;43(1):21-23.
16. Waters F, Collerton D, Ffytche DH, et al. Visual hallucinations in the psychosis spectrum and comparative information from neurodegenerative disorders and eye disease. *Schizophr Bull.* 2014;40(suppl 4):S233-S245.
17. Walther S, Strik W. Motor symptoms and schizophrenia. *Neuropsychobiology.* 2012;66:77-92. doi:10.1159/000339456.
18. Pappa S, Dazzan P. Spontaneous movement disorders in antipsychotic-naive patients with first-episode psychoses: a systematic review. *Psychol Med.* 2009;39:1065-1076.
19. Peralta V, Campos MS, De Jalón EG, Cuesta MJ. Motor behavior abnormalities in drug-naïve patients with schizophrenia spectrum disorders. *Mov Disord.* 2010;25:1068-1076.
20. Peralta V, Cuesta MJ. Motor features in psychotic disorders. I. Factor structure and clinical correlates. *Schizophr Res.* 2001;47:107-116.

21. Aleman A, Lincoln TM, Bruggeman R, et al. Treatment of negative symptoms: where do we stand, and where do we go? *Schizophr Res*. 2017;186:55-62.

22. Heinrichs RW, Zakzanis KK. Neurocognitive deficit in schizophrenia: a quantitative review of the evidence. *Neuropsychology*. 1998;12:426-445.

23. Kahn RS, Keefe RS. Schizophrenia is a cognitive illness: time for a change in focus. *JAMA Psychiatry*. 2013;70:1107-1112.

24. Nuechterlein KH, Barch DM, Gold JM, Goldberg TE, Green MF, Heaton RK. Identification of separable cognitive factors in schizophrenia. *Schizophr Res*. 2004;72:29-39.

25. Couture SM, Penn DL, Roberts DL. The functional significance of social cognition in schizophrenia: a review. *Schizophr Bull*. 2006;32(suppl 1):S44-S63.

26. Bowie CR, Reichenberg A, Patterson TL, Heaton RK, Harvey PD. Determinants of real-world functional performance in schizophrenia subjects: correlations with cognition, functional capacity, and symptoms. *Am J Psychiatry*. 2006;163:418-425.

27. Green MF. What are the functional consequences of neurocognitive deficits in schizophrenia? *Am J Psychiatry*. 1996;153:321-330.

28. Green MF, Kern RS, Braff DL, Mintz J. Neurocognitive deficits and functional outcome in schizophrenia: are we measuring the "right stuff"? *Schizophr Bull*. 2000;26:119-136.

29. Green MF, Nuechterlein KH, Kern RS, et al. Functional co-primary measures for clinical trials in schizophrenia: results from the MATRICS Psychometric and Standardization Study. *Am J Psychiatry*. 2008;165:221-228.

30. Medalia A, Choi J. Cognitive remediation in schizophrenia. *Neuropsychol Rev*. 2009;19:353-364.

31. Hurley K. *Schizophrenia: DSM-5 Definition*. 2018. Available at: https://www.psycom.net/schizophrenia-dsm-5-definition/.

32. Yogeswary K. Schizoaffective disorder: an overview. *Int J Clin Psychiatry*. 2014;2:11-15.

33. Bressert S. Brief psychotic disorder symptoms. *Psych Central*. 2018. Available at: https://psychcentral.com/disorders/brief-psychotic-disorder-symptoms/.

34. Overall JE, Gorham DR. The brief psychiatric rating scale. *Psychol Rep*. 1962;10:799-812.

35. Overall JE, Gorham DR. The Brief Psychiatric Rating Scale (BPRS): recent developments in ascertainment and scaling. *Psychopharmacol Bull*. 1988;24:97-99.

36. Kay SR, Fiszbein A, Opler LA. The positive and negative syndrome scale (PANSS) for Schizophrenia. *Schizophr Bull*. 1987;13:261-276.

37. Kumari S, Malik M, Florival C, Manalai P, Sonje S. An assessment of five (PANSS, SAPS, SANS, NSA-16, CGI-SCH) commonly used symptoms rating scales in schizophrenia and comparison to newer scales (CAINS, BNSS). *J Addict Res Ther*. 2017;8:324.

38. Mortimer AM. Symptom rating scales and outcome in schizophrenia. *Br J Psychiatry Suppl*. 2007;50:S7-S14.

39. Obermeier M, Schennach-Wolff R, Meyer S, et al. Is the PANSS used correctly? A systematic review. *BMC Psychiatry*. 2011;11:113.

40. Andreasen NC. Negative symptoms in schizophrenia. Definition and reliability. *Arch Gen Psychiatry*. 1982;39:784-788.

41. Andreasen NC. The Scale for the Assessment of Positive Symptoms (SAPS). The University of Iowa, Iowa City, 1984.

42. Haro JM, Kamath SA, Ochoa S, et al. The clinical global impression-schizophrenia scale: a simple instrument to measure the diversity of symptoms present in schizophrenia. *Acta Psychiatr Scand Suppl*. 2003;(416):16-23.

43. Kring AM, Raquel, Steven P. The Clinical Assessment Interview for Negative Symptoms (CAINS): final development and validation. *Am J Psychiatry*. 2013;170:165-172.

44. Kirkpatrick B, Strauss GP, Nguyen L, et al. The brief negative symptom scale: psychometric properties. *Schizophr Bull*. 2011;37:300-305.

45. American Occupational Therapy Association. Occupational Therapy Practice Framework: Domain and Process, 3rd ed. *Am J Occup Ther*. 2014;68(suppl 1):S1-S48.

46. Law MC, Baptiste S, Carswell A, McColl MA, Polatajko H, Pollock N. *Canadian Occupational Performance Measure Manual (COPM)*. 4th ed. Thorofare, NJ: Slack Inc; 2005.

47. Allen CK. *Occupational Therapy for Psychiatric Diseases: Measurement and Management of Cognitive Disabilities*. Boston, MA: Little, Brown and Company; 1985.

48. Allen Cognitive Level Screen and Large Allen Cognitive Level Screen Committee. *Allen Cognitive Level Screen-5 (ACLS-5), Large Allen Cognitive Level Screen-5 (LACLS-5), & NEW Disposable Large Allen Cognitive Level Screen (LACLS[D])* [Handout]. Allen Cognitive Group. 2016. Available at: http://allencognitive.com/wp-content/uploads/Info-2016-ACLS_5-LACLS_5-LACLS-D5-pdf.pdf.

49. Douglas A, Letts L, Eva K, Richardson J. Use of the cognitive performance test for identifying deficits in hospitalized older adults. *Rehabil Res Pract*. 2012;2012:638480.

50. Katz N. *Routine Task Inventory-Expanded (RTI-E)*. 2017. Available at: http://allen-cognitive-network.org/index.php/allen-cognitive-model/assessments/48-routine-task-inventory-expanded-rti-e.

51. Smith K. *Schizophrenia Medications*. 2018. Available at: https://www.psycom.net/schizophrenia-medications.

52. Laursen TM, Munk-Olsen T, Vestergaard M. Life expectancy and cardiovascular mortality in persons with schizophrenia. *Curr Opin Psychiatry*. 2012;25:83-88.

53. Ringen PA, Engh JA, Birkenaes AB, Dieset I, Andreassen OA. Increased mortality in schizophrenia due to cardiovascular disease–a non-systematic review of epidemiology, possible causes, and interventions. *Front Psychiatry*. 2014;5:137.

54. Haddad PM, Brain C, Scott J. Nonadherence with antipsychotic medication in schizophrenia: challenges and management strategies. *Patient Relat Outcome Meas*. 2014;5:43-62.

55. Mander H, Kingdon D. The evolution of cognitive-behavioral therapy for psychosis. *Psychol Res Behav Manag*. 2015;8:63-69.

56. Shimada T, Nishi A, Yoshida T, Tanaka S, Kobayashi M. Development of an individualized occupational therapy programme and its effects on the neurocognition, symptoms and social functioning of patients with schizophrenia. *Occup Ther Int*. 2016;23:425-435. doi:10.1002/oti.1445.

57. Deegan PE. Recovery as a self-directed process of healing and transformation. *Occup Ther Ment Health*. 2002;17 (3-4):5-21.

58. Bjørkedal ST, Torsting AM, Møller T. Rewarding yet demanding: client perspectives on enabling occupations during early stages of recovery from schizophrenia. *Scand J Occup Ther*. 2016;23:97-106.

59. Bejerholm U, Eklund M. Time use and occupational performance among persons with schizophrenia. *Occup Ther Ment Health*. 2004;20:27-47.

60. Bejerholm U, Eklund M. Construct validity of a newly developed instrument: Profile of Occupational Engagement in people with Schizophrenia, POES. *Nord J Psychiatry*. 2006;60:200-206.

61. Bejerholm U. Occupational balance in people with schizophrenia. *Occup Ther Ment Health*. 2010;26(1):1-17.

62. Vita A, Barlati S. Recovery from schizophrenia: is it possible? *Curr Opin Psychiatry*. 2018;31:246-255.

63. Zipursky RB, Reilly TJ, Murray RM. The myth of schizophrenia as a progressive brain disease. *Schizophr Bull*. 2013;39:1363-1372.

64. Lahera G, Gálvez JL, Sánchez P, et al. Functional recovery in patients with schizophrenia: recommendations from a panel of experts. *BMC Psychiatry*. 2018;18:176.

12

Substance Use Disorders

Nancy Carson

LEARNING OBJECTIVES

1. Identify the types of substance use disorders as defined by the *Diagnostic and Statistical Manual of Mental Disorders* (DSM–5).
2. Describe the symptomology of the different substance use disorders.
3. Understand the prevalence and risk factors for substance use disorders.
4. Recognize assessment methods for substance use disorders.
5. Discuss treatment approaches for substance use disorders, including psychopharmacology and psychotherapeutic approaches.
6. Articulate occupational therapy's role in the treatment of substance use disorders and co-occurring disorders.

INTRODUCTION

The Diagnostic and Statistical Manual of Mental Disorders, 5th Ed. (DSM-5) category of "Substance-Related and Addictive Disorders" includes the subcategories of substance use disorders, substance-induced disorders, substance intoxication and withdrawal, and substance/medication-induced mental disorders. Substance use disorder (SUD) refers to the use of alcohol or another substance in a manner that is unhealthy and disrupts daily life or results in distress.[1] SUDs are responsible for many problems that affect individuals and society. They create a significant burden that spans physical, mental, psychosocial, spiritual, economic, family, and legal domains.[2] Alcohol, tobacco, and illicit drug use are major global risk factors for disability and premature death.[3] In 2015, the number of disability-adjusted life-years (DALYs) attributed to alcohol consumption, tobacco smoking, and illicit drug use combined worldwide was 292.7. The combined mortality rate was 150.6 deaths/100,000 people.[4] In the United States in 2017, 18.7 million (7.6%) people aged 18 years or older had a substance use disorder and 8.5 million (3.4%) had both a substance use disorder and a mental illness.[5]

The resulting economic costs of SUDs are also significant and include costs associated with health care, law enforcement, and lost productivity.[6] The individual may also spend a considerable amount of money acquiring the substance, which may result in the family unit relying on public assistance or other financial aid from family or friends.[2] SUDs can also affect family members emotionally because they may feel anger, frustration, shame and guilt, or embarrassment due to the individual's behavior. Problems with relationships may develop as tension, conflict, violence, or abuse can result from substance use disorders. Divorce or the removal of children from the home may also occur, and the associated burdens on the spouse and children are significant. Alcohol use during pregnancy can cause birth defects and problems in child development, and children raised in homes where one or both parents are substance abusers are at an increased risk for emotional problems, such as poor behavioral or impulse control, poor emotional regulation, conduct or oppositional disorders, depression, anxiety, and the development of an SUD as they age.[2]

SUDs create a burden for society because they contribute to physical and mental disability, as well as deaths that result from accidents or diseases caused or worsened by substance use. Societal problems include housing instability, homelessness, unemployment, dependence on welfare, criminal behaviors, and incarceration. The societal costs create an enormous economic burden on the state and federal government and on insurance carriers or other payors who fund addiction treatment, health-related disorders, and social needs that are compromised because of the SUD.[2]

SUBSTANCE USE DISORDERS

There are nine categories of substances recognized in the DSM-5. All but one, caffeine, can result in an SUD. The remaining eight categories of substances include the following:

1. Alcohol
2. Tobacco
3. Cannabis
4. Hallucinogens
5. Inhalants
6. Opioid
7. Sedatives, hypnotics, or anxiolytics
8. Stimulants

There are 11 behaviors associated with SUDs. A person is diagnosed with a substance use disorder when two of these behaviors are displayed within a period of 12 months. These behaviors are categorized as impaired control, social impairment, risky use, or evidence of tolerance or withdrawal.[7] The behaviors associated with each category are summarized in Box 12.1.

There are four behaviors associated with impaired control. Consuming more of the substance than planned and not being able to stop, as well as worrying about stopping, indicate impaired control. Additionally, craving the substance and excessive time obtaining and using the substance are behaviors related to impaired control. Social impairment may be demonstrated by an inability to maintain responsibilities of home, work, or school. It may also manifest as a reduction in prior activities and the deterioration of personal relationships related to the substance use. As the individual spends more time and resources acquiring and using the substance, there is less time for prior responsibilities and activities. The effects of the substance use on the individual's overall functioning contributes to decreased role functioning and decreased quality of personal relationships.[7]

BOX 12.1	Behaviors Associated With Substance Use Disorders
Category	**Behavior**
Impaired control	Consuming more alcohol or other substance than originally planned
	Worrying about stopping or consistently failed efforts to control one's use
	Spending a large amount of time using drugs/alcohol, or doing whatever is needed to obtain them
	"Craving" the substance (alcohol or drug)
Social impairment	Use of the substance results in failure to "fulfill major role obligations" such as at home, work, or school.
	Giving up or reducing activities in a person's life because of the drug/alcohol use.
	Continuing the use of a substance despite its having negative effects on relationships with others (for example, using even though it leads to fights or despite people's objecting to it)
Risky use	Continuing the use of a substance despite health problems caused or worsened by it. This can be in the domain of mental health (psychological problems may include depressed mood, sleep disturbance, anxiety, or "blackouts") or physical health.
	Repeated use of the substance in a dangerous situation (for example, when having to operate heavy machinery or when driving a car)
Pharmacologic indicators (tolerance and withdrawal)	Building up a tolerance to the alcohol or drug. Tolerance is defined by the DSM-5 as "either needing to use noticeably larger amounts over time to get the desired effect or noticing less of an effect over time after repeated use of the same amount."
	Experiencing withdrawal symptoms after stopping use. Withdrawal symptoms typically include, according to the DSM-5: "anxiety, irritability, fatigue, nausea/vomiting, hand tremor or seizure in the case of alcohol."

From Horvath A, Misra K, Epner A, Cooper G. The diagnostic criteria for substance use disorders (addiction). Available at: http://www.amhc.org/1408addictions/article/48502-the-diagnostic-criteria-for-substance-use-disorders-addiction.

Risky use may include ignoring the negative effects of substance use on psychological and physical health. Despite health concerns that can be attributed to the use of the substance, the person continues use. Health and wellness problems may include difficulty sleeping, anxious or depressed mood, and problems with cardiovascular and respiratory functions. The effects will vary depending on the substance(s) being used and on the individual's prior overall health. Risky use also involves use of the substance in a dangerous situation or in a situation where compromising one's cognitive and physical skills may cause harm to self or others. Driving a car while under the influence of alcohol or illicit substances is the most well-known risky behavior; however, there are many other situations that can be compromised. For example, a health care professional who is under the influence of alcohol or illicit substances may not be able to provide optimal care to the patients receiving care and puts both the patients and their own career at risk.[7]

There are two pharmacologic indicators of substance use disorders, tolerance and withdrawal. Tolerance refers to the need to use more of the substance to obtain the same effect or getting a decreased effect with the same amount over time. Some people experience withdrawal symptoms when use of a substance is ceased. Examples of these symptoms include anxiety, irritability, hand tremor, and fatigue.[7]

Alcohol

Every year, 3 million deaths worldwide result from alcohol use. This accounts for 5.3% of all deaths, and 5.1% of the global burden of disease and injury is attributable to alcohol.[8] Over 75% of these deaths are men and, in the age group of 20 to 39 years, approximately 13.5% of the total deaths are alcohol-attributable.[8] The estimated global prevalence among the adult population in 2015 for heavy episodic alcohol use was 18.4%.[4] The number of DALYs attributed to alcohol use was 85 million years, and the mortality rate was 33 deaths/100,000 people.[4] It is the most widely used substance in the United States,[7] with 13% of the population 12 years of age and older over meeting the criteria for an alcohol use disorder (APA, 2015). Alcohol use disorders most commonly develop by the late 30s but may emerge at younger and older ages. Having multiple relatives with an alcohol use disorder increases the probability of someone developing an alcohol use disorder. Additionally, it is estimated that 10% to 20% of people drink more than the recommended moderation guidelines.[7] The recommended federal guidelines state that one drink per day for women and up to two drinks per day for men is considered the limit for moderate alcohol consumption. A drink is defined as 12 fluid ounces

of regular beer (5% alcohol), 5 fluid ounces of wine (12% alcohol), or 1.5 fluid ounces of 80 proof distilled spirits (40% alcohol). High-risk drinking is defined as the consumption of four or more drinks in 1 day or eight or more drinks per week for women and five or more drinks in 1 day or 15 or more drinks per week for men. Binge drinking is the consumption of four or more drinks for women and five or more drinks for men in a period of 2 hours. These excessive patterns of alcohol consumption are responsible for 88,000 deaths in the United States each year, including 1 in 10 deaths among working age adults (age 20–64 years).[9]

Tobacco

Tobacco use is a global public health epidemic. Tobacco use kills more than 7 million people a year worldwide. More than 6 million of those deaths are the result of direct tobacco use, with the rest the result of nonsmoker exposure to secondhand smoke. There are 1.1 billion smokers worldwide; approximately 80% reside in low- and middle-income countries.[10] The estimated global prevalence among the adult population in 2015 for daily tobacco smoking was 15.2%, and the number of DALYs attributed to tobacco smoking was 170.9 million years.[4] Mortality rates attributed to tobacco smoking were 110.7 deaths/100,000 populations, making tobacco smoking highest among harmful substance use for both DALYs and mortality.[4]

Tobacco use primarily consists of cigarette use but also includes cigarillos, cigars, pipes, and water pipes. Smokeless tobacco involves chewing tobacco, sniffing tobacco into the nose, or placing tobacco in the mouth between the cheeks and gums. Smokeless tobacco has health risks too but they are not as harmful and it's use is not as widespread as cigarettes. Cigarette addiction refers to the degree to which a person experiences a strong urge to smoke and may refer to the number of cigarettes smoked per day and the amount of time from waking to smoking the first cigarette of the day.[11] In 2016, approximately 15.5% of US adults smoked cigarettes, representing a decline of about 5% since 2005. Cigarette smoking is the leading cause of preventable disease and death in the United States and accounts for approximately 20% (>480,000 deaths) every year. This means that an estimated 37.8 million adults in the United States currently smoke cigarettes. More than 16 million Americans live with a smoking-related disease.[12]

Nicotine is the chemical contained in tobacco products; it is an extremely addictive substance. Almost everyone who smokes becomes addicted; therefore social smoking is generally rare. Although the health risks of tobacco use are well known, only a small number of people attempt to quit each year, and an even smaller percentage succeed. Addiction to nicotine results in very intense cravings, which can make quitting difficult.[7]

Cannabis

Marijuana comes from the *Cannabis sativa* or *Cannabis indica* plant, which contains the mind-altering chemical tetrahydrocannabinol (THC) and other similar compounds.[13] Marijuana is the most commonly used illegal substance worldwide[4] and in the United States.[13] The estimated global prevalence among the adult population in 2015 for cannabis use was 3.8%.[4] In the United States, more than 11 million young adults aged 18 to 25 years used marijuana in a given year,[4] and approximately 5% of people age 12 years and older meet the criteria for a cannabis use disorder.[7] Cannabis use disorders are more common in males than females.[7]

Marijuana can be smoked in hand-rolled cigarettes called "joints," in pipes or water pipes called "bongs," or in blunts (emptied cigars that have been partly or completely refilled with marijuana). Marijuana can also be inhaled through use of a vaporizer or mixed in food, such as brownies or cookies, or brewed as a tea.[13] When a person smokes or ingests marijuana, THC is absorbed, and it acts on specific brain cell receptors that ordinarily react to natural THC-like chemicals. The activation of more receptors creates the "high" that people feel. Other effects can include altered senses, altered sense of time, changes in mood, impaired body movement, difficulty with thinking and problem solving, and impaired memory. Marijuana also interferes with occupational functioning and daily routines. Regular cannabis use is associated with amotivational syndrome, a lack of ambition or desire to accomplish anything.[7] People who frequently use large amounts of marijuana report lower life satisfaction, poorer mental and physical health, more relationship problems, and less academic and career success.[13] When large amounts of marijuana are consumed, effects such as hallucinations, delusions, and psychosis may occur. Physically, marijuana use may cause breathing problems when smoked, increased heart rate, and intense nausea and vomiting.[13] Using large amounts of marijuana alone is not known to cause death; however, symptoms such as anxiety and paranoia, which can include delusions and hallucinations, can lead to emergency room visits.[13]

In recent years, cannabis has also been reported to be a known risk factor for the development of schizophrenia, although the exact neurobiologic process is not well understood. The incidence of psychosis in a cannabis-exposed and nonexposed population was found to be 31% and 20%, respectively. Cannabis exposure during the formative teenage years may be a factor that interacts with other factors, possibly causing schizophrenia.[14] In people diagnosed with schizophrenia, cannabis use can cause a worsening of symptoms of psychosis.[13]

Marijuana has been shown to have some medical benefits. It may reduce the side effects of chemotherapy and the weight loss that accompanies AIDS for some individuals. It is also believed to alleviate some forms of chronic pain; however, the medical use of marijuana remains controversial.[7] The term *medical marijuana* refers to treating symptoms of illness and other conditions with the whole unprocessed marijuana plant or its basic extracts. Currently, the US Food and Drug Administration (FDA) has not recognized or approved the medicinal use of marijuana. Clinical trials are being conducted with marijuana and its extracts to treat symptoms of illness and other conditions to determine its effectiveness. However, recreational marijuana is legal for adults older than 21 years in 10 states, and medical marijuana is legal in 33 states.[13]

Hallucinogens

Hallucinogens include a wide variety of substances that alter perception, thoughts, and feelings. They create euphoria and have psychedelic effects of visual and auditory perceptual distortions or hallucinations. Hallucinogens can be found in some plants and mushrooms or can be synthesized. Hallucinogens have been used for centuries, mostly for religious rituals.[15] Hallucinogens are taken orally, intravenously, nasally, or smoked. Some examples of hallucinogens include phencyclidine (PCP), D-lysergic acid diethylamide (LSD), and ketamine. PCP was developed as a general anesthetic for surgery decades ago and is no longer used due to its serious side effects. LSD is one of the most powerful mood-changing chemicals; it is made from lysergic acid found in a fungus that grows on rye and other grains. Ketamine is used as a surgical anesthetic for humans and animals, and veterinary offices are a source of much of the ketamine sold on the streets.[15] Hallucinogen use disorders are more common in men between the ages of 20 and 40 years. These disorders often lead to problems with roles and routines in daily life. Little regard for personal safety may be evident, and strong cravings for the substance can contribute to continued use.[7]

Inhalants

Inhalants refer to a wide variety of household products that contain hydrocarbons, such as glue, shoe polish, spray paints, cleaners, various aerosols, gasoline, and lighter fluid. These products produce vapors that are inhaled and cause intoxication. The vapors may be inhaled directly from a container, from a bag into which a substance has been placed, or from a rag soaked with a substance and then placed over the mouth or nose. More than 22 million Americans age 12 years and older have used inhalants.

Each year, approximately 750,000 people use inhalants for the first time. Inhalant abuse remains the least studied form of substance abuse, although research has increased in recent years.[16]

Inhalants are inexpensive, legal, and widely available. They are one of the first drugs used by young people. They produce significant psychoactive effects or euphoria, as well as dizziness, incoordination, slurred speech, lethargy, slowed reflexes, slowed thinking and movement, tremor, blurred vision, stupor or coma, generalized muscle weakness, and involuntary eye movement.[16] Chronic long-term use may result in serious complications such as brain damage, liver and kidney disease, and even death.[7]

Opioids

Prescription opioids are used to treat significant pain, and they are often prescribed following surgery or injury. The use of prescription opioids for the treatment of chronic noncancer pain, such as back pain or osteoarthritis, has increased in recent years, despite the risk of abuse or addiction.[17] The estimated global prevalence among the adult population in 2015 for opioid use was 0.37%.[4] As many as one in four patients receiving long-term opioid therapy is struggling with opioid addiction. The primary reason reported for prescription opioid misuse among US adult was to relieve physical pain.[18] Addiction and misuse of prescription opioids are concerning problems because drug overdose deaths continue to increase in the United States. The number of overdose deaths involving opioids (both prescription opioids and illegal opioids) increased 500% from 1999 to 2016. On average, 130 Americans die every day from an opioid overdose.[19] The most common drugs involved in prescription opioid overdose deaths include methadone, oxycodone (such as OxyContin), and hydrocodone (such as Vicodin).[20] Taking too many prescription opioids can stop a person's breathing and result in death.[17]

Heroin is an illegal opioid that has seen an increased use across the United States among men and women, most age groups, and all income levels.[20] Heroin is highly addictive and an overdose can cause slow and shallow breathing, coma, and death. More than 15,469 people died in 2016 from heroin abuse, sometimes with consumption of another substance. Nearly everyone who uses heroin also uses at least one other drug. Heroin is typically injected but can also be smoked and snorted. Injection also puts the person at risk for HIV, hepatitis C, and hepatitis B, as well as bacterial infections.[21]

Pharmaceutical fentanyl is a synthetic opioid pain reliever that is approved for treating severe pain.[20] It is typically used to treat advanced cancer pain because it is 50 to 100 times more potent than morphine. Most cases of fentanyl abuse in the United States are a result of illegally made fentanyl. It is often mixed with heroin and/or cocaine to increase its euphoric effects. The rate of overdose deaths involving synthetic opioids other than methadone, which includes fentanyl, doubled from 2015 to 2016. Roughly 19,400 people died from overdoses involving synthetic opioids other than methadone in 2016.[22]

Sedatives, Hypnotics, and Anxiolytics

Sedatives, hypnotics, and anxiolytic (SHA) substances affect the central nervous system to relieve anxiety, aid sleep, or produce a calming effect. Benzodiazepines are the main class of drugs in this category. Barbiturates are an older class of drugs that were used for these reasons but, due to a greater effect on respiratory depression and greater potential for death, they are seldom used today. All SHAs that are used have the potential to be fatal when overused or combined with alcohol or other drugs. These substances also often lead to tolerance and withdrawal, with females being at higher risk than males for abusing prescription drugs in this class. SHA addiction often occurs together with other drugs of abuse; for example, benzodiazepines may be used to slow oneself down after using cocaine.[7]

Stimulants

Stimulants include amphetamines and cocaine. The most commonly known amphetamine is methamphetamine, or "crystal meth." Other amphetamine drugs include dextroamphetamine and appetite suppressants.[7] The estimated global prevalence among the adult population in 2015 for amphetamine use was 0.77%.[4] Cocaine is a powerfully addictive psychostimulant drug made from the leaves of the coca plant native to South America.[23] It is the second most commonly used and trafficked illicit drug in the world after cannabis. The prevalence of cocaine use is particularly high among males between 15 and 34 years old. Of cocaine users, 5% will develop a substance dependence during the first year of use, and 20% will become dependent on cocaine in the long term. Cocaine addiction is a worldwide public health problem that has somatic, psychological, psychiatric, socioeconomic, and legal complications.[24] The estimated global prevalence among the adult population in 2015 for cocaine use was 0.35%.[4]

These drugs can be taken orally, intravenously, or nasally (snorted or smoked). Amphetamines may be prescribed for conditions such as obesity, narcolepsy, and attention-deficit/hyperactivity disorder. Exceeding the prescribed dose indicates a potential amphetamine use disorder. Stimulant intoxication produces feelings of euphoria, well-being, and confidence but can also result in paranoia, anxiousness, irritability, and depression. Dramatic mood swings and poor judgment may occur. Severe forms of amphetamine addiction may lead to significant weight loss and anemia. Skin picking may develop because amphetamine use can cause severely dry skin and itchiness. Amphetamine-induced psychosis can also develop, such as hallucinations that there are bugs crawling just below the surface of the skin.[7]

Although these stimulants create similar effects for the user, there are some major differences in how they work. Cocaine is derived naturally and is quickly removed from and almost completely metabolized in the body. Methamphetamine is a stimulant that is synthesized; crystal meth is made with the ingredient pseudoephedrine, which is found in many cold medicines. Making meth is a dangerous process because of the toxic chemicals involved and the potential for an explosion to occur during the process. Methamphetamine is metabolized much slower than cocaine, and a larger percentage of the drug remains unchanged in the body. Methamphetamine therefore remains in the brain longer and creates a stronger and longer lasting stimulant effect.

Both methamphetamine and cocaine increase levels of dopamine. Cocaine prolongs dopamine actions in the brain by blocking the reabsorption (reuptake) of the neurotransmitter by signaling nerve cells. At low doses, methamphetamine also blocks the reuptake of dopamine, but it also increases the release of dopamine, leading to much higher concentrations in the synapse, which can be toxic to nerve terminals.[23] In general, methamphetamine causes three times more release of dopamine than cocaine and has a half-life of 12 hours, whereas cocaine has a half-life of 1 hour. When these substances are smoked, methamphetamine produces a high for 8 to 24 hours, whereas cocaine produces a high for 20 to 30 minutes.[23]

Caffeine

Caffeine is the only substance listed in the DSM-5 that does not include a category for an SUD; diagnoses of caffeine intoxication and caffeine withdrawal are included. More than 85% of adults in the United States regularly consume caffeine. Caffeine is not considered a dietary nutrient; it functions as a stimulant. Caffeine occurs naturally in plants and is added to foods and beverages. Caffeinated beverages vary widely in their caffeine content. Most intake of caffeine in the United States is from coffee, tea, and soda. The Dietary Guidelines for Americans[9] define moderate caffeine consumption from coffee as three to five 8-oz cups/day or 400 mg/day, and states this can be incorporated into healthy eating patterns. Caffeine withdrawal can occur after suddenly stopping consumption of regular use and can occur with relatively small daily doses. Symptoms include headache, fatigue, difficulty concentrating, and irritable or depressed mood. Caffeine intoxication includes nervousness, restlessness, and psychomotor agitation. More serious effects include tachycardia and cardiac arrhythmia,

even death, following extremely high doses. The effects of caffeine intoxication can also result in difficulty with occupational performance.[7]

CO-OCCURRING DISORDERS OF MENTAL ILLNESS AND SUBSTANCE ABUSE

Concurrent SUDs and mental health disorders are common and are referred to as "co-occurring disorders." Co-occurring disorders were previously referred to as "dual diagnoses." Approximately 8.5 million adults in the United States had co-occurring disorders in 2017.[25] Past treatment almost always only addressed either the SUD or the mental illness; it was not common practice to treat both together. Recent research indicating the high prevalence of co-occurring disorders is a major concern for drug and alcohol and mental health services and underscores the need to address both disorders concurrently. Prevalence rates have been reported as 50% or more, depending on the location, methodology, and definitions used to define the disorders.[26]

People with mental health disorders are more likely than those without mental health disorders to have a concurrent SUD. Co-occurring disorders can be difficult to diagnose due to the variability and severity of symptoms that may occur in each disorder.[25] A number of reasons may explain the high rates of comorbidity. One disorder may influence the development of another disorder. For example, a person who consumes large amounts of alcohol may be more likely to develop depression. In some cases, substances may be used as a means of self-medication to relieve the distress of a mental disorder and, over time, an SUD develops. Other potential causes include the development of co-occurring disorders due to shared genetic predisposition of the disorders and socioeconomic factors, such as poverty or trauma.[26,27]

In many cases, people receive treatment for one disorder while the other disorder remains untreated. This may be due to inadequate screening, lack of provider understanding, an overlap of symptoms, or other urgent health issues that need to be treated. Integrated treatment is the best approach so that practitioners can address mental and substance use disorders at the same time, often lowering costs and leading to better outcomes.[25] There are core practice principles established for integrated treatment for co-occurring disorders. These include integrating treatment and training providers in both SUDs and mental illness disorders, providing staged treatment, motivational interventions, cognitive-behavioral therapy (CBT), and coordinated medication services (Box 12.2).

Individuals living with co-occurring disorders are likely to experience greater rates of relapse and more hospital readmissions resulting in potential treatment nonadherence.

BOX 12.2   Practice Principles of Integrated Treatment for Co-Occurring Disorders

Principle	Comments
1	Mental health and substance abuse treatment are integrated to meet the needs of people with co-occurring disorders.
2	Integrated treatment specialists are trained to treat both substance use disorders and serious mental illnesses.
3	Co-occurring disorders are treated in a stage-wise fashion, with different services provided at different stages.
4	Motivational interventions are used to treat consumers in all stages, but especially in the persuasion stage.
5	Substance abuse counseling, using a cognitive-behavioral approach, is used to treat consumers in the active treatment and relapse prevention stages.
6	Multiple formats for services are available, including individual, group, self-help, and family.
7	Medication services are integrated and coordinated with psychosocial services.

From Substance Abuse and Mental Health Services Administration. *Integrated Treatment for Co-Occurring Disorders: Training Frontline Staff.* DHHS Publ. No. SMA-08-4366. Rockville, MD: Center for Mental Health Services, Substance Abuse and Mental Health Services Administration, US Department of Health and Human Services; 2009.

Symptoms of mental disorders, including the positive symptoms of psychosis and greater levels of suicidal ideation, may worsen. The individual may experience increased interpersonal stressors and difficulties, social exclusion, greater risk for homelessness, and greater risk of physical disease or injury. The overall subjective quality of life may decline. The trauma of relapse and admission to an institutional setting alone can be distressing. Readmissions can result in increased medication and other treatment approaches, which can be traumatizing to the individual.[26] Co-occurring disorders are usually associated with poor treatment outcomes, leading to high levels of health service use. Despite the high rates of co-occurring disorders, they are often missed by clinicians practicing in either field and continues to be poorly understood. A better understanding of these comorbid disorders is needed to understand potential causal relationships among symptoms, disorders, and treatment.[27]

ASSESSMENT

All health care providers should be aware of the symptoms and criteria of SUDs. With the prevalence of these disorders, it is highly likely that practitioners will encounter individuals with diagnosed and undiagnosed SUDs, regardless of the treatment setting. Occupational therapists may treat individuals who have health conditions resulting from substance abuse. In pediatric populations, the child may have a health condition associated with or resulting from a parent or caregiver's SUD. During the occupational therapy evaluation process, the individual's occupational performance is assessed, and factors that support or hinder occupational performance are identified. Taking into consideration the prevalence of SUDs, it becomes clear that screening for SUDs is important. Occupational therapists have the skills and training to address healthy occupational performance patterns. When a client has a diagnosed SUD, this may include supporting abstinence and working with the individual to establish healthy coping skills. For clients who may be undiagnosed or at risk for an SUD, it is important to establish therapeutic rapport so that optimal support can be provided, and the individual can be referred for appropriate treatment within the interprofessional team.

A survey of occupational therapy practitioners across all practice settings has found that most of those practitioners outside the mental health setting did not routinely assess or treat SUDs.[28] In primary care settings, many physicians do not feel prepared to recognize and help patients with SUDs due to a lack of time and adequate training. There is uncertainty regarding treatment effectiveness, perceived patient resistance, discomfort with discussing substance abuse, and a fear of losing patients.[29] Detecting substance abuse problems is a challenge for primary care providers and a challenge for other members of the health care team. The National Institute on Drug Abuse provides a resource guide[30] for clinicians to screen adult patients in general medical settings. Because these disorders consistently rank among the 10 leading preventable risk factors for years of life lost to death and disability, screening is essential for improved outcomes.[31] Screening must be done appropriately, with the right questions asked to disclose the presence of risky behavior associated with an SUD. There are suggested approaches to screening patients in the health care environment, and practitioners are encouraged to work with the interprofessional team to determine who will perform these screenings.[29] A simple initial screen can be incorporated into the client interview by asking about tobacco, alcohol, and drug use using a routine and nonjudgmental approach. Start with open-ended questions such as, "Tell me about your alcohol use." Integrating questions when appropriate can elicit an honest answer; the question may be asked when assessing occupational performance related to socialization and leisure activities or when assessing overall wellness habits and routines. There are also several short substance abuse screening instruments available. One is the four-item CAGE or CAGE-AID (adapted version that also includes drug abuse) included in a health status questionnaire. The questions on the CAGE-AID are as follows[32]:

1. Have you ever felt you should cut down on your drinking or drug use?
2. Have people annoyed you by criticizing your drinking or drug use?
3. Have you ever felt bad or guilty about your drinking or drug use?
4. Have you ever had a drink or used drugs first thing in the morning to steady your nerves or to get rid of a hangover?

Directions for administration and scoring are available on the *Substance Use Screening and Assessment Database*,[33] a resource created by the Alcohol and Drug Abuse Institute Library at the University of Washington. The database is extensive, including over 1000 instruments; more than 50 of these instruments have validity and reliability information provided as well. There is also a resource guide available from the National Institute on Drug Abuse (NIDA)[30] that provides in-depth information on screening for health care practitioners. Included in the guide is the NIDA Quick Screen and the NIDA-modified ASSIST, two tools to guide the screening process. Additionally, the Substance Abuse and Mental Health Services Administration[34] website also provides resources for screening tools.

A model was developed following an Institute of Medicine recommendation for community-based screening for health risk behaviors, including substance use. The Screening, Brief Intervention, and Referral to Treatment (SBIRT) model[35] is an evidence-based approach used for the identification, reduction, and prevention of misuse and abuse of substances. Clients are screened for risky substance use behaviors using standardized screening tools; for those clients screening positive, the health care professional provides brief information, advice, and feedback to address the concerns. Clients needing additional or more comprehensive interventions are provided a referral to treatment. Information on SBIRT and additional resources are provided on the SAMHSA website.[35] The Massachusetts Department of Public Health, Bureau of Substance Abuse Services also provides a guide for the use of the SBIRT model, which is available on the Internet.[36]

In evaluating individuals with substance use disorders, the occupational therapist will use the Occupational Therapy Practice Framework[37] to guide the evaluation process and determine how the individual's occupations, roles, and routines are affected by the disorder. The Canadian Occupational Performance Measure[38] may be used to guide the interview process and skilled observation of the client's behaviors during the interview and, while engaged in occupations, will provide additional information. As stated throughout this chapter, SUDs interfere with occupational performance because negative behaviors associated with the substance use replace behaviors that were healthy or previously meaningful to the client. Maladaptive habits and routines develop to support the SUD, and these become ingrained in the individual's daily life. Abstaining from the use of the substance creates a void in the person's routine and may require a different environmental context. The occupational therapist evaluates the client's occupational performance and assesses the factors that support or restrict success in meaningful occupations.

An example of an assessment tool developed by an occupational therapist is the Life History Questionnaire (LHQ).[39] It is a self-report tool developed to measure the extent of occupational dysfunction attributable to substance abuse. It contains 70 items, one unifying construct, and eight subscales. It was found "to be valid and reliable for measuring the extent of occupational dysfunction and specific areas of strengths and weaknesses."[39] It is designed to assist practitioners in selecting intervention strategies for their clients. The eight factors, or subscales, are the following:

1. Occupational disruption
2. Habits and routines
3. Social environment
4. Family disapprobation
5. Residual strengths
6. Self-medicating behaviors
7. Physical environment
8. Readiness for change

THERAPEUTIC MANAGEMENT

There are a variety of approaches that may be implemented to treat or manage SUDs. The treatment or approach selected will depend on the type of SUD being addressed, as well as any comorbidities. Social, economic, and environmental factors associated with the substance abuse should also be considered to improve outcomes.[29] The National Institute on Drug Abuse has identified 13 principles of effective treatment for drug addiction that provide a comprehensive overview for health care professionals addressing SUDs[40]:

1. Addiction is a complex but treatable disease that affects brain function and behavior.
2. No single treatment is appropriate for everyone.
3. Treatment needs to be readily available.
4. Effective treatment attends to multiple needs of the individual, not just their drug abuse.
5. Remaining in treatment for an adequate period of time is critical.
6. Behavioral therapies—including individual, family, and group counseling—are the most commonly used forms of drug abuse treatment.
7. Medications are an important element of treatment for many patients, especially when combined with counseling and other behavioral therapies.
8. An individual's treatment and services plan must be assessed continually and modified as necessary to ensure that it meets their changing needs.
9. Many drug-addicted individuals also have other mental disorders.
10. Medically assisted detoxification is only the first stage of addiction treatment and by itself does little to change long-term drug abuse.
11. Treatment does not need to be voluntary to be effective.
12. Drug use during treatment must be monitored continuously because lapses during treatment do occur.
13. Treatment programs should test patients for the presence of HIV/AIDS, hepatitis B and C, tuberculosis, and other infectious diseases as well as provide targeted risk reduction counseling, linking patients to treatment if necessary.[40]

Approaches generally follow one of three models. The medical model focuses on the physiologic causes of addiction, with pharmacology as the primary method of treatment to address symptoms and change behavior. The psychological model focuses on therapeutic approaches to address emotional factors or learned patterns of maladaptive behavior. The sociocultural model focuses on changing the social, physical, and cultural environments to promote self-help and social support.[29] Occupational therapy approaches for SUDs incorporate components of the psychological and sociocultural models to address the occupational performance deficits that may result from an SUD.

Pharmacotherapy

There are effective pharmacotherapy options for individuals with SUDs. The use of these medications has three broad objectives: (1) the management of acute withdrawal syndromes through detoxification; (2) reduction of cravings and urges to use illicit drugs; and (3) prevention of relapse and return to drug use.[41] Although there are FDA-approved medications to treat tobacco, alcohol, and opioid dependence, there are currently no FDA-approved medications to treat cocaine, methamphetamine, and cannabis dependence, despite urgent clinical need and extensive research.[42,43]

Nicotine replacement therapies are more effective for tobacco cessation than stopping abruptly, with no pharmacologic assistance. Types of replacement approaches include the transdermal nicotine patch, nicotine gum, nicotine lozenge, nicotine vapor inhaler, and nicotine nasal spray. They replace the nicotine obtained from smoking to prevent withdrawal symptoms, including anger and irritability, depression, anxiety, and decreased concentration.[42] The first-line treatment is a combination approach using the patch plus gum or lozenges.[43] Additionally, bupropion SR (Zyban) and varenicline (Chantix) are recommended by the FDA as effective first-line therapies for tobacco cessation.[42] Bupropion is a medication that is an atypical antidepressant. It was originally developed and approved as an antidepressant and then later found also to help people quit smoking. It can be used at the same dose for cigarette smoking or depression treatment or for both simultaneously. Varenicline is a nicotine partial agonist that reduces the craving for cigarettes. Both are prescription medications.[44]

Benzodiazepines are the standard of care for the treatment of alcohol detoxification to address alcohol withdrawal effects.[43] Benzodiazepines can improve treatment outcomes but should only be used on a short-term basis because physical tolerance of these medications can occur rapidly, resulting in dangerous interactions if patients using the medication resume alcohol consumption.[42] Naltrexone is a medication used to block the effects of opioids that has also been used with alcohol use disorders. It works by interfering with opioid receptors and blocking the rewarding aspect of drinking, therefore reducing craving.[42,44] Naltrexone has been shown to reduce the frequency and intensity of drinking, reduce the risk of relapse to heavy drinking, and increase abstinence.[42] Acamprosate is a relapse prevention medication that is believed to affect the brain's glutamate receptors and reduce cravings.[43,44] It is most effective when given after the cessation of acute withdrawal. It acts to decrease cravings to alcohol that are caused by a desire to feel relief from withdrawal symptoms.[42]

Disulfiram (Antabuse) is the first FDA-approved medication for alcohol dependence. It works by inhibiting the enzyme that converts acetaldehyde to acetate in the breakdown of alcohol.[42] As acetaldehyde builds up, this results in an unpleasant reaction that includes sweating, nausea, vomiting, facial flushing, tachycardia, hyperventilation, shortness of breath, and hypotension if a person consumes alcohol when taking the medication.[42,44] This serves to extinguish an addictive behavior through negative reinforcement and behavioral counterconditioning. The knowledge of a negative reaction leads to refraining from drinking and assists the individual to achieve an initial period of abstinence.[42]

The most effective pharmacotherapies for opiate use disorders are agonist therapies, including methadone and buprenorphine.[42,43] Agonist medications suppress opioid cravings by blocking the ability of other opioids to bind to the receptors. Medications with similar actions to those of the abused drug but that have different pharmacokinetic profiles are used.[42] The evidence indicates that opioid agonist therapy, with methadone or buprenorphine, improves outcomes in multiple domains.[43] Methadone, a pure agonist, has been used for more than 40 years in the treatment of opioid addiction. Federal guidelines require methadone to be administered through regulated maintenance programs. These programs also offer chemical dependency counseling, and some offer additional mental health services to address overall psychosocial health. Methadone is highly effective in preventing undesirable outcomes, and individuals addicted to opiates such as heroin no longer experience peaks of euphoria or the negative effects of withdrawal, such as anxiety, agitation, diarrhea, and insomnia.[43] The individual is no longer motivated to engage in drug-seeking behaviors and, with this prevention of reinforcement and absence of aversive effects, methadone maintenance is an extremely effective long-term treatment for opioid dependence.[42]

Buprenorphine is an opioid partial agonist and is often formulated with naloxone as an abuse deterrent.[43] Buprenorphine/naloxone (Subutex) is used to treat opiate dependence in outpatient office-based practices. It has significantly less regulatory requirements compared to methadone. Common opioid side effects, including sedation, constipation, and nausea, can be seen with buprenorphine.[42,43]

Naltrexone, an opioid receptor antagonist, can also be used for the treatment of opioid use disorder.[43] Naltrexone blocks dopamine and unlike agonist therapies, naltrexone has been used as a relapse prevention strategy. Patients addicted to opioids cannot get high from opioids while on naltrexone, making it more likely that they will not want to use opioids and remain abstinent. Additionally, naltrexone

has some benefits over replacement therapies, including no risk of overdose and no addictive potential; however, there are some problems with treatment retention.[42]

As stated earlier, more than 115 individuals die in the United States every day from opioid overdoses. Naloxone (Narcan) is an effective and safe antidote to opioid-related overdoses, including heroin and fentanyl, and is essential in preventing fatal opioid overdoses. However, awareness of its benefits remains limited in some areas. Naloxone is a competitive opioid receptor antagonist that can reverse the neuroinhibitory effects of opioids, thereby temporarily stopping opioid overdose–induced respiratory depression or allowing additional time for essential medical intervention. Naloxone is an effective emergency treatment that can be used by emergency personnel or family and friends of persons known or suspected to have had an overdose.[44]

In considering pharmacotherapy for SUDs, it is important to determine the client's goals because complete abstinence may not be a realistic goal for all clients, despite recommendations from the health care community. A nonjudgmental discussion is essential to assess the patient's ability and desire for making a change in substance use patterns. Once the patient has agreed to address the negative substance use, treatment options can be discussed. Medication-assisted treatment versus behavioral treatment should be explained, along with methods for combining approaches to maximize outcomes. Also, some clients may only agree to undergo detoxification as opposed to ongoing treatment, despite evidence that supports it. Because of client resistance and, in some cases, the lack of a therapeutic alliance for prescribers to address concerns effectively, pharmacotherapy is considered to be underused in the treatment of SUDs.[43]

PSYCHOTHERAPY

There are a variety of psychotherapeutic approaches that can be used to treat SUDs and support recovery. These approaches can be delivered in a variety of settings and programs. Psychotherapeutic approaches may include individual and group counseling, which can include CBT, contingency management, motivational interviewing, and motivational enhancement therapy. Settings and programs include inpatient and residential treatment, intensive outpatient treatment, partial hospital programs, recovery support services, and 12-step programs. Peer support may also be used to support recovery.[45]

Counseling focuses on skill building to stop substance use and promote adherence to a recovery plan. Individual counseling focusing on specific needs and outcomes, and group counseling provides social reinforcement for achieving and maintaining recovery.[45] CBT focuses on recognizing and stopping negative thinking and behavior related to the substance use. It may also increase awareness of the stressors, situations, and feelings that lead to substance use and assist the individual with identifying appropriate ways to manage these stressful events.[45] Cognitive-behavioral therapy approaches are covered in more detail in Chapter 6. Contingency management is a type of behavioral therapy that provides incentives to reinforce positive behaviors or changes. It often involves giving vouchers that can be exchanged for goods or services when the individual passes routine drug testing. Contingency management has been extensively tested and evaluated in the context of substance misuse treatment.[46]

Motivational interviewing (MI) is discussed in Chapter 2. It is a therapeutic interaction style that promotes a collaborative and empathetic communication style for the therapist in motivating patients to engage in behavior change. MI evokes internal motivation while emphasizing intrinsic strengths and resources. It was designed specifically for substance use clients but has been applied successfully in other populations seeking behavior change.[47] Motivational enhancement therapy (MET) combines MI with psychological counseling. It is supportive and intended to create insight for apprehensive or defensive patients. A commitment to a specific plan to engage in treatment and focus on recovery is the desired outcome. It is generally used early on to engage people in treatment.[45] MET is targeted at the ambivalence to change that is present in some individuals who may enter the health care setting to address an SUD, but they do not demonstrate or state a desire for making changes in their lives.[47]

Treatment can be provided in inpatient or residential settings that are designated as specialty SUD treatment facilities or within specialized units located in broader health care hospitals or behavioral health facilities. The focus is typically on detoxification and intensive treatment, including transition to a community-based setting or program as soon as possible. If inpatient treatment is not deemed necessary or is not a viable option financially or otherwise, an alternative treatment delivery mode is partial hospitalization or intensive outpatient treatment. Treatment spans multiple days and sessions a week to provide intensive treatment for the individual. Treatment may then be transitioned to fewer outpatient sessions, as appropriate.[45]

There are also a variety of recovery support services that can be used with treatment or as stand-alone approaches for individuals unable to participate in clinical rehabilitation programs. These are typically nonclinical services provided by peers or individuals in recovery who can use their own experiences to help others working toward recovery. Peer supports are an integral component of the SUD treatment system. Self-help or support groups such as Alcoholics Anonymous and other 12-step programs for substance abuse provide peer support for stopping substance use. Clubhouses, specialized living situations, and drop-in centers are available in some geographic locations and use peer-to-peer services, mentoring, and coaching to assist individuals in changing to a lifestyle without alcohol and drugs.[45]

The type of service or program through which treatment is provided will depend on several factors. These include the type of substance use and severity of the substance use problem, motivation to stop using the substance, support or lack of support in the sociocultural environment, cognitive functioning, and whether co-occurring mental illness is present. In the early stages of recovery, separation from social and cultural components of the individual's environment may be necessary to promote long-term abstinence. This may occur through hospitalization followed by temporary relocation to a semicontrolled or monitored sober community, such as a halfway house where the individual can live with other people in recovery. This may be a court-mandated treatment if the individual has committed a crime. A halfway house provides social support from other residents who are in recovery and participation in group activities, shared meals, and tasks reinforces efforts to remain abstinent. Ongoing support after leaving a residential program or halfway house is highly encouraged for relapse prevention. It is also important to screen for co-occurring mental illness and provide appropriate treatment when indicated.[47]

OCCUPATIONAL THERAPY APPROACHES

Understanding the neurobiology of addiction provides implications for occupational therapy practice.[48] The neurobiologic factors underlying the addiction process involve the brain's reward system, also known as the mesocorticolimbic system, a set of interrelated structures of the cerebral cortex, midbrain, and limbic system. Substance use promotes the release of pleasurable neurochemicals in this system. Chronic substance abuse can create long-lasting changes in the structure and function of the mesocorticolimbic system, resulting in tolerance or the decreased ability for the substance to provide the same effect. This results in powerful cravings for the substance and sensitization or increased pleasure from the substance when ingested after periods of abstinence, thus leading to an escalating cycle of use and abuse. Understanding the difficulty in breaking the addiction cycle promotes increased empathy and understanding on the part of the occupational therapist and leads to the development of more effective occupational therapy interventions.

Additionally, a model of "addiction as occupation" has been presented in the literature.[49] This suggests that the activities supporting the addiction constitute an occupation that provides meaning to the individual. When the individual is no longer engaging in substance use, the absence of this as an occupation must be considered. Failure to do so promotes relapse because the individual is experiencing an occupational loss by not engaging in occupations that were previously significant in everyday life. "Occupational therapists understand individuals as being deeply embedded in the context of their occupational lives, which shape not only their surroundings but also their personal identities, values, and personal roles. In this way, occupation contributes to what individuals perceive as meaningful, how they relate to others, and how daily life is structured."[49] Occupational therapy's role when working with individuals in recovery is to assist the individual in identifying, exploring, and establishing healthier occupations that are meaningful and can take the place of the addiction. In exploring the occupational lives of people with addiction, seven themes related to occupational meaning emerged: (1) connection; (2) locus of control; (3) penetration; (4) identity; (5) motivation; (6) coping and escape; and (7) habituation. These themes indicate that addiction provides habits and routines, and addiction increases feelings of social connectedness and comfort. There is a belief that one is predisposed to addiction and that addiction provides an identity. Engaging in addiction is enjoyable, and it is a way of coping with life; however, one is able to fulfill other roles when abstaining.[49] Although other professions may address behavioral and occupational deficits associated with addiction-related disorders, occupational therapy's unique approach is the facilitation of real activities in natural environments to engage people in occupations that are meaningful and enjoyable.[48] It may be the reestablishment of old occupations, reframing occupations away from a focus on addiction to a focus on healthy living, or the establishment of new occupations to support recovery.

Occupational therapy practitioners work with individuals with SUDs in defined treatment programs, as well as in many other practice areas. As stated earlier, co-occurring disorders of mental illness and SUD are high, with prevalence rates reported as 50% or more.[26] Additionally, the prevalence of these disorders in the general population is high, making it likely that practitioners will encounter individuals with diagnosed and undiagnosed SUDs, regardless of the treatment setting. Having knowledge and expertise in evidence-based approaches provides the practitioner with the tools to address an SUD and positively affect the overall occupational performance of the individual. Examples of effective SUD interventions from other disciplines that fit within the domain of occupational therapy or can be adapted to facilitate occupational engagement and participation consistent with the Occupational Therapy Practice Framework[37] include brief interventions, CBT, motivational strategies, and 12-step programs.[50]

Brief interventions include use of alcohol and drug screening questionnaires as part of the occupational profile to identify individuals who have alcohol and/or drug use problems. When identified, brief interventions may include assessing readiness for change and providing brief interventions in the form of motivational interviewing targeted to identify the potential for behavioral change and how it can positively affect occupational performance.[50] CBT includes addressing distorted thinking related to substance use, development of coping skills and application to occupational performance, and facilitation of problem solving to address changes in occupational performance activities and contexts that occur when an individual is no longer using alcohol and/or drugs.[50]

Motivational strategies are selected to match the readiness for change stage of the individual. The stages include precontemplation, contemplation, preparation, action, and maintenance. Evaluation of occupational habits and dysfunctions to increase awareness of the substance use on occupational performance would be implemented during the precontemplation stage. Identifying and exploring resources for making changes to support recovery would be implemented during the preparation stage.[50] Facilitating the incorporation of the 12 steps identified in 12-step programs to positively impact occupational performance is another example of an effective SUD intervention that can be adapted to facilitate occupational outcomes.[50]

The most common intervention provided by occupational therapists and reported in the literature is a life skills approach for maintaining abstinence.[51] The type of setting and program varies; examples include a halfway house treatment setting,[39] transitional living center,[52] peer support community program for adults in permanent supportive housing,[53] and intensive residential program at an alcohol and drug abuse center.[54] Additional interventions cited in the literature include a parenting program for women with an SUD,[55] the development of time management skills to maintain a routine for supporting abstinence,[56] and a theater-based community engagement project for veterans recovering from SUDs.[57]

SUMMARY

Although the development of a conceptual framework for understanding how addiction affects a person's occupational performance and the assertion of addiction as an occupation has been presented in the literature, there have been few rigorous studies to support occupational therapy's role in addiction treatment.[58] A systematic review of occupational therapy in the treatment of addiction has identified 16 theoretic and professional role studies, 8 qualitative and 14 quantitative studies. All studies had low levels of evidence.[58] There is a need for occupational therapy practitioners working in the field of addiction to conduct rigorous research and disseminate findings to validate occupational therapy's role in addiction treatment.

The evidence thus far suggests that occupational therapy provides a component to treatment that is missing in many treatment programs. The following quote summarizes the powerful contribution of occupational therapy in supporting recovery for individuals with SUDs[39]:

> On entering treatment, clients experience gaps in their routines that were formerly filled by substance use, and the absence of a new routine can trigger relapse. Extensive repetition of new replacement habits and patterns of task performance, along with contextual change, is required to make the transition to recovery. Much of current substance abuse treatment focuses on changing the person and his or her thinking and commitment to change, which are important. The strength of occupational therapy is its focus on the performance and contextual elements that have great potential to promote long-term recovery.

CASE STUDY 12.1

David is a 52-year-old man who sustained bilateral upper extremity (UE) second- and third-degree burn injuries 3 months ago in an accidental explosion at the factory where he works. He also has first- and second-degree burns to his chest, neck, and face. He spent several weeks in the hospital and is now being seen as an outpatient three times a week. His therapy sessions are covered by workman's compensation. He is divorced, has no children, lives alone, and socializes rarely. He has a brother and cousin who live close by, and he sees them occasionally. He is currently out of work due to his injuries.

Occupational Profile

The Canadian Occupational Performance Measure (COPM) is administered to structure the interview process, gather information, and assess the client's self-perception of occupational performance. David presents with a flat affect, is nonverbal most of the time, and does not initiate conversation; however, he will answer questions willingly.

Client's concerns: When asked to identify his primary concerns, he states that his decreased hand function is his major concern. He is worried that he won't be able to return to work if he does not recover fully from his injuries.

Successful occupations: He states that he is an excellent machinist and enjoyed his work most of the time. He is unable to identify any other occupations.

Barriers: He states that his injuries are his primary barrier. He indicates that it may be difficult to resume working, even if he recovers his hand function, but he is unable to articulate why he feels that way. When asked what he would like to do if he does not resume working, he states that he doesn't know.

Supports: He states his brother and cousin are supportive of him and have helped maintain his home and took care of his dog while he was hospitalized. They continue to support him and invite him to do things with them but he is not always interested in what they have planned. He states that he tends to be more of a "loner."

Occupational history: He has worked for his current employer for the past 18 years; prior to that, he worked various machinist jobs.

Values and interests: He states that he values being independent. His stated hobbies are watching TV, walking his dog, and drinking beer.

Daily life roles and routine: When asked to describe a typical day, he is unable to recount how he spends most of the day.

Analysis of Occupational Performance

Occupations and performance skills: David is able to complete his ADLs and live independently, although he requires extra time to complete tasks, and he modifies some activities due to limitations in strength, coordination, and sensation.

Client factors: He answers questions freely about his use of alcohol and states that he drinks every night to relax. Although his behavior never indicates that he is intoxicated during therapy sessions, he self-reports drinking up to 10 beers every night and occasionally consuming liquor. He also reports that he was prescribed pain medication after the accident, and he continues to use the medication occasionally.

Interventions and Rationale

Occupational therapy sessions are primarily focused on increasing overall UE functioning, including therapeutic exercises and functional activities to address his limited

CASE STUDY 12.1—cont'd

strength, coordination, and sensation, with the goal of returning to his prior level of function so he can return to work as a machinist. After several weeks, the therapist has established trust with David, and he engages more in conversation during his therapy sessions. When he initiates a comment regarding alcohol use and use of pain medication, the therapist uses the CAGE brief screen[32] to ask questions in a nonjudgmental manner. When asked "Have you ever felt you should cut down on your drinking or use of pain medication?" he responds that he has felt that way occasionally. When asked "Have people annoyed you by criticizing your drinking or use of pain medication?" he responds no because he seldom socializes. When asked "Have you ever felt bad or guilty about your drinking or use of pain medication?" he responds not really. When asked "Have you ever had a drink first thing in the morning to steady your nerves or to get rid of a hangover?" he hesitates before answering and then states, "not first thing in the morning." When asked to clarify what he means, he reveals that over the past few months he has started drinking earlier and earlier each day.

The therapist engages David in conversation using a MI approach by asking open-ended questions, providing affirming responses and reflective listening, and summarizing as appropriate. Conversations take place while David is engaged in functional activities. The therapist looks for change statements indicating potential desire or willingness to change. The discussion develops gradually over several sessions, and he eventually states that his alcohol use is concerning to him; he realizes that being out of work and at home most of the time has escalated his drinking to the point that he no longer feels he is able to control it. He is very resistant to a drug treatment program, and then he does not want to talk about it for several sessions. The therapist follows his lead and waits until he does start talking about drinking again. The therapist uses a MI approach to facilitate discussion regarding what he can do to address his alcohol and pain medication usage and is surprised when he states that he has a neighbor who goes to Alcoholics Anonymous groups. He recently talked to the neighbor when walking his dog and the neighbor invited him to go with him to a meeting, and he agreed. He went to one meeting, and he liked it and he is considering going again.

During his therapy sessions, the therapist has been introducing different functional activities to address David's physical performance skills. He expressed interest in doing minor repairs on his home; therefore, his therapy sessions include small woodworking projects to address fine motor skills and the ability to use tools in a safe manner. He enjoys making bird feeders and putting them in his backyard. He reports enjoying bird watching, which reminds him of spending time with his father when he was young. He reports that he no longer uses pain medications and is trying to limit his alcohol consumption. The therapist continues to assist in identifying occupations that can replace "addiction as occupation" and to engage him in therapeutic conversation using a supportive motivational approach.

CASE STUDY 12.2

Annie is a 25-year-old woman with a history of heroin use. She has been in an inpatient treatment facility for treatment twice in the past 3 years. She also has a history of alcohol and tobacco use. Several months ago, she began a relationship with a man she met through a friend. He does not use illegal drugs and he supports her abstinence from heroin. She is unemployed and is living with her new boyfriend; 3 weeks ago, she found out she was pregnant. She started attending a program at the community mental health center for pregnant women with a history of substance use disorders. The program includes a weekly group therapy session facilitated by a clinical counselor, and a weekly life skills session facilitated by an occupational therapist.

Occupational Profile

Participants complete a nonstandardized questionnaire that includes questions about current occupations, habits and routines, social environment, prior experience with infants and children, and expectations of parenting. There is no time allotted for individual interviews, so during the first session, participants are asked to identify their primary concerns and have the opportunity to discuss their concerns with others and identify what skills they would like to learn during the class sessions. Participants can attend sessions throughout their pregnancy and then transition to another class for mothers and infants. Class size is limited to eight participants, and the session is facilitated by one occupational therapy practitioner. Annie completes the

Continued

CASE STUDY 12.2—cont'd

questionnaire and provides substantial comments and information. She is very engaged in class sessions. She reveals both in the questionnaire and during the first session that she has dealt with anxiety for the past 10 years, describing herself as the type who worries about everything. She admits to alcohol and drug use as a coping mechanism.

Client's concerns: She is concerned that she will not be able to abstain from alcohol and tobacco use while pregnant, and she is also concerned that she may resume heroin use in the future. She is not confident in her ability to maintain long-term abstinence, and she worries about being a good mother.

Successful occupations: She is currently unemployed; she finished her last treatment program 6 months ago and moved in with her mother. She was not confident in looking for a job, and her mother had encouraged her to take time to think about what she wants to do. She met her boyfriend a month later and claims it was "love at first sight." She moved in with him 3 months ago when her mother decided to move. She currently takes care of the home and cooks meals; her boyfriend works full time as a service technician for a heating and air conditioning company and works as an Uber driver one or two evenings a week to make some extra money. She is independent in activities of daily living (ADLs).

Barriers: She reports that her lack of confidence and anxiety are barriers. She worries about the financial costs of raising a child and her lack of income.

Supports: Her boyfriend is supportive. Her mother is supportive but recently moved to another city with her new boyfriend. She has an older brother but does not see him much, and she does not know her father. She has a few friends but has distanced herself from them recently as they continue to use illegal drugs at times.

Occupational history: She dropped out of high school but did complete her GED. She has worked as a cashier, office manager, waitress, and sales clerk.

Values and interests: She values family and wants to be a good mother. She indicates that she is interested in pursuing a business degree and would like to eventually work for a company in a management role. She also states that she is interested in learning more about financial management careers.

Daily life roles: She currently identifies as a girlfriend, daughter, and mother-to-be.

Current and past routines: She feels like she has a lot of free time currently. She reports a lot of variation in her routine when she was using drugs but she currently maintains a fairly stable routine.

Client's priorities and desired targeted outcomes: She would like to develop skills for maintaining abstinence and would like to learn parenting skills. She would also like to identify coping mechanisms for her anxiety, and she would like to investigate some career options.

Analysis of Occupational Performance

There is no time allotted for evaluation outside of the weekly group session. Annie reports having an anxiety disorder as well as an SUD. Her support mechanisms are limited because her boyfriend works long hours, her mother has moved to another city, and she no long has contact with her former friends. Her insight and readiness to change appear to be very positive. She is independent in ADLs and independent ADLs. She reports low confidence for long-term abstinence but is committed to working toward it. She reports being anxious about her parenting skills and thinks that she lacks positive coping mechanisms for anxiety overall.

Interventions and Rationale

Occupational therapy intervention consists of the weekly life skills group sessions. The format is educational and uses a CBT approach that incorporates skill building. Each session focuses on an aspect of parenting skills while also addressing mechanisms for maintaining abstinence. Annie participates in the group sessions with the following outcomes:

- An educational component is provided in all sessions and may include reviewing typical infant behavior, such as sleep-wake routines, feeding routines, and monthly developmental milestones. Breastfeeding versus bottle feeding is discussed in one session, and skills such as changing diapers, bathing infants, and soothing fussy babies are practiced or simulated in other sessions. Participants are encouraged to discuss their concerns about their ability to care for their infant during each session.
- Self-monitoring of anxiety is introduced in the first session and discussed in each subsequent session so that participants can identify triggers and physical and mental reactions to stress.
  - After the first two sessions, Annie begins to identify potential triggers, including boredom, during which she feels like she focuses on negative things that could happen to her. These include an inability to care for her baby properly, experiencing a relapse, her boyfriend leaving her, and developing financial problems. She also identifies her tendency to think of herself as a failure for having used heroin and having to go to a treatment center twice. Her focus on negative

CASE STUDY 12.2—cont'd

thinking results in feelings of anxiety. She then has trouble sleeping and concentrating on using her time productively to prepare for the birth of her baby.

- Positive coping mechanisms are discussed and practiced, including deep breathing, guided imagery, progressive muscle relaxation, mindfulness meditation, and sensory modulation strategies.
  - Annie practices mindfulness meditation and, although she has difficulty with it at first, she is intrigued with what she reads about it, and includes it in her daily routine, varying her approach and her environment to experiment with what works best. She also finds music to be calming and, at times, she finds upbeat music to be a great distraction when she is engaged in negative thinking.
- Occupation as addiction is discussed, and the need for healthy routines is addressed. This includes identification of positive activities and occupations, included proactively in daily routines and to be used as participants become more aware of personal triggers.
  - Annie begins to verbalize and practice additional coping mechanisms. She develops a daily routine, including positive activities to fill her time to alleviate boredom. She likes to read so she starts going to the local library 1 day a week. She checks out fiction books as well as parenting books. She also becomes interested in organic foods and healthy eating and begins reviewing

recipes online. She makes a goal to try one new healthy recipe a week, and she finds that she enjoys cooking. She would like to find a part-time job but doesn't find anything right away so she volunteers at a food bank one morning a week. She says that she would like to find something she could do from home to earn some money, and she dedicates some time to researching potential home-based opportunities.

Annie attends weekly sessions consistently and is very engaged. She feels more in control of her anxiety as the weeks go by, and she feels more prepared to be a mother and more aware of how to deal with her negative thinking and anxiety. She stopped alcohol and tobacco use when she found out she was pregnant, and she does not use heroin any more. She does report still having the desire to use and how difficult it can be at times to resist it. Also, she has started attending a 12-step program several times a week and finds that is helping her to remain abstinent. She also reports some tension in her relationship with her boyfriend. She admits that their relationship evolved quickly, and they are still learning a lot about each other. Most of the tension has developed around discussions related to child rearing. She is also concerned because he does use alcohol at least once a week and smokes cigarettes. He states he plans to quit smoking when the baby is born and he will not drink around her or the baby. She is committed to the relationship and believes that he is too and is optimistic that they will work it out.

SUGGESTED LEARNING ACTIVITIES

1. Review at least two of the drug and alcohol use screening tools on the Substance Abuse and Mental Health Services Administration website (available at: https://www.integration.samhsa.gov/clinicalpractice/screeningtools#sample%20screening%20forms) and at least two of the instruments in the Substance Use Screening and Assessment Instruments Database managed by the Alcohol and Drug Abuse Institute, University of Washington (available at: http://lib.adai.washington.edu/instruments).

2. Review module 4 of the evidence-based SAMHSA publication *Integrated Treatment for Co-Occurring Disorders* (available at: https://store.samhsa.gov/system/files/trainingfrontlinestaff-itc.pdf). Read the three vignettes and complete the exercises at the end of the module.

3. To learn more about the opiate crisis, read *Dreamland: The True Tale of America's Opiate Epidemic.*[59]

REFLECTION QUESTIONS

1. What do you think of the concept of "occupation as addiction" and the implications for treatment from the perspective of the occupational therapy practitioner?

2. Considering co-occurring disorders, what do you think are the most challenging issues to address in the health care system?

3. How can occupational therapy be a part of the solution in the opioid crisis?

4. How comfortable are you in addressing substance use disorders with clients across practice settings?

REFERENCES

1. American Psychiatric Association. *Diagnostic and Statistical Manual of Mental Disorders.* 5th ed. Washington, DC: American Psychiatric Association; 2013.
2. Daley DC. Family and social aspects of substance use disorders and treatment. *J Food Drug Anal.* 2013;21(4):S73-S76.
3. Lim SS, Vos T, Flaxman AD, Danaei G, Shibuya K, Adair-Rohani H, et al. A comparative risk assessment of burden of disease and injury attributable to 67 risk factors and risk factor clusters in 21 regions, 1990–2010: a systematic analysis for the Global Burden of Disease Study 2010. *Lancet.* 2012;380:2224-2260.
4. Peacock A, Leung J, Larney S, Colledge S, Hickman M, Rehm J, et al. Global statistics on alcohol, tobacco and illicit drug use: 2017 status report. *Addiction.* 2018;113:1905-1926.
5. Substance Abuse and Mental Health Services Administration. *Key Substance Use and Mental Health Indicators in the United States: Results from the 2017 National Survey on Drug Use and Health.* HHS Publ. No. SMA 18-5068, NSDUH Series H-53. Rockville, MD: Center for Behavioral Health Statistics and Quality, Substance Abuse and Mental Health Services Administration; 2018.
6. Rehm J, Mathers C, Popova S, Thavorncharoensap M, Teerawattananon Y, Patra J. Global burden of disease and injury and economic cost attributable to alcohol use and alcohol-use disorders. *Lancet.* 2009;373:2223-2233.
7. Horvath A, Misra K, Epner A, Cooper G. The diagnostic criteria for substance use disorders (addiction). Available at: https://www.gracepointwellness.org/1408-addictions/article/48502-the-diagnostic-criteria-for-substance-use-disorders-addiction.
8. World Health Organization. *Global Status Report on Alcohol and Health 2018.* Geneva: World Health Organization; 2018.
9. US Department of Health and Human Services; US Department of Agriculture. Dietary Guidelines for Americans 2015–2020. 8th ed. Available at: http://health.gov/dietaryguidelines/2015/guidelines.
10. World Health Organization. Tobacco Fact Sheet 2018. Available at: https://www.who.int/news-room/fact-sheets/detail/tobacco.
11. West R. Tobacco smoking: Health impact, prevalence, correlates and interventions. *Psychol Health.* 2017;32(8):1018-1036.
12. Centers for Disease Control and Prevention. Current cigarette smoking among adults in the United States. Available at: https://www.cdc.gov/tobacco/data_statistics/fact_sheets/adult_data/cig_smoking/index.htm.
13. National Institute on Drug Abuse, National Institutes of Health, US Department of Health and Human Services. Marijuana. 2018. Available at: https://d14rmgtrwzf5a.cloudfront.net/sites/default/files/drugfacts-marijuana.pdf.
14. Shrivastava A, Johnston M, Terpstra K, Bureau Y. Cannabis and psychosis: neurobiology. *Indian J Psychiatry.* 2014;56(1):8-16.
15. National Institute on Drug Abuse, National Institutes of Health, US Department of Health and Human Services. Hallucinogens. Available at: https://d14rmgtrwzf5a.cloudfront.net/sites/default/files/hallucinogens_df_1_2016.pdf.
16. National Institute on Drug Abuse, National Institutes of Health, US Department of Health and Human Services. Inhalants. Available at: https://d14rmgtrwzf5a.cloudfront.net/sites/default/files/drugfacts-inhalants.pdf.
17. Centers for Diseases Control and Prevention. Prescription opioids. Available at: https://www.cdc.gov/drugoverdose/opioids/prescribed.html
18. Han B, Compton WM, Blanco C, Jones CM. Correlates of prescription opioid use, misuse, use disorders, and motivations for misuse among US adults. *J Clin Psychiatry.* 2018;79(5):4-14.
19. Centers for Diseases Control and Prevention. Understanding the epidemic. Available at: https://www.cdc.gov/drugoverdose/epidemic/index.html.
20. Centers for Diseases Control and Prevention. Opioid basics. Available at: https://www.cdc.gov/drugoverdose/opioids/index.html.
21. Centers for Diseases Control and Prevention. Heroin. Available at: https://www.cdc.gov/drugoverdose/opioids/heroin.html.
22. Centers for Diseases Control and Prevention. Fentanyl. Available at: https://www.cdc.gov/drugoverdose/opioids/fentanyl.html.
23. National Institute on Drug Abuse, National Institutes of Health, US Department of Health and Human Services. Cocaine. Available at: https://d14rmgtrwzf5a.cloudfront.net/sites/default/files/drugfacts-cocaine.pdf.
24. Karila L, Petit A, Lowenstein W, Reynaud M. Diagnosis and consequences of cocaine addiction. *Curr Med Chem.* 2012;19(33):5612-5618.
25. Substance Abuse and Mental Health Services Administration. *Integrated Treatment for Co-Occurring Disorders*: Training Frontline Staff. DHHS Publ. No. SMA-08-4366. Rockville, MD: Center for Mental Health Services, Substance Abuse and Mental Health Services Administration, US Department of Health and Human Services; 2009.
26. Cleary M, Thomas SP. Addiction and mental health across the lifespan: an overview of some contemporary issues. *Issues Ment Health Nurs.* 2017;38:(1):2-8.
27. Lai HM X, Cleary M, Sitharthan T, Hunt GE. Prevalence of comorbid substance use, anxiety and mood disorders in epidemiological surveys, 1990–2014: a systematic review and meta-analysis. *Drug Alcohol Depend.* 2015;154:1-13.
28. Thompson K. Occupational therapy and substance use disorders: are practitioners addressing these disorders in practice? *Occup Ther Health Care.* 2007;21:3:61-77,
29. Tenegra JC, Leebold B. Substance abuse screening and treatment. *Prim Care.* 2016;43:217-227.
30. National Institute on Drug Abuse, National Institutes of Health, US Department of Health and Human Services. Screening for Drug Use in General Medical Settings Resource Guide. Available at: https://www.drugabuse.gov/sites/default/files/resource_guide.pdf.
31. Murray CJ, Atkinson C, Bjalla K, Birbeck G, Burstein R, Chou D, et al. The state of US health;1990-2010 burden of diseases, injuries, and risk factors. JAMA. 2013;310:591-606.
32. Brown RL, Rounds, LA. Conjoint screening questionnaires for alcohol and other drug abuse: criterion validity in a primary care practice. *Wis Med J.* 1995;94(3):135-140.

33. Alcohol and Drug Abuse Institute. Substance use screening & assessment instruments database. Available at: http://lib.adai.washington.edu/instruments.

34. Substance Abuse and Mental Health Services Administration. Screening tools. Available at: https://www.integration.samhsa.gov/clinical-practice/screening-tools#sample%20screening%20forms.

35. Substance Abuse and Mental Health Services Administration. SBIRT: screening, brief intervention, and referral to treatment. Available at: https://www.integration.samhsa.gov/clinical-practice/sbirt.

36. Massachusetts Department of Public Health, Bureau of Substance Abuse Services. SBIRT: A step-by-step guide for screening and intervening for unhealthy alcohol and other drug use. Available at: https://www.masbirt.org/sites/www.masbirt.org/files/documents/toolkit.pdf.

37. American Occupational Therapy Association. Occupational therapy practice framework: Domain and process, 3rd. edition. *Am J Occup Ther.* 2014;68(Suppl 1):S1-S51.

38. Law MC, Baptiste S, Carswell A, McColl MA, Polatajko H, Pollock N. *Canadian Occupational Performance Measure Manual.* 4th ed. Thorofare, NJ: Slack; 2005.

39. Martin LM, Triscari R, Boisvert R, et al. Development and evaluation of the Lifestyle History Questionnaire (LHQ) for people entering treatment for substance addictions. *Am J Occup Ther.* 2015;69:6903250010.

40. National Institute on Drug Abuse, National Institutes of Health, US Department of Health and Human Services. Principles of drug addiction treatment: a research-based guide (3rd ed.) Available at: https://d14rmgtrwzf5a.cloudfront.net/sites/default/files/675-principles-of-drug-addiction-treatment-a-research-based-guide-third-edition.pdf.

41. O'Brien CP. Anticraving medications for relapse prevention: a possible new class of psychoactive medications. *Am J Psychiatry.* 2005;162(8):1423-1431.

42. Douaihy AB, Kelly TM, Sullivan C. Medications for substance use disorders. *Soc Work Public Health.* 2013;28(3-4):264-278.

43. Klein JW. Pharmacotherapy for substance use disorders. *Med Clin North Am.* 2016;100:891-910.

44. Adams JM. Increasing naloxone awareness and use: the role of health care practitioners. *JAMA.* 2018;319(20):2073-2074.

45. Substance Abuse and Mental Health Services Administration. Treatment for substance use disorders. Available at: https://www.samhsa.gov/treatment/substance-use-disorders.

46. Petry NM. Contingency management: what it is and why psychiatrists should want to use it. *Psychiatrist.* 2011;35(5):161-163.

47. Medina J. Treatment of Substance Use Disorders (SUDs). Psych Central. 2018. Available at: https://psychcentral.com/disorders/addictions/substance-use-disorders-treatment.

48. Gutman SA. Why addiction has a chronic, relapsing course: the neurobiology of addiction. *Occup Ther Ment Health.* 2006;22(2):1-29.

49. Wasmuth S, Crabtree JL, Scott PJ. Exploring addiction-as-occupation. *Br J Occup Ther.* 2014;77(12):605-613.

50. Stoffel VC, Moyers PA. An evidence-based and occupational perspective of interventions for persons with substance-use disorders. *Am J Occup Ther.* 2004;58:570-586.

51. Amorelli CR. Psychosocial occupational therapy interventions for substance-use disorders: a narrative review. Occup Ther Ment Health. 2016;32(2):167-184,

52. Boisvert R. Enhancing substance dependence intervention. *OT Pract.* 2004;9(10):11-16.

53. Boisvert RA, Martin LM, Grosek M, Clarie AJ. Effectiveness of a peer-support community in addiction recovery: participation as intervention. *Occup Ther Int.* 2008;15(4):205-220.

54. Peloquin SM, Ciro CA. Self-development groups among women in recovery: client perceptions of satisfaction and engagement. *Am J Occup Ther.* 2013;67:82-90.

55. Knis-Matthews L. A parenting program for women who are substance dependent. *Mental Health Spec Interest Sect Q.* 2003;26:1-4.

56. White S. Let's get organized: An intervention for persons with co-occurring disorders. *Psychiatr Serv.* 2007;58(5):713.

57. Wasmuth S, Pritchard K. Theater-based community engagement project for veterans recovering from substance use disorders. *Am J Occup Ther.* 2016;70:7004250020.

58. Rojo-Mota G, Pedrero-Pérez EJ, Huertas-Hoyas E. Systematic review of occupational therapy in the treatment of addiction: Models, practice, and qualitative and quantitative research. *Am J Occup Ther.* 2017;71:7105100030.

59. Quinones S. *Dreamland: The True Tale of America's Opiate Epidemic.* New York: Bloomsbury Press; 2015.

13

Neurocognitive Disorders

Nicole Maxham

LEARNING OBJECTIVES

1. Identify the various disorders that are categorized as neurocognitive disorders (NCDs).
2. Understand the importance of early detection of delirium and implications for older adults.
3. List and briefly identify assessment tools used in practice with cognitive-related disorders.
4. Be able to identify and explain common treatment interventions, approaches, and models used with individuals diagnosed with NCDs.

NEUROCOGNITIVE DISORDERS AND NEW CHANGES

Neurocognitive disorders (NCDs) is an umbrella term used to describe a wide variety of diagnoses, disorders, and diseases that create a change in an individual's mental function, specifically cognition.[1] The disease that people most quickly attribute to changes in cognition is dementia, or Alzheimer disease. However, there are several conditions and diseases which can have implications on an individual's cognitive status. The new DSM-5 took what was formerly called dementia, delirium, amnestic, and other cognitive disorders in the DSM-IV and created the new category, neurocognitive disorders (NCDs).[1] Most notable, the DSM-5 puts dementia within the category titled major neurocognitive disorder.[1] However, the term, dementia, is still used in literature, in practice, and throughout writings. In addition to Alzheimer disease and dementia, other disorders that cause changes in cognition include vascular-related incidents such as cerebrovascular accident (CVA) or aneurysm. Other conditions that can present with symptoms related to impaired cognition include Lewy Body dementia, Parkinson disease, traumatic brain injury (TBI), infectious diseases including the human immunodeficiency virus (HIV) and acquired immune deficiency syndrome (AIDS), substance or medication abuse, and Huntington disease.

As indicated in this list, there are a lot of diseases, conditions, and etiologies that can lead to a diagnosis of neurocognitive disorder and cause changes in cognition. One thing all of these NCDs have in common is that they cause a gradual decline in cognitive status, opposed to being developmental in nature. In other words, individuals with NCDs are not born with a cognitive dysfunction; rather, it is acquired through time as part of the disease process or from an external cause such as TBI or infection. However, regardless of the cause, the symptoms are quite similar and impact multiple areas of the brain. The areas of the brain most impacted are those responsible for complex attention, executive functioning, learning and memory, language, proprioception and motor skills, and social skills.[2]

When an individual's complex attention is impacted, practitioners will see changes in a person's processing speed, and three areas of attention: sustained, divided, and selective attention.[2] Sustained attention is the ability to stay focused and involved on a task for a period of time. An individual who is having difficulty with sustained attention would present as the patient who gets distracted easily, or can only attend to a task for a few minutes at a time. When working with these individuals, it may be easier to break tasks into smaller, more manageable parts to ensure success with the session and to help minimize frustration. Divided attention, more commonly known as multitasking, is the ability to carry out more than one task at the same time, such as being able to hum a song while doing homework.[3] A patient that has a difficult time with multitasking will perform best when there are minimal distractions in the environment, such as having an organized work space and eliminating extraneous sounds and visual stimuli. Selective attention refers to the ability to select and focus on one particular stimulus or task while multiple pieces of stimuli are happening at one time.[3] Similar to divided attention, people who have difficulty with selective attention will perform best in environments that limit extraneous stimuli.

Executive functioning is one of the most complex aspects of cognition, as many aspects of daily life are controlled and impacted by one's executive functioning skills. This is because executive functioning skills, which reside in the frontal lobe of the brain[4] are directly responsible for an individual's social behavior, emotional regulation and self-awareness, and working memory, and one's ability to learn societal rules, plan, make decisions, and respond to and correct errors.[5] From a caregiver or therapist point of view, when the executive dysfunction develops, the client may present as having a change in personality, mood, or social skills.[5] For example, the person who used to be very social and outgoing may become reclusive or seem awkward in social situations, where at baseline this was not the case. This same individual may find it difficult to execute, or initiate, the tasks of everyday living, because their ability to plan, use their working memory, and stay organized is impaired.[5] For people that live with executive dysfunction, it may be useful to use lists, planners, check-off sheets, or calendars in order to stay organized, break projects into smaller more manageable tasks, and plan for the future. For individuals whose social skills are impacted, it would be beneficial to participate in social groups run by either an occupational therapy practitioner or mental health professional to help recognize, correct, and develop typical social skills and behaviors.

Another area most commonly impacted by NCDs is an individual's learning and memory. For many individuals with difficulties related to memory, it is often short-term memory (STM) that is impacted the most.[6] In other words, these people will have the most difficulty remembering new and recent events. These individuals may also repeat themselves multiple times within the same conversation and have a difficult time tracking and remembering items despite using a list or a visual cue. One way that occupational therapy practitioners and caregivers can assist these individuals, is to teach compensatory strategies such as list making and use of visual aids such as calendars. During therapy sessions, or in group settings, these individuals may need occasional reminders, or verbal cues, to stay on task, or may need to reread written directions.[7]

Language centers are another area of the brain that may be impacted with a diagnosis of an NCD. People who have difficulties surrounding language may present with difficulty with word finding.[8] A way that many people compensate for word-finding difficulty is to begin using broad, general terms rather than being specific. For example, "I wonder where the *thing* that goes here might be," or they will point to what they want and say, "Can you hand me that *thing* over there?" because they cannot think of the word that they want. Some people will have difficulty with both expressive and receptive language, meaning they have a hard time not only saying what they want and need, but they also have a hard time understanding what others are saying to them.[8]

When people with an NCD have difficulty with motor skills and proprioception, they often think of Parkinson disease. However, there are many NCDs where both gross and fine motor movements and old skills learned through repeated muscle memory become difficult.[5] This is true for all NCDs, including Parkinson disease, depending on the stage and severity of the disease process. For example, a person with rather advanced dementia may forget how to braid hair despite the fact that they used to do their hair every day. From a proprioception and perception standpoint, these individuals may have a hard time remembering to use landmarks to get around, or they get lost easily. For example, this would be the individual who could easily get lost if they took a walk around their neighborhood, and wouldn't be able to find their way home. Important things to remember when planning treatment sessions or groups for individuals with difficulty in motor planning and proprioception skills is that they might need more time and it may be more difficult to attend to spatial tasks. A way to compensate would be to use maps or have written directions to find new places. You may see people try to compensate by following others in a crowd when in an unfamiliar place. Unfortunately, this behavior puts the individual at a higher risk of getting lost if they are not concentrating on their surroundings or if the people they are following aren't going where they need to go.

People with various NCDs may display changes in their social skills and behaviors.[5] As is true with most symptoms related to NCDs, the severity of these changes depends on many factors and variables. Some people will not experience any changes in social skills and behaviors, whereas others may seem like an entirely different person to loved ones and regular caregivers. On a milder side of the spectrum, family and caregivers may notice a slight change of personality; however, the person is still able to function within social norms. For example, family members might describe their loved one as being "different" or "off," yet in a typical social setting, other people who may not be as familiar with that individual would not notice anything different. On the contrary, some people may display negative behaviors that do not align with social norms, often behaving without regard for others. These are the people who might scream, swear, act out, be physically aggressive, or say mean and hurtful things. They may also speak inappropriately or behave in ways that would make others typically feel uncomfortable. These same people may appear impulsive by making decisions without thinking of consequences or the safety of oneself or others. This of course needs to be taken into consideration when planning groups and even one to one therapy treatment sessions, because it is the occupational therapy practitioner's job to ensure that everyone involved is safe and also feels comfortable. Depending on the person and the severity of their behavioral changes, they may be easily redirected, or on the other extreme, need to be removed from a group situation. Many times, it is best to try and redirect the person back to the task with a verbal cue, or reframe their negative thoughts into those that are more appropriate with simple rewording or paraphrasing.

TYPES OF NEUROCOGNITIVE DISORDERS

Alzheimer Disease

Similar to other neurocognitive disorders, Alzheimer disease is known to cause physical changes to the structures within the brain and is progressive in nature. Typically, the hippocampus is the region most impacted with this disease process, as it is the center of learning and memory in the brain,[9] and often is what attributes to the hallmark symptom of memory loss in these individuals. Individuals with Alzheimer disease experience both short-term and long-term memory loss, language difficulties including word finding and aphasia, changes in executive functioning, and, in some cases, personality.[9]

There are three stages of Alzheimer disease: early, middle, and late.[9] Of course, every individual is unique and needs to be addressed on a case by case basis. However, the disease is progressive in nature; thus, regardless of the individual, symptoms typically start as mild and progress to severe. Symptoms vary depending on the individual and which stage they present with (Box 13.1). However, symptoms range from repeating oneself, forgetting or misplacing commonly used items, difficulty with word finding, getting lost easily, wandering, changes in behavior or personality, forgetting how to use everyday objects or objects that were once familiar to the individual, and, with severe dementia, the individual will forget how to complete self-care tasks, or activities of daily living (ADLs), including washing, dressing, and even eating and speaking.[7] Depression and anxiety may also be

> ### BOX 13.1   Common Behavioral and Mood Changes That Can Be Seen in the Early to Late Stages of Alzheimer Disease.[9]
>
> | Early Stage | Late Stage |
> | --- | --- |
> | Irritability | Anger |
> | Anxiety | Agitation and aggression |
> | Depression | Behavioral outbursts |
> | | Restlessness |
> | | Hallucinations |
> | | Delusions |
> | | Sleep difficulty |

present in patients with Alzheimer disease.[9] This finding is not surprising for many people. For those diagnosed earlier in life, the thought of losing memories can be frightening and saddening. Additionally, losing the ability to be independent and feel like a burden on loved ones is stressful and negatively impacts the patient's perception of their own quality of life. All of these sudden and difficult life changes can lead to depression and other mental health changes. Furthermore, the stress and anxiety of constantly feeling lost and confused, especially for those patients who have difficulty with orientation, puts those with Alzheimer disease at a higher risk for anxiety disorders.[9] Often, these symptoms are treated pharmaceutically; however, it is important to be aware of the signs and symptoms of depression and anxiety, so that these observations can be communicated to the interdisciplinary team for early treatment.

Parkinson Disease

When people think about the progression and symptoms of Parkinson disease, they do not always think of the cognitive changes that can occur. Most people know the classic signs of Parkinson disease including tremors, bradykinesia, rigidity or tone abnormalities, and difficulty with gait and balance.[9] Many of these symptoms are due to the pathophysiological nature of the disease, as it impacts the dopamine-producing neurons in the substantia nigra of the brain. These neurons are responsible for the brain's movement centers.[9] However, Parkinson disease is still a neurodegenerative disorder, thus symptoms beyond physical impairments can be seen. Cognitive, behavioral, and mood abnormalities caused by changes within the brain's physiology can occur and include apathy, increased depression and anxiety, sleep disturbances, and changes in perceptions of senses including taste or smell.[9] As the disease progresses, memory, attention, insight, safety, planning, and motor sequencing are impacted, making it increasingly difficult to safely and independently participate in ADLs.[9]

CASE STUDY 13.1 Parkinson–Josh*

Josh is an 85-year-old male living in an apartment in an assisted living facility. The nursing staff have noticed that Josh is needing more assistance with his ADLs and has had a number of falls in the past month. Additionally, Josh is requiring well beyond two hours of care and assistance from nursing staff per day. At his level of assisted living, the nursing staff is only able to provide up to two hours of care a day. As a result, you are asked to evaluate and treat Josh for strategies related to ADLs and to see if this level of assisted living is appropriate with implementation of environmental modifications and compensatory strategies to decrease falls in his apartment.

On the day of the evaluation, you first check in with nursing staff to make sure that Josh is in his apartment and knows that you are coming. You find out from the nurse that Josh was notified that occupational therapy would be coming by, and that he is in the apartment. When you knock on the door, there is no answer, however you can hear movement behind the door. You knock again and are greeted by a disheveled older adult, who looks confused as to why you are there even after an introduction. He hesitantly lets you into his apartment. You notice that there is clutter, including clothes, tissues, and papers on the floor and around the surfaces of the apartment. Josh is walking with a shuffled gait, and has forgotten his rolling walker in the bathroom. Josh sits down on the couch and repeatedly asks you who you are, and why you are visiting him, despite already introducing yourself and the purpose of your visit at the door. He insists to you that he does not need any assistance for self-care, and that he is fully independent throughout the day, never needing assistance from nursing staff. When you ask him about his recent falls, he does not recall falling, but does admit that he has very poor eyesight making it hard to find things in his apartment.

Over the course of a few days, and in collaboration with the interdisciplinary team and Josh's family, the decision is made to have Josh move to another area of the assisted living facility where residents can have more individualized care around the clock. This move is temporary at first, and is being viewed as a trial, to see if Josh performs better with more support from staff. While in his new apartment, Josh has an additional two falls within a week, due to his shuffling gait, even with a rolling walker. As a result, the interdisciplinary team asks that physical therapy starts working with Josh to address balance and gait training. While collaborating with physical therapy to address the goals of improved balance and gait, you and Josh create occupational therapy goals that also address

balance and safety related to his various occupations. Josh is particularly concerned with his mobility on and off the unit, particularly getting to dinner as he recently had a fall in the dining room. Also of concern is transfer training, safe rolling walker use in the bathroom, bedroom, and hallways, environmental modifications to address decreased eyesight and coordination, and strategies to improve independence and performance in all areas of self-care to increase overall quality of life. What are some possible treatment interventions Josh's occupational therapist should use?

Intervention: To address Josh's decreased eyesight and difficulty with planning and organization, labels were placed around the apartment. All labels were large, with dark large font, on high contrast neon paper, and were laminated for longevity. Josh and the occupational therapist worked together to find places for all of his clothing items, bathroom products, and office supplies. All shelves and drawers were labeled with the name of the contents in each. How do you think this impacted Josh and his independence?

Outcome: Labels worked to increase Josh's independence with ADLs and instrumental activities of daily living (IADLs) in several ways. First, Josh was able to independently locate and retrieve items without having to ask for nursing staff to find things for him. This also helped to address his anxiety. Through working with Josh, the occupational therapist realized that a lot of his anxiety was related to not being able to find items in his room, because he thought that people had come into his room and taken them. The labels also helped Josh to keep his room clean and organized, by decreasing clutter on surfaces, and most importantly the floor, which decreased his risk of falling. The labels in the bathroom and closet, specifically, helped increase independence with self-care, in that Josh was able to independently choose his own clothing, and set up his own supplies for sink level bathroom hygiene.

Intervention: In addition to labels, bright colored tape was placed around the grab bars and rails around the toilet in the bathroom. While working with Josh, the occupational therapist realized that the bars in the bathroom and the wall they were attached to were both white. This made the grab bar more difficult to see on the wall, and put Josh at a high risk of falling due to unsafe transfers on and off the toilet. In addition to the rails, a strip of bright colored tape is placed on the floor directly in front of the toilet, to show Josh where his feet should be before he sits down on the toilet.

Continued

Outcome: With new, brightly colored rails, Josh is able to see the grab bars and differentiate between the bars and the walls. As a result, Josh is better able to steady himself on and off the toilet while using the grab bars, despite his coordination difficulties. In addition to the rails, the strip of bright-colored tape on the floor has made Josh more aware of his foot placement for transfers and his falls in the bathroom have decreased.

Intervention: Due to Josh's diagnosis of Parkinson disease, Josh also has difficulty with cognition. Specifically, Josh has a hard time remembering names of caregivers and staff, times and dates of important appointments, the location of his apartment in the building, telephone numbers, family members' birthdays, and the daily activities on the unit. Josh and the occupational therapist work together to brainstorm cognitive aids that Josh will enjoy using and can easily implement into his lifestyle and apartment.

Outcome: The occupational therapist works with Josh to implement using a notepad for note taking when he is off the unit. For example, if Josh makes plans with another resident off the unit, he can write it down and find the note later. In conjunction with the notepad, Josh started using a calendar on his computer to keep track of important dates and reminders that he had written on his notepad. Staff on the unit were trained in the importance of daily updates to Josh's communication board in his room, listing the names of the staff working with him that day, and if applicable, any appointments that day. Josh also was given a monthly calendar to hang in his room that listed the times and locations of all activities that were planned for the unit to increase his social interactions, and find more leisure occupations beyond his apartment. Josh was given a small sign to have taped to the seat of his rolling walker with the room number of his apartment so that he could ask for assistance to get back to his apartment if he got lost on the unit. In general, these cognitive strategies helped Josh to feel less anxious, as he knew that he could always find his way back to his apartment, or be able to give an accurate location if he needed help. He knew if and when he had appointments, and who would be taking him, and by being more organized, he self-reported feeling less confused.

*Name changed for confidentiality.

Frontotemporal Lobar Degeneration

This NCD is unique in that it tends to start showing symptoms earlier than those diagnosed with Alzheimer disease or another NCD.[9] Frontotemporal lobar degeneration is caused by progressive nerve cell loss in the brain's frontal or temporal lobes.[9] The significance of the earlier onset is that in the working individual, there may be implications for the occupations of work, leisure, and social pursuits, as behavioral and social regulation are likely to be impaired. This makes it difficult for others who are unaware of the diagnosis, as they may wrongfully assume that the individual is otherwise healthy and not understand that the person with the NCD is having difficulty regulating social and behavioral responses. For occupational therapy practitioners, it may be beneficial to look at ways to change the environment for working individuals or teach caregivers ways to best assist the client, so as to promote as much independence as possible. For younger people in particular, they may be easily embarrassed or feel as though they are taking a lot of time from their loved ones if they need a lot of assistance.

Lewy Bodies

NCD with Lewy bodies has a motor component as well as a cognitive component, similar to the symptoms seen in Parkinson disease. In other words, these individuals experience not only a cognitive decline but also a functional decline related to motor coordination skills.[9] Similar to Alzheimer disease, people with Lewy body dementia experience changes within their brain. This particular type of NCD is caused by abnormal deposits that damage brain cells and progressively gets worse with time, similar to other NCDs.[9] Due to the interaction of both the cognitive and motor skills, these individuals are more prone to have difficulty earlier on in the disease process with functional skills related to ADLs and mobility, as compared with an individual without motor coordination impairments.[9] This is not to say that people with cognitive impairments related to NCD will not also experience deficits with motor coordination as the disease progresses; however, these difficulties might not develop or emerge until later in the disease process, when the individual has difficulty with motor planning.

Vascular Neurocognitive Disorders

The most common cerebrovascular event seen by occupational therapists are strokes or CVAs, but can include any condition that impacts blood flow to or within the brain.[9] When treating patients who are diagnosed with any vascular neurocognitive disorder, it is helpful to have an understanding of the anatomy of the brain and the functions of the various areas of the brain. The benefit in knowing brain anatomy is that when imaging and scans can detect the area of the brain impacted, therapists can make some assumptions as to what deficits they may see in their client. For example, damage to the frontal lobe during a vascular insult would have a much different outcome than damage in the occipital lobe. Since the brain is complex, and cerebrovascular events can take place in any area of the brain, each patient will present differently and need to be treated on a case by case basis. Additionally, the degree to which the patient's cognition is impacted and the rate of progression are also dependent on the area of the brain that is affected and how severe the damage is.[9] The brain is quite resilient and with skilled occupational therapy, patients have been known to make phenomenal progress in functional skills, often with implementation of compensatory strategies. Another complexity when treating patients with a vascular neurocognitive disorder is that there are often physical impairments that follow a cerebrovascular incident.[9] Most commonly, people will experience fluctuations in muscle tone and strength, and visual perceptual skills may be impaired, which could also be a focus of occupational therapy intervention.[9]

Traumatic Brain Injury

Traumatic brain injury (TBI) is diagnosed when damage is caused to the brain by an external, mechanical force.[9] TBIs are very common after vehicle accidents where there is a lot of force applied to the brain, an object makes contact with the brain, or the brain rapidly moves within the skull. Neurocognitive changes after a TBI include difficulty with complex attention, executive functioning, learning and memory, delayed information processing, or typical social skills.[9] The severity of the deficits seen in a TBI vary greatly depending on the area of the brain involved, the severity of the damage, and how the damage impacts the physiological structure of the brain. For example, in the event that a foreign object enters the skull and damages brain structures, there may be other deficits present in addition to the cognitive changes that would be seen in a neurocognitive disorder. These damaged areas not only could lead to a deficit in cognition, but also a deficit in other functional skills based on the area of the brain involved. Similar to a vascular neurocognitive disorder, if multiple areas of the brain are impacted from trauma, there may be several functional deficits that could be the focus of skilled occupational therapy intervention. The progression of treatment depends on the individual and includes past medical history specifically related to prior brain injuries, as repeated TBIs or brain injuries can slow the progression of healing or impact the severity of the deficits seen in the individual. For this reason, individuals need to be treated

on a case by case basis and should be treated with an individualistic approach.

WHAT IS DELIRIUM?

Delirium is unique and quite different than the confusion and behavioral changes seen in diseases such as Alzheimer disease.[9] Delirium is an acute change that occurs suddenly and causes changes in a person's cognition and behavior. The biggest difference between the cognition changes and behavioral disturbances seen in delirium compared to Alzheimer disease,[9] for example, is that delirium is not permanent and happens suddenly, within 24–48 hours.[10] Patients who are diagnosed with delirium have symptoms that cannot be explained by another disorder or diagnosis, such as dementia or Parkinson disease. In many cases, the cause of the sudden change can be found through medical testing ordered by a physician, performed in a laboratory, including blood work and urine analysis, which often can determine subtle acute changes in the body that the patient cannot verbalize.[10] In most cases, delirium is resolved with either a correction or change in medications, treatment with an antibiotic following an infection, such as a urinary tract infection (UTI), or stabilization of metabolic levels within a patient's body.[10]

Delirium and the Occupational Therapy Practitioner

As an occupational therapy practitioner, it is important to know the signs and symptoms of delirium because it can tell a lot about the patient. As delirium is often a result of a metabolic or acute change within the body,[10] a sudden, drastic change in a patient's memory, cognition, or behaviors could be the first sign that something is medically wrong, even if the patient is unaware of it. Since delirium is an early detection method that something is wrong, it is important to communicate these findings to the interdisciplinary team and those involved with the care and treatment of the patient. In most cases, blood work or urine samples will be obtained to rule out common bacterial infections such as a UTI or the start of an infection elsewhere in the body.[10] In most cases, when lab values come back abnormal, they are easily corrected with administration of antibiotics that stop the infection process.[10] Once the medications have had a chance to metabolize within the body and the infection begins to clear, the patient's symptoms begin to subside. Interestingly, most people are unaware that they are in a delirious state. Even after treatment, they might not recall the things that they said or did, or their perception of the events may differ from reality.

Delirium and the Older Adult

When delirium occurs in an older adult, it should be a red flag for all health care professionals. In many older adults, a common symptom of a UTI is delirium.[10] It is not clear as to why older adults can become delirious when experiencing a UTI; however, it is important to know that older adults can be impacted in this way to ensure prompt treatment. In many cases, particularly in hospitals or skilled nursing facilities, where families and primary caregivers are not around the patient 24 hours, an occupational therapy practitioner or nurse may be the first person to notice a change in the patient. When communicating with the interdisciplinary team, it is important to document in both verbal and written format the changes that you notice. Important details to include are new or worsening behaviors, confusion, impaired STM, not recognizing familiar people or objects, saying things that do not make sense, or becoming easily distracted during tasks. In an acute care setting, where the population is generally more sick and susceptible to infections or worsening conditions, it is important to be prompt and accurate in reporting to the team to ensure the health and safety of the patient.

CASE STUDY 13.2   Delirium—Jean*

Jean is a pleasant and fiercely independent 90-year-old female living in an apartment in the assisted living facility where you are the occupational therapist. Jean recently experienced a fall on ice that resulted in a fracture in her wrist and neck. You are asked to evaluate and treat her for safety and independence with ADL, as well as implementation of a home exercise program for her broken wrist. She wears a collar on her neck and a wrist cock-up splint on her left arm and has strict non-weight bearing precautions on her left upper extremity. After building rapport and working together for many weeks, you know Jean very well. One day you knock on Jean's apartment door. She tells you to come in and you notice that she has papers strewn around her apartment and she seems quite sleepy, as evidenced by her slouching on the couch when you enter the room. Normally, Jean is upright, alert, and watching the news and she keeps her papers in organized piles. You take mental note, but continue with the session. You ask Jean where the exercise handouts are located that she normally keeps on a stand in her living room, but she is unable to tell you where they are. She blames it on people coming into her room in the middle of the night; however, you find out from nursing staff that nobody was in Jean's room that night. You also notice that Jean is not wearing her wrist splint and it is in the bed. When questioned, she admits to you that she was "woozy" in the night and tried to put her wrist splint on her foot. When she realized the split was not fitting she gave up. When you provide Jean with an extra copy of her hand exercises she has difficulty performing them correctly. Jean typically can follow the drawings and written directions with only minimal verbal cues and encouragement. Today she cannot perform any of them without hand over hand tactile cues, explicit one-step verbal commands, and you have to stop her from performing tasks and positions that compromise her non-weight bearing precautions. You ask Jean if she is feeling okay, or if something is wrong, but she attributes her behaviors to poor sleep from having to wear her neck collar. You tell her you are concerned and that you will check in with her nurse, but that you will be back tomorrow. You document your concerns in the computer and verbally communicate with nursing staff your concerns and that you are worried she might have a UTI as her symptoms have occurred within a 24-hour time period.

When you go into work the next morning you read that Jean fell in the middle of the night and needed assistance. When you see Jean for her appointment, she tells you that she did fall, but that it occurred in front of her doctor and nurse, when in fact it happened in the middle of the night and was unwitnessed. During today's session, Jean continues to be confused, her apartment is still unkempt, and she continues to need a lot of assistance for her exercises. You again report your concerns to the team. Later that same day, Jean falls again in her apartment, this time in the living room while talking on the telephone. This second fall along with your voiced concerns prompts staff to run lab work, and Jean is diagnosed with a UTI. Jean is prescribed antibiotics. It takes 48 hours for the delirious symptoms to subside. However, Jean makes a dramatic turn for the better and after 4 days is back to her baseline. When discussing the events with Jean afterward, she has no recollection of her behavior or cognitive changes. However, she is grateful that you and the team found a solution and prevented the risk of more falls. Jean's story is one seen all too often in health care settings, where a simple infection can cause drastic changes in thinking and processing, and often leads to safety concerns. If left untreated, it could cause serious harm.

*Name changed for confidentiality.

EVALUATION

Cognition Screens for the OT Practitioner

The Montreal Cognitive Assessment

The Montreal Cognitive Assessment (MoCA) is great tool to use in any practice setting. Many occupational therapists like to use the MoCA because it is quick, usually taking 10 minutes or less, user friendly, scripted, and free online. Its effectiveness has been compared to the Mini-Mental State Exam (MMSE) and it has been found to be just as accurate, and in some cases better than, the MMSE, showing that it is a quick screen that is reliable to use.[11] Occupational therapists can use this assessment in several different ways. It can be used to get a baseline score when working with an individual with a known NCD diagnosis. This way, whenever caregivers notice a change, the MoCA can be administered again to see if the score has in fact dropped, indicating a decline in cognition. A second way that this screen can be used is to quickly get a score to support a sudden change from normal cognitive functioning. For example, in the Jean case study, a MoCA would have been a great assessment to use because the patient did not have a diagnosis of an NCD, but was showing symptoms that would indicate a deficit. By administering the MoCA, the occupational therapist could show the interdisciplinary team that an individual is not at their typical level of functioning if they typically do not present with impaired cognition. In these situations, it is not uncommon for the MoCA to be readministered after treatment, to see if the change in cognition was due to delirium or another temporary factor.

The Saint Louis University Mental Status Exam

The Saint Louis University Mental Status (SLUMS) Exam is very similar in format to the MoCA[11] in that it is also a pen-and-paper test that asks questions to assess cognitive deficits, specifically orientation, memory, attention, and executive functions, and can be used as a way to track cognitive changes over time.[12] The test goes through a series of 11 questions that target different aspects of cognition. In addition to targeting orientation, memory, attention, and executive functions, questions used in the SLUMS target delayed recall, numeric calculation and registration, immediate recall, and visual spatial skills, all of which are areas that can be impacted with a diagnosis of an NCD.[12] Similar to the MoCA, the SLUMS can be used in a variety of settings, is quick and easy to administer, and can be used as a baseline score or as a quick screen to assess a sudden change in memory or behavior of a client. One study[12] found the SLUMS to be slightly better at detecting mild NCD as compared with the MMSE. However, more research is needed to compare the two assessment methods.[12]

The Mini–Mental State Exam

The MMSE is another pen-and-paper exam that asks questions to assess various areas of cognition.[13] This screen also uses a script and provides the occupational therapist or evaluator with detailed scoring criteria.[13] Like the SLUMS and MoCA, the MMSE can be used as a baseline or a quick screen to quickly determine cognitive changes in patients. Many practitioners like using pen-and-paper tests with a score because they help support the observations noted during therapy sessions in a quantifiable way. However, the MMSE has been found to be less accurate in detecting more subtle or small changes in cognition versus a more obvious decline compared with other standardized assessments.[14]

The Kettle Test

The Kettle Test (KT) is the most unique assessment when compared with the other assessments described, as it is not a pen-and-paper test. Rather, the occupational therapist observes the client as they participate in a functional skill related to making tea. The KT outlines the specific steps and set up of the test, as well as materials needed and scoring methods as the individual progresses through the assessment.[15] The individual is asked to make two hot beverages, one for the therapist and one for the client, using at least two different ingredients.[16] While the client is making the beverages, the practitioner is assessing thirteen areas of performance.[15] Not only is this test functional, it is also a great way to observe other areas of concern when working with people with NCDs. For example, working with a kettle and hot liquids takes a lot of concentration, safety awareness, insight, and judgment, all within a task the client would have to do if living on their own. With a pen-and-paper test, a practitioner may not be able to make these observations. Small to moderately significant correlations were found when the validity of the KT was compared with the MMSE and the Clock Drawing Test,[17] illustrating the validity of the assessment in practice.[16]

TREATMENT CONSIDERATIONS

As an occupational therapy practitioner, the symptoms caused by NCDs could impact sessions and treatment approaches in several ways. Clients may experience difficulty with planning, decision-making, attention span or focus, word finding and naming familiar people and objects, sequencing and planning daily tasks or ADLs, impaired social skills, and impaired performance with IADLs.[9] Understandably, these symptoms play a significant role in a client's independence and quality of life. For an occupational therapy practitioner, the treatment needs to be client centered and focused on maintaining as much independence as possible either through implementation of compensatory techniques, adaptations, modifications, or caregiver training. One common practice is to observe the individuals either at home or in the most natural context possible.[7] This way, as the occupational therapy practitioner, you can recommend changes to improve independence, such as creating new routines, modifying existing routines, adding adaptive equipment, or making changes to the environment.[7] However, it is important to remember that depending on the stage of the NCD, it may be more difficult to implement new changes, due to impaired STM, which will impact carryover between sessions.[9] During treatment sessions, occupational therapy practitioners may notice that the client responds better to certain types of cueing, perhaps verbal, written, or tactile, which can be taught to primary caregivers to make daily routines easier.[7] In the next section, common models used in practice to help guide occupational therapy practitioners as they work with individuals with various NCD diagnoses are discussed.

Fostering Independence

Regardless of diagnosis or ability, one of the most important focuses of occupational therapy intervention is fostering safety and independence in meaningful occupations. Using this as a basis for treatment, the Model of Human Occupation (MOHO)[18] focuses on what is most important to the client. Keeping that in mind, it is important for occupational therapy practitioners to modify activities the person once enjoyed to provide mental stimulation and promote the highest level of independence while working within the just right challenge,[7] that is, making sure activities are still enjoyable, safe, and not too hard or easy. It is important for those with NCDs to stay engaged, particularly if they tend to have difficulties regulating behaviors or to wander when bored or agitated. By focusing on what is most important to the client and modifying occupations as needed, the person can still participate in the occupations they enjoy the most. One challenge that occupational therapy practitioners may experience is trying to determine what occupations are the most meaningful for a client, particularly if the client has difficulty with expressive language. In this scenario, it may be best to interview primary caregivers to get a better understanding of what occupations were of high importance to the client before they started to decline. In the event that the client lives in a facility, such as a skilled nursing facility, it may be beneficial to interview staff to determine what occupations the individual is having the most difficulty doing, or is not participating in to the fullest extent. This could include leisure occupations and ADLs.

One activity that occupational therapy practitioners can suggest early on, shortly after a diagnosis of an NCD, is creating a journal or memory book. In this way, individuals can document their hobbies, interests, and achievements, and include pictures of family and friends earlier in the disease process. The idea is that by capturing this information earlier in the disease process, individuals can have a voice in occupations that are most meaningful, and what occupations are of the most importance regarding maintaining independence. In theory, if an individual is unable to voice their wants and needs, such as in a late-stage NCD, occupational therapy practitioners and caregivers can use the memory book or other memory aid, as a tool to guide sessions, and to ensure the best quality of life and satisfaction with perceived independence.

Mental Health and Well-Being

Intervention with people who have NCD can address occupations beyond ADLs, including leisure occupations. This is important because as it becomes more difficult to remember how to sequence tasks, or how to participate in social situations, some individuals may withdraw from occupations they formerly loved. This can lead to increased incidence of depression and anxiety within this population. The Kawa Model[19] is perhaps the most unique of all the models mentioned throughout the treatment section of this chapter in that it can be used in several different ways in practice, making it quite versatile particularly when used in a health and wellness context. The key feature of this model is that it is a visual aid to help clients map out their obstacles and barriers to success in occupations. The visual components consist of the water, riverbanks, rocks, driftwood, and the spaces in between all of these areas where the water flows.[20] Water represents the client's life flow through time, space, or situation, riverbanks are support systems, rocks are occupational obstacles, or things that impede the client's ability to participate, driftwood is personal attributes of the client, and the gaps between everything where the water passes represents the water's ability to pass despite challenges.[20]

In many instances, using the Kawa Model is helpful when starting a therapeutic relationship with a client, as it is a fun and interactive way to address obstacles and barriers to success. Additionally, using the model as an interactive component in a treatment session can help with stress reduction, as art has been known to decrease stress and anxiety in study participants.[21] Additionally, this model is helpful for people who may have a hard time identifying resources and support systems during times of stress or difficulty. In other words, the client can see that despite their rocks, or obstacles, there are still spaces where the water flows, and they have support from their riverbanks. This is crucial when working with individuals with NCDs who might be expressing signs and symptoms of depression and anxiety as their disease progresses.[9]

Environment and Context

Naturally, one of the first areas of treatment that comes to mind when working with NCD populations is the environment and context in which occupations are performed. The main reason for this is that occupational therapy practitioners want to ensure both safety and independence in the most natural contexts possible. There are various ways in which occupational therapy practitioners can implement models into practice that target the environment and how the individual interacts with their surroundings. One such model is the Person-Environment-Occupation-Performance (PEOP) model. Many occupational therapy practitioners use the PEOP model in practice when assessing the environment in which occupations are performed. For example, it may be necessary to modify the environment by removing dangerous items, or figure out solutions to safety hazards, such as flammable liquids, stairwells, medications, and appliances.[7] Other environmental considerations include throw rugs, clutter, furniture, and access to familiar objects.[7] An important thing to remember is that due to impaired STM, if caregivers or therapists move commonly used items out of their familiar spots, this could create more confusion, making signs and labels necessary for finding objects. It is also important to remember adequate lighting for walking pathways, particularly for individuals who may get up frequently in the night or wander.[7] Increasing lighting and decreasing clutter and obstacles, drastically lowers the chance of falls in people with NCDS, and is especially important when working with older adults to prevent a broken bone or acute injury.

Similar to the PEOP model, there are three components of the Occupational Adaptation (OA) model: the patient or person, the environment, and the interaction between the person and environment.[22,23] Similar to PEOP, when occupational therapy practitioners use the OA model, they are focusing on how all of these factors interact during participation in an occupation.[23,24] Furthermore, if there is an obstacle in one of the three domains inhibiting participation, it is up to the occupational therapy practitioner to make adaptations to the occupation, or make suggestions to caregivers, to foster success. An example of an OA may be having large, clearly written signs, with high contrast, and explicit step-by-step directions. This enables the client to maintain their independence with basic ADL and IADL tasks such as dressing, washing, and making a snack.[7] Other forms of OA may include implementing adaptive equipment such as communication devices or high-contrast tableware to promote independence. However, due to STM deficits, implementing new adaptive equipment

into a routine may be difficult for an adult with an NCD to remember between sessions, resulting in poor carryover.

The tables in Box 13.2 give more detail and additional resources to the models mentioned in the treatment section of this chapter, and can be used as a quick reference tool.

Caregiver Education

One area that can be easily overlooked when working with an NCD population is the importance of quality caregiver education and training. Unfortunately, NCDs are progressive in nature, and STM, new learning, and various aspects of cognition are impacted and will continue to deteriorate with time. As mentioned earlier, occupational therapy practitioners always try to keep sessions as client-centered as possible and give as much autonomy and control to the client. However, when clients reach a point in their disease process where new learning is no longer possible, or there is no longer any carryover of techniques addressed in sessions, it is beneficial to consider switching to a caregiver education approach.

Topics that can be addressed in training with caregivers include verbal cues to guide the patient, how to sequence or simplify a task, or break a task into smaller parts, keep patients engaged, redirect and channel negative behaviors or outbursts, make environmental modifications to foster safety, operate equipment, and what resources are available for respite services for caregivers to prevent burnout. A lot of focus is on the patient and how much their lives are changing; however, these changes can be just as difficult for loved ones or caregivers. Furthermore, without adequate training, occupations can be unsuccessful and stressful for both the caregiver and the patient. In other words, if a caregiver is not aware of the best ways to foster independence and safety, occupations become increasingly more difficult to perform. This can result in caregivers needing to provide more assistance than necessary, or lead to an increase in negative behaviors in the patient as a result of increased frustration or uncertainty during a task. Fortunately, there are many online resources and reading materials for caregivers, which can serve as visual reminders for how to best serve the individual even after the therapist has left at the end of the session.

Despite how much training and education an occupational therapy practitioner provides a caregiver, it is important to validate and acknowledge the burden of caregiving in both a physical and mental context. In this way, it is equally important to provide resources and connections for caregivers to seek respite services. Many families seek daytime services for individuals. These programs are great in that they provide respite, but they also ensure the individual has the opportunity to participate in programs that are specifically designed

(text continues on p. 201)

BOX 13.2   The Following Tables Give More Detail and Additional Resources to the Models Mentioned in the Treatment Section of This Chapter, and Can Be Used as a Quick Reference Tool

Model of Human Occupation (MOHO)[18]

Theorists, Authors, Contributors:	Gary Kielhofner, DrPH, OTR, FAOTA
Core constructs, principles, and/or assumptions:	Subsystems: 1. Volition • Personal causation, values, interests 2. Habituation • Roles and habits 3. Performance capacity • Objective and subjective parts[18] Environment: • Occupation occurs in meaningful environments • Includes place, objects, social context, and community • Environmental factors work together to either create constraints or empowerment[18]
Highlights:	• Can be used as a model or as a frame of reference • Used across the life span and interprofessionally • User-friendly website with continuing-education opportunities, programs, and products • About 30 years old and widely used • Largest number of research-based publications[25] • Several assessments have been created using MOHO as a guiding model[26] • Significant evidence in all areas of practice • A continually evolving, open system[18]
Critical analysis/Evidence:	Haglund and Kielberg (1999)[10] evaluated if MOHO followed the values and beliefs of OT, if it supported the intervention process, and if it was consistent with the regulations and societal values in Sweden. The last question was important because of the extensive use and popularity of the model outside of the practice and the United States. In conclusion,[27] they felt as though the model needed further development in order to support intervention and assessment in OT. They felt as though there needed to be a greater focus on the environmental aspects of OT and the therapy process.[27] Despite the findings that suggest a lack of environmental factors, MOHO is still published in over 200 peer-reviewed research articles[27] and is very commonly used and recognized internationally and in and out of the practice of OT. Over 80% of OT's use the model and even more are familiar with the model. The model is great when evaluating the internal, motivating factors that give patients their drive, or volition.

BOX 13.2 The Following Tables Give More Detail and Additional Resources to the Models Mentioned in the Treatment Section of This Chapter, and Can Be Used as a Quick Reference Tool—cont'd

Person-Environment-Occupation-Performance (PEOP) Model

Theorists, Authors, Contributors:	Carolyn Baum & Charles Christiansen

Core constructs, principles, and/or assumptions:	Components:
	1. Person: intrinsic factors
	2. Environment: extrinsic factors
	3. Occupation: meaningful activity
	4. Performance: success in task and personal satisfaction with task
	  • Occupational performance (OP) is the outcome
	Intervention includes:
	Occupations/purposeful activities and contextualism[28,29]
	Five intervention strategies:
	1. Establish/restore
	2. Adapt/modify
	3. Alter
	4. Prevent
	5. Create
	(Brown, 2014)[5]
	Assumptions:
	  • Relationship between people, environments, and occupations are unique and dynamic
	  • Environment is a major factor in successful and satisfying OP
	  • Change the environment, not the person
	  • OP changes as occupations, environments, and people change
	  • OT starts by identifying what occupations the person wants or needs to learn
	  • OT promotes self-determination and the inclusion of people[28]

Highlights:	• Top-down approach with focus on function and participation • Applicable to individuals, organizations, and populations • Health and well-being measured by ability to participate in occupational roles • Can be client-centered[30] • Christiansen, a contributor to the model, is also the executive director of the American Occupational Therapy Foundation (AOTF)
Critical analysis/Evidence:	• Used in occupational science and health promotion[31]; identified and evaluated the evidence based research that supports the PEOP model. Despite being a well-known model, and being implemented into measurable tests such as the activity card sort, pediatric activity card sort, and the kitchen task assessment, the model has only three research articles that have evaluated the effectiveness of the PEOP model.[31] In those three studies the focus was on stroke survivors and children with developmental coordination disorder.[31] More studies should be done to test the effectiveness of this model in other populations.

Continued

BOX 13.2   The Following Tables Give More Detail and Additional Resources to the Models Mentioned in the Treatment Section of This Chapter, and Can Be Used as a Quick Reference Tool—cont'd

Kawa Model[19]

Theorists, Authors, Contributors:	Dr. Michael Iwama, PhD, OTC
Core constructs, principles, and/or assumptions:	Elements[20]: 1. Mizu (water): client's life flow through time, space, or situation 2. Torimaki (environment): where the sides of the river meet the bottom of the river. Includes family, finances, social networks, home, work, school 3. Iwa (rocks): circumstances that impede client's river flow 4. Ryuboku (driftwood): attributes of the client. Includes personal attributes, character, personality, special skills, immaterial objects, and assets 5. Sukima (spaces and gaps between obstructions): water, or life, can still flow through despite the challenges, which is where OT and occupation come into play Assumptions[19,20]: • Integration of earth and self are inseparable • Judgment and interpretation of truth are situational • Disability is only negative when viewed through the lens created by social consequences
Highlights:	• Uses images of nature • Evolved from grounded theory with a focus on the fluid elements of shared experiences and meaning[19] Japanese cultural elements: • Decentralized self (less individualized) • Temporal orientation • Shared experience • Dependency and interdependency • Collective agency[19] • Allows the client to express views about health and lifestyle changes[32] • Originates from the Eastern philosophy, making the model culturally relevant
Critical analysis/Evidence:	• Often used more as a therapeutic technique • However, determined to be a more effective tool compared with traditional interviewing during an occupational profile[32] • Easily understood and utilized by clients.[20] Studies conducted by Nelson[25] with indigenous Australian people highlight the conflict that many experience when using the Kawa Model. The model is a way for therapists, and other health care providers, to guide their practice and interventions with clients. However, sometimes the model is best used as a therapeutic activity to help engage clients, rather than as a guide for practice. This is not to say that the model is not effective. When used as a way to engage clients in occupation and start conversation between therapist and client, the drawing of the river was quite therapeutic.[32] Therapists were able to use the model and incorporate it into an activity to build rapport with clients and understand their cultural differences,[32] which suggests that perhaps this model is better used when there are barriers that are preventing therapy with a client.

for people with cognitive impairments. Furthermore, having the activities in a designated building ensures the individual is in a safe environment. This is of particular importance for families who worry about the safety of their loved when left home alone. Most of these programs are run during daytime business hours, which allows for working families to resume their occupations of work or leisure without having to worry about loved ones.

In the end, the occupational therapist needs to work collaboratively with the interprofessional team, client, and client caregivers to determine the necessary supports and treatments that will work best for the client and their families. In this way, the occupational therapist is able to facilitate as much functional independence as possible while maintaining safety and quality of life for those living with NCDs.

SUGGESTED LEARNING ACTIVITIES

1. Check out the American Occupational Therapy Association page for quick and simple tips and tricks and worksheets to implement in practice when working with individuals with NCDs. https://www.aota.org/
2. Interview a caregiver or nursing staff member on a memory care unit to discuss the progressive mental, behavioral, and cognitive changes they have observed in a patient or relative.
3. Volunteer a few hours at an adult day center to get a firsthand experience of interacting with people who present with NCDs and/or cognitive deficits.

REFLECTION QUESTIONS

1. If you were working with an older adult who seemed different than their baseline regarding behaviors and typical functional level, who would be the first person you address on the interdisciplinary team? What details would you communicate? Why is it so critical to identify sudden behavioral, cognitive, or physical changes as soon as possible?
2. Which frame of reference or treatment approach do you think you will use in practice most often? What are the pros and cons, or limitations to this model? Do you envision yourself using multiple treatment approaches?
3. What techniques or strategies could you use when working with a patient who presents with behavioral challenges secondary to NCD? How would you try to maintain the therapeutic relationship with the individual? What recommendations would you make to staff and/or a caregiver working with an individual who displays negative behaviors or is being unsafe?
4. What are some common ways to adapt the individual's environment to optimize their level of independence and decrease dependence on a caregiver? In what ways can you modify the environment to decrease risk of injury? In what ways can you communicate and work with a client with NCD during an ADL session, to promote maximal independence?

REFERENCES

1. American Psychiatric Association. *Diagnostic and Statistical Manual of Mental Disorders*. 5th ed. Washington, DC: American Psychiatric Association; 2013.
2. Jahn H. Memory loss in Alzheimer's disease. *Dialogues Clin Neurosci*. 2013;15:445-454.
3. Hahn B, Wolkenberg FA, Ross TJ, et al. Divided versus selective attention: evidence for common processing mechanisms. *Brain Res*. 2008;1215:137-146.
4. Alvarez JA, Emory E. Executive function and the frontal lobes: a meta-analytic review. *Neuropsychol Rev*. 2006;16:17-42.
5. Diamond A. Executive functions. *Ann Rev Psychology*. 2013; 64:135-168.
6. MacDuffie KE, Atkins AS, Flegal KE, Clark CM, Reuter-Lorenz PA. Memory distortion in Alzheimer's disease: deficient monitoring of short- and long-term memory. *Neuropsychol*. 2012;26:509-516.
7. American Occupational Therapy Association. Alzheimer's Disease Tip Sheet. 2011. Available at: https://www.aota.org/About-Occupational-Therapy/Patients-Clients/Adults/Alzheimers.aspx.
8. Ferris SH, Farlow M. Language impairment in Alzheimer's disease and benefits of acetylcholinesterase inhibitors. *Clin Interv Aging*. 2013;8:1007-1014.
9. Alzheimer's Association. Alzheimer's Disease and Dementia. 2018. Available at: https://www.alz.org/alzheimers_disease_1973.asp.
10. Hamby JR. Altered mental status. In: Smith-Gabai H, ed. *Occupational Therapy in Acute Care*. Bethesda, MD: American Occupational Therapy Association; 2011:589-592.
11. Nasreddine ZS, Phillips NA, Bédirian V, et al. The Montreal Cognitive Assessment, MoCA: a brief screening tool for mild cognitive impairment. *J Am Geriatr Soc*. 2005;53:695-699.
12. Tariq SH, Tumosa N, Chibnall JT, Perry MH III, Morley JE. Comparison of the Saint Louis University mental status examination and the mini-mental state examination for

detecting dementia and mild neurocognitive disorder—a pilot study. *Am J Geriatr Psychiatry*. 2006;14:900-910.

13. Folstein MF, Folstein SE, White T, Messer MA. *Mini-Mental State Exam, User's Guide*. 2nd ed. Lutz, FL: PAR; 2010.

14. O'Bryant SE, Humphreys JD, Smith GE, et al. Detecting dementia with the mini-mental state examination (MMSE) in highly educated individuals. *Arch Neurol*. 2008;65:963-967.

15. Hartman-Maeir A, Armon N, Katz N. *Kettle Test Protocol*. Jerusalem: School of Occupational Therapy, Hadassah and Hebrew University of Jerusalem; 2005.

16. Hartman-Maeir A, Harel H, Katz N. Kettle Test—a brief measure of cognitive functional performance: reliability and validity in stroke rehabilitation. *Am J Occup Ther*. 2009;64:592-599.

17. Hartman-Maeir A, Katz N, Armon N. Validity of a cognitive–functional observation (the "Kettle Test") in an elderly sample with suspected dementia. Paper presented at: the Israeli Society for Occupational Therapy Annual Conference; July, 2004; Haifa.

18. Kielhofner G. *Model of Human Occupation: Theory and Application*. 4th ed. Philadelphia: Lippincott Williams & Wilkins; 2008.

19. Iwama MK. *The Kawa Model: Culturally Relevant Occupational Therapy*. New York: Reed Elsevier; 2006.

20. Tupe D. Emerging theories. In: Boyt Schell BA, Gillen G, Scaffa ME, eds. *Willard and Spackman's Occupational Therapy*. 12th ed. Philadelphia: Lippincott Williams & Wilkins; 2014:557-562.

21. Stuckey HL, Nobel J. The connection between art, healing, and public health: a review of current literature. *Am J Public Health*. 2010;100:254-263.

22. Schkade JK, Schultz S. Occupational adaptation: toward a holistic approach to contemporary practice, Part 1. *Am J Occup Ther*. 1992;46:829-837.

23. Schultz SW. Theory of occupational adaptation. In: Boyt Schell BA, Gillen G, Scaffa ME, eds. *Willard & Spackman's Occupational Therapy*. 12th ed. 2014:527-540).

24. Schkade JK, Schultz S. Occupational adaptation: Toward a holistic approach to contemporary practice, Part 2. *Am J Occup Ther*. 1992;46:917-926.

25. Lee J, Kielhofner G. *Achieving best practice: using evidence linked to occupation-based models*. PowerPoint presentation. Chicago: University of Illinois at Chicago; 2009.

26. Lee SW, Taylor R, Kielhofner G, Fisher G. Theory use in practice: a national survey of therapists who use the model of human occupation. *Am J Occup Ther*. 2008;62(1):106-117.

27. Haglund L, Kiellberg A. A critical analysis of the Model of Human Occupation. *Can J Occup Ther*. 1999;66:102-108.

28. Brown C. Ecological models in occupational therapy. In: Boyt Schell BA, Gillen G, Scaffa ME, eds. *Willard and Spackman's Occupational Therapy*. 12th ed. Philadelphia: Lippincott Williams & Wilkins; 2014:494-504.

29. Loukas KM. Occupational performance in natural environments: Dynamic contexts for participation. In: Jacobs K, MacRae N, Sladyk K, eds. *Occupational Therapy Essentials for Clinical Competence*. Thorofare, NJ: Slack, Inc.; 2014:149-158.

30. Christiansen C, Baum CM. *Occupational Therapy: Enabling Function and Well-being*. 2nd ed. Thorofare, NJ: Slack, Inc.; 1997.

31. Lee J. Achieving best practice: a review of evidence linked to occupation-focused practice models. *Occup Ther Health Care*. 2010;24:206-222.

32. Nelson A. Seeing white: a critical exploration of occupational therapy with Indigenous Australian people. *Occup Ther Int*. 2007;14:237-255.

14

Other Psychiatric Diagnoses

Nancy Carson

LEARNING OBJECTIVES

1. Identify the types of feeding and eating disorders, personality disorders, dissociative disorders, and somatic symptoms and related disorders as defined by the *Diagnostic and Statistical Manual of Mental Disorders* (5th edition; DSM-5).
2. Describe the symptomology of the different disorders.
3. Recognize assessment methods for these disorders.
4. Discuss treatment approaches, including psychopharmacology and psychotherapeutic approaches.
5. Articulate occupational therapy's role in the treatment of these disorders.

INTRODUCTION

This chapter reviews some of the psychiatric disorders identified by the American Psychological Association (APA) in the DSM-5 that have not been covered in previous chapters. They include feeding and eating disorders, personality disorders, dissociative disorders, somatic symptom and related disorders, sleep-wake disorders, and neurodevelopmental disorders. The impact on occupational functioning and the role of the occupational therapy practitioner (OTP) for diagnoses in each of these categories will be discussed.

FEEDING AND EATING DISORDERS

Eating disorders are serious illnesses that are characterized by severe disturbances to a person's eating behaviors.[1] Eating disorders affect at least 30 million people of all ages in the United States,[2,3] and all eating disorders have an elevated mortality rate.[4] Common eating disorders include binge eating disorder and bulimia nervosa. Anorexia nervosa is a less common disorder but is very serious. Anorexia nervosa has the highest mortality rate of any psychiatric disorder. The estimated mortality rate is approximately 10%, with one in five of those deaths resulting from suicide.[5] It is a life-threatening disorder because of the effects of weight loss and starvation on body systems. An individual diagnosed with anorexia nervosa restricts caloric intake, resulting in body weight that is significantly low for age, gender, and physical stature. The reduced body weight may occur because of restriction or binge eating and purging. The individual is extremely fearful of gaining weight and exhibits an impaired self-experience of weight or body shape.[6] There is a strong desire to be thin, and a distorted body image leads to a belief that one is overweight, even when severely malnourished.[1]

An individual diagnosed with bulimia nervosa exhibits recurrent episodes of binge eating in which the person eats a large amount of food within a 2-hour period and experiences a sense of lack of control during the episode. Compensatory behaviors—such as self-induced vomiting, inappropriate use of laxatives or diuretics, fasting, or excessive exercising—may also be exhibited. The binge eating and inappropriate compensatory behaviors both occur, on average, at least once a week for 3 months.[1,6] These compensatory behaviors are usually done in private, resulting in feelings of shame and disgust. People with bulimia nervosa may weigh in the normal range for their weight or be slightly overweight. Like people with anorexia, they usually fear gaining weight, strongly desire to lose weight, and are intensely dissatisfied with their body shape and size.[1] See Table 14.1 for a list of the symptoms of anorexia nervosa and bulimia nervosa.

TABLE 14.1   Symptoms of Eating Disorders.

Anorexia Nervosa	Bulimia Nervosa
Dramatic weight loss and preoccupation with weight, dieting, food, counting calories and fat grams	Evidence of binge eating indicated by the disappearance of large amounts of food or presence of numerous empty food containers attributed to the individual
Failure to maintain a body weight appropriate for age, height, and build; denial that extreme thinness is a problem; cessation of menstruating	Evidence of purging behaviors, including frequent trips to the bathroom after meals, frequent vomiting, and/or use of laxatives or diuretics
Refusal to eat certain foods, such as carbohydrates, fats, or certain food groups or only eating certain low-calorie foods	Hiding food and eating rapidly and alone
Skipping meals and even preparing elaborate meals for others but refusing to eat them	Drinking excessive amounts of water or noncaloric beverages, and/or excessive use of mouthwash, mints, and gum
Dressing in layers or loose bulky clothes to hide weight loss or stay warm	Dental problems, such as enamel erosion, cavities, discoloration of teeth from vomiting, and tooth sensitivity
Difficulty concentrating, dizziness, fainting, muscle weakness, dry skin and hair	Calluses on the back of the hands and knuckles from self- induced vomiting
Extreme focus and talking about food, calories and weight; making comments about being fat; frequent mirror checking	
Excessive and rigid exercise regime that is maintained despite weather, fatigue, illness, or injury	
Complaining about constipation or stomach pain; abnormal laboratory findings	
Difficult emotions around eating, mood swings, becoming distant from friends	

Adapted from references 1 and 43.

A binge eating disorder is defined by episodes of binge eating without the use of inappropriate compensatory behaviors. As a result, people with binge eating disorder often are overweight or obese. Binge eating disorder is different from overeating, which may occur occasionally is not associated with a lack of control. Binge eating disorder is less common but is much more severe than overeating. The median age of onset for binge eating disorder is 21 years, and the median age of onset for both bulimia nervosa and anorexia nervosa is 18 years.[2]

Feeding and eating disorders also include avoidant-restrictive food intake disorder, pica, rumination disorder, and other specified feeding or eating disorders.[6] Avoidant-restrictive food intake disorder is the persistent failure to meet appropriate nutritional and/or energy needs, as indicated by failure to achieve expected weight gain, significant nutritional deficiency, or the need for nutritional supplementation as a result of the restricted food intake. This behavior cannot be explained by medical, environmental, or cultural factors.[6] Pica is the recurrent ingestion of non-nutritive substances for at least 1 month at an age for which this behavior is developmentally inappropriate.[6] Rumination disorder is the repeated regurgitation of food, in which the regurgitated food is rechewed, reswallowed, or

spit out, for a period of at least 1 month.[6] Other specified feeding or eating disorders include the presence of feeding or eating behaviors that are clinically or functionally concerning, but criteria for a specific feeding and eating disorder are not met. Night eating syndrome is included in this diagnosis; it includes recurrent episodes of night eating and/or excessive nighttime eating.[6]

In people diagnosed with anorexia, comorbid mood disorders occur 33% to 50% of the time, and comorbid anxiety disorders, including obsessive-compulsive disorder and social phobia, occur approximately 50% of the time. In people diagnosed with bulimia and binge eating disorder, nearly 50% have a comorbid mood disorder, more than 50% have comorbid anxiety disorders, and nearly 10% have a comorbid substance use disorder, with alcohol being the substance misused.[7]

Therapeutic Management

There are various approaches in the treatment of eating disorders. The provision of services for treatment will vary based on the symptom severity, insurance coverage, available programs, and other individual needs. Treatment may be provided through outpatient or intensive outpatient providers, partial hospitalization, residential programs, or inpatient hospitalization. Hospitalization may be required if the individual is medically unstable, with acute health risks or coexisting medical problems, or if the individual is psychiatrically unstable, with rapidly worsening symptoms or is suicidal and unable to contract for safety.[8]

Treatment interventions may be pharmacologic, nutritional, physical, neurologic, or psychotherapeutic. Interventions need to be individualized because approaches will vary, depending on the symptom severity and stage of recovery. Pharmacologic approaches may include the use of the antipsychotic medication olanzapine for weight gain in individuals with anorexia nervosa. Research studies have indicated that olanzapine's effect on the salience network,[9] as well as the antihistaminergic effect of olanzapine at the hypothalamic histamine H1 receptor, result in weight gain.[10] Olanzapine may be prescribed for use in inpatient treatment for individuals not gaining sufficient weight during hospitalization. Nutritional approaches may include low-energy-density dietary counseling,[11] nutrition education, nutritional planning, and monitoring nutritional choices.[8] Physical approaches may include reducing excessive exercising[1] and incorporating physical activity, such as yoga.[11] Neurologic approaches may include transcranial magnetic stimulation or deep brain stimulation.[11]

Examples of evidence-based psychotherapeutic approaches include cognition-focused, emotion regulation, exposure-based, motivation enhancement, integrative, and family-based approaches.[11]

Cognition-Focused Approaches

Cognition-focused approaches include cognitive-behavioral therapy (CBT) and cognitive remediation (CR). CBT is presented in Chapter 6 and CR in Chapter 7 of this text. CBT focuses on modifying distorted beliefs and attitudes that maintain the eating disorder behavior, such as distorted thinking related to the meaning of weight, shape, and appearance.[8] It is believed that anorexia nervosa is associated with a rigid cognitive style and deficits in cognitive flexibility.[12] CR addresses thought processes rather than content and targets rigid thinking processes related to eating behaviors that are considered a core component of anorexia nervosa.[8] Research studies have indicated some improvement in cognitive flexibility following CR in an inpatient program for individuals diagnosed with anorexia nervosa.[13]

Emotion Regulation Approaches

There has been increased interest in treatment that targets affect regulation. Empiric support of the role of emotion in binge eating has suggested that eating alleviates negative emotions, and therefore binge eating is maintained through negative reinforcement.[14-16] Emotion regulation approaches

include acceptance and commitment therapy (ACT), dialectic behavior therapy (DBT), and mindfulness-based interventions.[8,11]

The focus of ACT is on actions as opposed to emotions and thoughts. It is believed that maladaptive behaviors regulate emotional states[17]; therefore the individual accepts personal thoughts and feelings and focuses on actions and behaviors. The individual is encouraged to identify personal values and commit to actions that embody these values. The emphasis is on accepting a certain degree of negative emotion as a part of life and focusing primarily on living an authentic life through goal-directed behavior.[8] Components of ACT may include mindfulness, acceptance, willingness, defusion, values clarification, and committed action.[11] Although ACT for eating disorders has been implemented, there has been minimal empiric support for its efficacy.[18]

Another approach for the treatment of eating disorders is DBT, which was originally developed for the treatment of borderline personality disorders. DBT has since been used for developing skills to replace maladaptive eating disorder behaviors.[8] DBT includes components of CBT and Buddhism and focuses on teaching distress tolerance, emotion regulation, interpersonal effectiveness, and mindfulness.[19] Distress tolerance can help one cope with crises effectively by using distraction and self-soothing. Identifying emotions can make one less emotionally vulnerable, and interpersonal effectiveness can be beneficial in learning how to ask for help.[19] Mindfulness skills can help reduce judgmental thinking. Research has suggested that individuals with eating disorders have poor interoceptive awareness,[20] leading to decreased awareness of internal mood states. They may be at risk of using binge eating as a coping strategy for elevated distress associated with intense affective experiences. Mindfulness has been incorporated into DBT and CBT approaches, and pilot data have suggested that mindfulness training may be a promising treatment for eating disorders.[21] DBT promotes acceptance, as well as behavior change, which works well in the recovery process and allows for the individual to challenge the all or none thinking typical of an eating disorder. There is evidence for the efficacy of DBT in reducing binge eating.[22,23]

Exposure-Based Approaches

Exposure with response prevention (ERP) for the treatment of anorexia nervosa proposes that individuals assume maladaptive behaviors to avoid negative feelings and emotions.[24] Furthermore, these maladaptive behaviors are maintained through negative reinforcement. ERP involves increased exposure to the aversive stimuli while preventing avoidance behaviors, which in theory decreases the experience of negative emotions. Modified ERP has been found to be effective in the treatment of bulimia nervosa[24-26] and shows promise for the treatment of anorexia nervosa.[27,28]

Dissatisfaction with one's own body is a component of both bulimia nervosa and anorexia nervosa. Mirror and body image exposure use mirrors to view one's own body in an effort to decrease body dissatisfaction. A small body of evidence has indicated positive results with this approach.[29,30]

Motivation Enhancement

Motivational interviewing, which was discussed in Chapter 2, can also be used as an adjunct to CBT or by itself in the treatment of eating disorders to address ambivalence and promote readiness to change. Adaptations of motivational interviewing for eating disorders have been addressed in the literature,[31-33] and there is some evidence that suggests a reduction in ambivalence toward treatment with motivational enhancement approaches.[34,35]

Integrative Approaches

Integrative approaches include enhanced CBT (CBT-E),[36] which focuses on the relationship between cognitive and behavioral symptoms of eating disorders. The approach can be personalized and can be used for treatment with all types of eating disorders. Another approach is integrative cognitive-affective therapy (ICAT) for the treatment of bulimia nervosa.[37] ICAT is primarily an emotion-focused therapy and may include other components, such as motivational interviewing, mindfulness, cognitive therapy, behavior therapy, and interpersonal therapy. Interpersonal psychotherapy is an evidence-based treatment for bulimia nervosa and binge eating disorder that incorporates the social and interpersonal context by focusing on problem areas such as grief, interpersonal role disputes, role transitions, and interpersonal deficits. Improvement in these areas have been linked with symptom reduction.[8] ICAT is comprised of four phases: (1) increasing motivation and attending to emotion; (2) modifying eating behavior and managing urges for binge eating; (3) identifying precipitants of negative emotional states; and (4) relapse prevention and healthy lifestyle promotion.[37] Both CBT-E and ICAT have been found to be effective in reducing bulimic behaviors.[37]

Family-Based Treatment

Family-based treatment includes all family members to help reestablish healthy eating, restore weight, and diminish negative compensatory behaviors. There is a focus on refeeding and full weight restoration, instead of focusing on the cause of the eating disorder. This approach has been shown to be effective for adolescents with anorexia and bulimia.[8] There is evidence that progress made during hospitalization or residential treatment is often lost after transitioning home.[38] This indicates the need to include the family and social environment when providing treatment for eating disorders, and research supports the efficacy of family-based treatment (FBT).[39,40]

Occupational Therapy Approaches

The overall goal of occupational therapy with clients with eating disorders is to improve one's overall functioning through the use of meaningful occupations. In constructing the occupational profile, the OTP looks for disruptions in daily performance patterns and habits resulting from the eating disorder. For example, excessive exercising in a highly structured routine or excessive attention to body image and weight may be revealed.[41] Eating disorders can result in occupational performance issues in many areas of functioning.[42] Self-care can be negatively affected by body image problems. Attention, concentration, and memory may be impaired due to malnutrition and negatively affect work and school responsibilities. Obsessive behavior related to exercise, weight checking, grocery shopping, and food routines can consume one's time and create social isolation.[43] Difficulty socializing or eating with others may become more difficult, especially in food-related situations, and difficulty having fun and identifying enjoyable activities can prove difficult.[44]

A focus on tasks and activities related to food behaviors can provide important information. For example, working with an individual during meal preparation and cooking provides an opportunity to observe the client's relationship with food and to discuss one's feelings regarding enjoyment and satisfaction with eating patterns and routines. The OTP must be empathic and understanding of the individual's difficulty with expressing thoughts, and emotions because feelings of shame related to the behaviors may be present. The individual may have a history of hiding maladaptive behaviors, feeling out of control, and may be resistant to treatment. It is necessary to understand how the maladaptive behavior is meeting the individual's needs to help the person develop health-promoting occupations that can replace them.[41]

OTPs provide services as part of a multidisciplinary team. Occupational therapy treatment sessions may be structured as individual sessions or groups. Example of individual session topics offered currently at one treatment facility include body image, leisure, life skills, use of supports, return to school, return to work, employment, cognition, time management and routine, life roles, coping skill use, sensory tools, and socialization skills. Groups focus on skill acquisition or skill generalization.[45]

At another facility, the OTP meets with the individual to discuss their daily routine and interests. Occupational therapy assists the person in rebalancing activities into a healthier and more balanced pattern by developing the skills needed to live a more balanced life. The occupational therapists lead a range of groups focusing on lifestyle rebalance, social skills, and therapeutic media. Leisure group provides an opportunity for each patient to develop appropriate physical activities and access community resources. The social eating group is used to facilitate a graded approach to eating and progresses to meals out in the community. It may include meal planning, shopping, and cooking skills, as appropriate. The creative art group provides a creative outlet, an opportunity to develop interests and hobbies, and allows for the therapist to observe and address motivation, communication, and social interaction in a nonthreatening environment.[46]

One more current example of occupational therapy intervention in a well-established eating disorders treatment program illustrates the role of occupational therapy in inpatient, partial hospitalization, and intensive outpatient settings. The occupational therapists provide services to empower individuals to acquire healthy, valued, and age-appropriate roles. There are three primary goals for occupational therapy at this facility[47]:

1. To provide a safe setting where the person with an eating disorder may engage in multisensory activities via doing
2. To provide the patient with a setting where the verbal insights learned in psychotherapy can be converted into new behaviors
3. To practice habits that create or reinforce healthy roles and occupations

Engaging in multisensory activities provides accurate sensory input that challenges and competes with the distorted thoughts and beliefs experienced by individuals with eating disorders. The focus on healthy sensory experiences provides an opportunity to discover or reconnect with enjoyable and satisfying activities and occupations.[47] Occupational therapy provides a safe environment in which to assimilate information learned in therapeutic counseling sessions and experiment with "healthier behaviors related to choice, decision-making, asking for help, setting realistic expectations, tolerating imperfection, feelings of achievement and competence, and problem solving."[47]

Examples of purposeful activities practiced through individual and group occupational therapy sessions include the following[47]:

- Planning and preparing snacks and meals
- Meal pacing
- Grocery shopping
- Clothes shopping
- Leisure and hobby exploration
- Socializing with peers during group games
- Planting and caring for plants and vegetables
- Money management and budgeting
- Time management skills
- Goal setting
- Developing volunteer and employment opportunities
- Becoming familiar with one's own sensory preferences

The focus of occupational therapy is to assist the individual in establishing and/or returning to meaningful occupations and roles that are satisfying and support recovery.[47]

During occupational therapy treatment, there may be times when symptoms of an eating disorder are evident, and an eating disorder is suspected, but services being rendered are for a different health issue. Further exploration of eating behavior by asking about food consumption, meal routines, eating preferences, and body image may provide more information indicating a possible eating disorder or disordered eating behaviors. If warranted, suggesting a consult with a nutritionist would provide more insight into eating behaviors.

PERSONALITY DISORDERS

The DSM-5 category of personality disorders includes the diagnosis of general personality disorder, which serves as the overarching category under which 10 specific personality disorders are defined.[6] To diagnose a personality disorder, a person must exhibit at least two of four core features: rigid, extreme, and distorted thinking patterns; problematic emotional response patterns; impulse control problems; or significant interpersonal problems. These features deviate from cultural norms and are pervasive and inflexible, stable over time, and lead to distress or impairment.[6,48] The onset of a personality disorder occurs in adolescence or early adulthood, and the symptoms cannot be explained more appropriately by another disorder.[48]

The 10 personality disorders are grouped into three clusters according to types of symptoms that are present. Cluster A disorders are characterized by odd or eccentric behavior, cluster B by dramatic and overly emotional behavior, and cluster C by anxious fearful thinking and behavior.[6] The four core features combine in a different way for each specific personality disorder. The individual must meet the minimum criteria required for that disorder, and the symptoms must cause functional impairment and/or subjective distress.

Cluster A Disorders

Cluster A includes paranoid personality disorder, schizoid personality disorder, and schizotypal personality disorder. The common features of these personality disorders are social awkwardness and social withdrawal. There is a predominance of distorted thinking in each of these disorders.[49,50]

The paranoid personality disorder is characterized by a pervasive distrust and suspiciousness of other people. People with this disorder will keep their distance from others because they assume that they may take advantage of them or humiliate or harm them in some way. They misinterpret other people's comments and behaviors and feel threatened, hold grudges, and exhibit pathologic jealously. As a result, they do not form close relationships with others.[49,50]

An individual with schizoid personality disorder presents as being detached socially with a restricted emotional range. They may be oblivious to social cues inattentive, and nonresponsive to praise or criticism from others. They do not form close relationships and tend to be socially isolated. They usually choose solitary activities and do not seem to take pleasure in life activities.[49,50]

People with schizotypal personality disorder are acutely uncomfortable in social settings and have great difficulty in establishing and maintaining close relationships with others. They tend to be socially isolated and reserved and may have excessive social anxiety associated with paranoid fears rather than negative judgments about self.[50,51] This disorder differs from schizoid personality disorder in that they also experience perceptual and cognitive distortions and/or eccentric behavior.[50] They may see or hear things that others do not see or believe because they interpret stimuli or facts inconsistently with cultural norms.[51] They may be unusually superstitious or have incorrect interpretations of causal incidents, believing them to have specific meaning for them. Vague, circumstantial, metaphorical, or overelaborate thinking and speech and inappropriate or constricted affect may be observed.[51]

Cluster B Disorders

Cluster B includes borderline personality disorder, narcissistic personality disorder, histrionic personality disorder, and antisocial personality disorder. The common features of these personality disorders are impulse control and emotional regulation, with a tendency toward dramatic and erratic behavior.[49,52]

People with antisocial personality disorder demonstrate a pattern of disregarding or violating the rights of other people and often exhibit hostility, aggression, deceit, and/or manipulation. They have a tendency to act on impulses and place themselves in dangerous situations that can result in accidents and legal difficulties. Many individuals with antisocial personality disorder have exhibited hostile or deceitful behaviors, such as hurting or intimidating others or stealing or destroying property, during childhood and may have been previously diagnosed with conduct disorder.[49,52]

The individual with a histrionic personality disorder craves being the center of attention. A pattern of excessive emotion and attention-seeking behavior is observed. The individual may dress flamboyantly and engage in excessive flirting or seductive behavior. Exaggerated emotional responses such as crying excessively over seemingly minor situations or being overly or inappropriately affectionate may be observed. Despite the display of emotion, the depth of emotion is lacking, with the perception of being shallow and insincere evident to others. Because of this, it is difficult for people with histrionic personality disorder to establish intimate relationships, despite being uncomfortable being alone.[49,52]

Narcissistic personality disorder is fueled by a strong sense of entitlement. This sense of entitlement results from a grandiose sense of self-importance and leads to a lack of empathy for other people. There is a belief of superiority in beauty, intelligence, power, or talent as compared with others, and this leads to a disregard for those around them. Individuals with narcissistic personality disorder take advantage of others and may appear arrogant and condescending. They value status and are self-absorbed and preoccupied with dreams of immense success, power, and attention, yet they do not necessarily engage in constructive activities to achieve these goals. When confronted with the realization that they are not superior to others, they may feel devastated or angry and may take these feelings out on others. They can be very manipulative in gaining attention from those around them. The need for attention and admiration, along with their lack of empathy, results in troubled and/or superficial relationships.[49,52]

Borderline personality disorder is the most well-known personality disorder; it has been widely studied and reported on in the literature. People with borderline personality disorder exhibit a pattern of instability in personal relationships. They experience a poor self-image and unstable intense emotions, along with a strong propensity for impulsive behavior. They have a black or white all or nothing perspective on life, as well as toward self and others. They misinterpret the actions and behaviors of others and are prone to angry outbursts and unstable emotional reactions. They have a fear of abandonment and may have repeated suicide attempts. They may engage in risky sexual behavior and self-injurious behavior. They may also abuse alcohol, use illegal substances, or binge eat to feel better emotionally in the moment. Frequent changes in jobs, relationships, and living environment can result from the difficulty in interpersonal relationships.[49,52]

Cluster C Disorders

Cluster C includes avoidant personality disorder, dependent personality disorder, and obsessive-compulsive personality disorder. The common features of these personality disorders are anxiety and fearfulness.[49,53] People with avoidant personality disorder experience excessive shyness along with feelings of inadequacy and a hypersensitivity to criticism. They think that they are not good enough and are socially inhibited. They fear that others will criticize or reject them; therefore they avoid social situations and have few if any close relationships. Social inadequacy negatively affects developing a satisfying social network and can negatively affect career advancement.[49,53]

The core feature exhibited in dependent personality disorder is submissive and clingy behavior. The individual has difficulty making independent decisions and living independently. Being alone is frightening, and there is a strong desire to be taken care of and supported by others. In a relationship, conflict is avoided for fear of being abandoned, and this increases the risk of being subjected to manipulation and abuse. When a relationship ends, they immediately look for another person to provide support to them and take care of them.[49,53]

Obsessive-compulsive personality disorder is not the same as obsessive-compulsive disorder; this is a separate category of disorders in DSM-5 (see Chapter 10). A person with obsessive-compulsive personality disorder can be described as stubborn, rigid, and controlling. A pattern of preoccupation with orderliness, rules, and perfection is observed. The person may be driven at work to do everything perfectly and dislike delegating to others because of the fear that the other person may do a substandard job. However, the focus on perfection often results in a lack of efficiency and an inability to see the big picture, resulting in failure to complete tasks. Social relationships may be neglected as the person focuses on work, or relationships may deteriorate due to the rigid and controlling behavior exhibited.[49,53]

To be diagnosed with a personality disorder, the traits associated with the specific personality disorder must be observed consistently and within various contexts; the traits should be considered the norm for the person's behavior over the long term. Children and teenagers are not typically diagnosed with personality disorders because they are still developing personality traits. Adults may inconsistently display behaviors associated with a personality disorder; however, this does not constitute this diagnosis. Furthermore, these traits must cause functional impairment, defined as problems in interpersonal relationships at work, school, or home, as well as subjective distress, meaning that the symptoms create distress for the individual. The individual may experience embarrassment, shame, or other painful emotional distress as a result of the personality disorder.[49] A systematic review and meta-analysis of personality disorders in the Western countries has found a 12.16%

TABLE 14.2 Prevalence of Personality Disorders.[54]	
Cluster	Prevalence
Cluster A	
Paranoid	3.02 (1.44–5.31)
Schizoid	2.82 (0.57–6.62)
Schizotypal	3.04 (1.21–5.64)
Any cluster A	7.23 (2.37–14.42)
Cluster B	
Borderline	1.90 (0.85–3.34)
Histrionic	0.83 (0.36–1.48)
Antisocial	3.05 (2.10–4.16)
Narcissistic	1.23 (0.43–2.40)
Any cluster B	5.53 (3.20–8.43)
Cluster C	
Avoidant	2.78 (1.74–4.06)
Dependent	0.78 (0.37–1.37)
Obsessive-compulsive	4.32 (2.16–7.16)
Any cluster C	6.70 (2.90–11.93)
Any personality disorder	12.16 (8.02–17.02)

Adapted from Volkert J, Gablonski T, Rabung S. Prevalence of personality disorders in the general adult population in Western countries: systematic review and meta-analysis. *Br J Psychiatry.* 2018;213:709-715.

prevalence rate for any personality disorder and prevalence rates for DSM clusters A, B, and C to be from 5.53% to 7.23%. Prevalence was highest for obsessive-compulsive personality disorder, at 4.32%; dependent personality disorder had the lowest rate, at 0.78% (Table 14.2).[54]

Excess medical morbidity and mortality are associated with personality disorder. Comorbid mental health problems are high in individuals diagnosed with personality disorder. These mental health problems include depression, anxiety, substance use, suicidal behavior, and suicide. Despite high levels of service use, these comorbid conditions are difficult to treat.[55]

Therapeutic Management

Historically, personality disorders have been considered difficult to treat by mental health professionals due to a reluctance of individuals to seek therapy, along with poor response and engagement from individuals who do seek treatment.[56] Medications do not specifically treat personality disorders; however, psychotropic medications, including antidepressants, antipsychotics, and mood stabilizers, are prescribed for individuals diagnosed with a personality disorder with greater frequency than most other diagnostic groups, in part due to comorbid diagnoses with other mental health disorders.[57] Pharmacotherapy is beneficial for the treatment of maladaptive personality symptoms, with most evidence presented for borderline and schizotypal personality disorders and, to a lesser degree, avoidant and antisocial personality disorders.[57] There is evidence to support pharmacotherapy for the reduction of impulsivity and aggression, which are most characteristic of borderline and antisocial personality disorders, psychotic-like symptoms and cognitive deficits characteristic of schizotypal personality disorders, and social anxiety characteristic of avoidant personality disorder.[57] There is limited evidence for psychotherapeutic approaches across the range of personality disorders except for borderline personality disorder and, to a lesser extent, antisocial personality disorder.[55] Specialist treatments with evidence of effectiveness in borderline personality disorder include DBT,[55,56] CBT,[56] cognitive analytic therapy, schema-focused therapy, mentalization-based treatment, and transference-focused therapy.[55] DBT and CBT are the most well-known approaches, with the most evidence support.[56]

DBT is based on cognitive behavioral approaches. It is grounded in a biosocial theory of personality disorder in which a dysfunction in the emotional regulation system develops and negatively affects interpersonal relationships and self-worth. It is thought to develop as a result of an invalidating environment and lack of appropriate response to a child's emotional needs during childhood.[56] DBT is the only evidence-based treatment for borderline personality disorder (BPD). It has also been shown to be effective for other psychiatric disorders, including mood disorders, posttraumatic stress disorder, and eating disorders. DBT consists of four parts—a skills training group, individual psychotherapy, telephone consultation, and a therapist consultation team. Treatment is targeted at the core symptoms of BPD, including an unstable sense of self, tumultuous relationships, fear of abandonment, emotional lability, impulsivity, and self-injurious behaviors. The skills training group teaches psychosocial skills that address core mindfulness, interpersonal effectiveness, emotion regulation, and distress tolerance.[58] There is also a focus on validation technique to build self-acceptance.

Core mindfulness teaches the individual to focus on the present and thus control their mind; the practice is grounded in Zen Buddhism. Interpersonal effectiveness focuses on assertive communication of personal needs in relationships and communicating effectively and with respect to self and others. Emotional regulation increases an awareness and understanding of emotions and strategies to deal appropriately with emotions. Distress tolerance

focuses on managing personal response to stressful events in healthy ways.[56] There are many different variations of CBT approaches for individuals with personality disorders, but the core features are similar (see Chapter 6).

Individuals with antisocial personality disorder are usually reluctant to commit to treatment. There is a lack of robust evidence for specific interventions for treatment, but there is some evidence for group-based cognitive and behavioral interventions targeted at reducing offensive antisocial behavior.[59] Those individuals with antisocial personality disorder who are dangerous may present in the criminal justice system, and forensic psychiatry services will be needed. Treatment usually includes anger management and violence reduction approaches; close monitoring and supervision is required in these programs.[55]

Implications for Occupational Therapy

There is little research on occupational therapy and personality disorders. However, given the prevalence of personality disorders, it is highly likely that OTPs will encounter individuals with diagnosed personality disorders or presenting with symptoms during service provision for occupational functioning deficits. When working with the individual who demonstrates maladaptive behaviors associated with a personality disorder, the ability to recognize and respond appropriately to these behaviors will enhance occupational therapy services.

An article in the occupational therapy literature has explored social participation of people with cluster B personality disorders[60]; it found more difficulty and dissatisfaction with social roles as compared with daily activities for the 31 participants who were inpatients or attending a day treatment program. Interpersonal relationships and fitness were the least satisfying areas of life, and difficulties with work, school, and leisure were acknowledged. Personal care was the most satisfying and least problematic life habit indicated.

Another article in the occupational literature focused on women with BPD and examined their perception of their daily occupations and adaptation to daily life.[61] This was a qualitative study; d the resulting theme revealed "having few organized daily activities and poor personal causation prevent changes in adaptation to daily life."[61] Competency versus incompetency to perform and positive self-image versus lack of self-image were the categories that emerged from the data to support the overall theme.

In another article, the Model of Human Occupation was used to guide treatment for women with BPD in an inpatient setting.[62] The Model of Human Occupation Screening Tool (MOHOST) was used for assessment and to explore how the BPD symptoms affected occupational performance. For example, motivation may be affected by feelings of abandonment and emptiness, severe dissociative symptoms, paranoid ideation, and/or suicidal behavior leading to difficulty with process and motor skills and negatively affecting occupational performance. A pattern of intense and unstable relationships and impulsivity can also negatively affect occupational engagement. When emotionally dysregulated, individuals with BPD exhibit maladaptive behaviors and experience difficulty in the areas of volition, habituation, and personal causation, leading to decreased and unsatisfactory participation in daily occupations. Multiple treatment pathways were provided; these included activities of daily living (ADLs), crafts, and horticultural and culinary activities. The pathways focused on participation and commitment to the treatment process and everyday activities and active engagement in meaningful occupations.[62]

When working with individuals with personality disorders, the Occupational Therapy Practice Framework (OTPF)[63] guides practice. Some methods to support individuals with personality disorders include education and understanding of the disorder to support self-empowerment. Encouraging a healthy lifestyle that includes physical activity, avoidance of alcohol and illegal substances, and provision of routine medical care is also important. Stress management techniques, opportunities for emotional expression, and supportive family and social relationships should also be fostered.

DISSOCIATIVE DISORDERS

Dissociation is a mental process in which a person experiences a disconnection in thoughts, memories, feelings, actions, or sense of identity.[6] Daydreaming or difficulty recalling familiar actions when lost in thought are examples of mild dissociation that are normal experiences. More severe types of dissociation resulting in functional problems and distress are referred to as "dissociative disorders," and they are frequently associated with past trauma.[6] The five core symptoms of dissociative disorders are as follows[64]:

- Amnesia—recurrent memory problems, often described as "losing time"; these gaps in memory can vary from several minutes to years.
- Depersonalization—a sense of detachment or disconnection from one's self. This can include feeling like a stranger to yourself, feeling detached from your emotions, feeling robotic or like you are on autopilot, or feeling like a part of your body does not belong to you.
- Derealization—a sense of disconnection from familiar people or one's surroundings—for example, close relatives or your own home may seem unreal or foreign.

- Identity confusion—an inner struggle about one's sense of self or identity, which may involve uncertainty, puzzlement or conflict.
- Identity alteration—a sense of acting like a different person some of the time.

There are three types of dissociative disorders—dissociative identity disorder, dissociative amnesia, and depersonalization-derealization disorder. Dissociative identity disorder was previously referred to as "multiple personality disorder" from 1980 to 1994 in the DSM-3.[65] In 1994, it was renamed "dissociative identity disorder" (DID). This disorder is associated with childhood experiences of physical and sexual abuse. Approximately 90% of individuals diagnosed with DID are victims of childhood abuse and neglect. Criteria for diagnosis include the existence of two or more distinct identities accompanied by changes in behavior, memory, and thinking. Memory is affected by ongoing gaps in everyday events, personal information, and/or past traumatic events. These occurrences are not considered cultural or religious practices. Self-injurious and suicidal behaviors are common among individuals with dissociative identity disorder.[6]

Depersonalization-derealization disorder involves an ongoing or episodic sense of detachment or being outside of one's self. Depersonalization is defined as observing one's actions, feelings, thoughts, and self from a distance, and derealization is described as viewing other people and things around one's self as detached and dreamlike. Depersonalization and derealization may be experienced separately or together.[66] Symptoms of this disorder may include any or all of the following symptoms: numbing of emotions and bodily senses, altered bodily perceptions, distorted sense of time, feeling detached from self, and feeling that things are unreal.[64] The person recognizes that the experience is not real and feels distressed by the experience.

Dissociative amnesia is memory loss that is more severe than normal forgetfulness and that cannot be explained by a medical condition. The memory loss is usually related to a traumatic or stressful event, such as childhood emotional abuse and neglect. The individual may or may not be aware of the memory loss.[66] Dissociative amnesia is the most common dissociative disorder.[64] The three types of dissociative amnesia are localized amnesia, selective amnesia (which may occur along with localized amnesia), and generalized amnesia. Localized amnesia, the most common type of dissociative amnesia, is the failure to recall events during a specific period of time. Selective amnesia is the inability to remember a specific aspect of an event or some events within a period of time. Generalized amnesia is the most severe and rarest type of dissociative amnesia. It may involve the complete loss of a person's identity in addition to all memories of their past.[64,66] Other forms of dissociative amnesia can also occur; people with generalized amnesia may also lose semantic knowledge (previous knowledge about the world) and procedural knowledge (forgetting well-learned skills). Systematized amnesia is amnesia for a category of information (e.g., no memory of family, no memory of a specific person, or childhood sexual abuse). Continuous amnesia is the inability to form new memories. Microamnesias are also typical in dissociative disorders; the amnesia is for a very brief period of time.[64]

Dissociative amnesia can also occur with dissociative fugue. A fugue occurs when there is sudden and unexpected travel away from home or work. The person may act in a way that is purposeful, with a specific goal, or may present as wandering. It is associated with identity confusion or assumption of a new identity and may last for days, weeks, or longer.[64]

Therapeutic Management

Psychotherapy is the treatment of choice for DID. It focuses on integration of the different elements of identity by assisting the individual in remembering and coping with past traumatic experiences. Common types of therapy include CBT, DBT, and hypnosis. There are no medications for the treatment of DID, although they may be used to treat coexisting conditions such as depression.[66]

Because dissociation disorders are frequently associated with past trauma, OTPs working with individuals with dissociative disorders should use a trauma-informed care approach. This can include a wide range of sensory-based treatments, body-oriented approaches, and occupation-focused interventions to assist the individual in feeling grounded and safe. Understanding what trauma is and the impact of trauma on the individual is necessary to provide meaningful and individualized care. Trauma-informed care is interdisciplinary and evidence-based, with resources available for practitioners to develop effective skills in the provision of trauma- informed care. An in-depth discussion of trauma-informed care is provided in Chapter 17.

SOMATIC SYMPTOMS AND RELATED DISORDERS

Somatic symptom and related disorders refer to a group of disorders in which the person experiences physical symptoms and/or pain that is not directly associated with a specific physical cause or the expected intensity of an existing medical disorder. Generally, people who have a somatic symptom and related disorder have normal medical test results, or the results do not support the person's symptoms. This category includes somatic symptom disorder, illness anxiety disorder, conversion disorder, and factitious disorder.

Somatic Symptom Disorder and Illness Anxiety Disorder

Somatic symptom disorder is the presence of one or more somatic symptoms, such as pain or weakness, that result in distress to the individual and/or difficulty with daily functioning. The symptoms are generally not well defined by a medical condition or explained by organic pathology. When there is a medical condition that correlates with the symptoms, it is inconsistent with the magnitude of symptoms and distress that is reported, and treatment of the condition does not relieve the symptoms or distress. Excessive thoughts, feelings, and behaviors related to the somatic symptoms are present for at least 6 months. They are accompanied by a high level of anxiety and are disproportionate and persistent in relation to the symptoms. Somatic symptom disorder (SSD) presents on a continuum of mild to severe, depending on the number and extent of the psychobehavioral symptoms that are present or the severity of the somatic symptoms. Illness anxiety disorder (IAD) is diagnosed when an individual is preoccupied with having a serious illness, despite the absence of any somatic symptoms or physical distress.[67]

The causes of SSD and IAD are unknown and are most likely complex. They may involve genetic factors, adverse childhood experiences, attachment insecurity, developmentally induced difficulty in emotion recognition and regulation, and cultural factors. Organic illnesses, stressful work conditions, and adverse life events are considered precipitating factors for bodily distress that along with predisposing personality aspects, may contribute to SSD and IAD.[67]

The diagnosis is made after determining the presence or absence of the relevant diagnostic criteria and should be considered for patients with persistent physical symptoms. A thorough physical and mental evaluation provides the basis for an accurate diagnosis, along with consideration of lifestyle factors and use of legal and illegal substances. The individual's overall functioning, expectations, beliefs, and illness behavior are also considered, along with any patterns of dysfunctional health care utilization.[67]

Conversion Disorder

Conversion disorder, also called "functional neurologic symptom disorder," is a mental disorder in which symptoms affecting voluntary motor or sensory function are not attributed to a neurologic or medical disorder; rather, they are caused by an unconscious conflict or psychological stressor.[68] Other names for conversion disorder include psychogenic disorder and nonorganic disorder.[69] It can be difficult to diagnose conversion disorder. A thorough history, including the presence of clinical symptoms without corresponding organic disease, is required for an accurate diagnosis. One or more symptoms of altered voluntary motor or sensory function must be present and must evoke significant distress or impairment in social or occupational functioning. A sudden serious illness, accompanied by a lack of appropriate concern and a history of psychological problems that improve when physical symptoms emerge, are typical signs of conversion disorder. Some common examples of conversion symptoms include blindness, paralysis, dystonia, anesthesia, difficulty walking, and hallucinations.[68] The individual with conversion disorder is not pretending to have these symptoms; to this person, the symptoms are real, uncontrollable, and distressing. In contrast, malingering behavior occurs when the individual intentionally exhibits the symptoms of a physical or neurologic disorder for personal or financial gain.[68]

Conversion disorder is a common condition, especially in neurologic and rehabilitation services.[70,71] One study has found it to be the second most common reason for seeing a neurologist.[70] Understanding the cause of conversion disorder can be helpful in conceptualizing the role of occupational therapy in treatment. There can be multiple predisposing, precipitating, and perpetuating factors that play a role in the onset of conversion disorder. Predisposing factors can include emotional and personality disorders, stressful life events, history of psychological trauma, and genetic vulnerability. Precipitating factors can include physical injury, illness, and panic attacks. Perpetuating factors can include abnormal illness belief, secondary gain from illness, and receiving health benefits due to illness. Some individuals present with a history of psychological trauma, and others present without psychological risk factors. Some individuals appear to develop conversion disorder after experiencing a physical injury and some do not. Although there may be a precipitating psychological or physical event at onset, there is no typical or consistent pattern in the development of this disorder; therefore it is important to consider all psychological, physical, and risk factors when evaluating and treating conversion disorder.[69]

Factitious Disorder

Factitious disorder (FD) is a mental disorder characterized by intentional fabrication of illness, injury, or impairment. The individual presents with physical symptoms that require further medical examinations, tests, or procedures and may even include hospital admission. The individual may exaggerate existing physical or medical symptoms, pretend to have symptoms, lie about a medical condition, or engage in self-injury to produce medical concerns. The ability to access in-depth medical information on the Internet provides the opportunity to research and present with a wide range of medical disorders, some of which may

be very complex. There is no obvious benefit or ulterior motive for the individual from this fabrication, and therefore it can be difficult to diagnose. It may be that the behavior is an attempt to receive attention from others or may provide a sense of power and excitement when the person is successful in manipulating and controlling health care providers and others.[72] Factitious disorders are considered rare but may be underdiagnosed; prevalence estimates range from 0.5% to 2%.[73] To diagnose FD, an extensive series of medical tests are usually conducted, and the lack of an organic explanation for the patient's problems is documented.[72] It is a challenge to understand the extent of the individual's volitional control over symptoms versus the potential of psychopathology that may exist beyond volitional control.[73] More than two-thirds of individuals with FD also meet the criteria for a personality disorder,[74] and many individuals have experienced childhood adversity, have co-occurring somatoform disorders, and have substance abuse or mood disorders.[75] The term "Munchausen's syndrome" was identified in 1951[76] and refers to a severe and chronic form of FD.[72] The individual typically presents with a history of numerous medical visits that are often with different health care providers, vague symptoms that do not improve and are inconsistent following testing and/or treatment, vast knowledge of medical terminology and diagnoses, and a desire to engage in medical tests and procedures.[77] Munchausen's syndrome by proxy was defined in 1977[78]; it is defined as the imposed presentation of false illness or injury by one person on another person. It is most commonly associated as being inflicted by a parent or caregiver on a child.

Therapeutic Management

Psychotherapy is an established treatment approach for SSD; however, it can be difficult for the individual to accept that there is no organic cause for the symptoms or that the experience of symptoms in the presence of an organic cause is disproportionate in nature. Therefore it may be difficult to believe that psychotherapy will be beneficial. Health care professionals should strive to build a therapeutic relationship with the patient by listening attentively to physical complaints and providing feedback on the emotional aspects that are exhibited. Next, encouraging the individual to consider the possibility of psychosocial, as well as biologic context factors, can be approached, and framing the approach to coping with the symptoms should be advocated.[67]

Occupational therapy can focus on incorporating supportive behaviors and coping mechanisms into basic and instrumental ADLs. These may include relaxation techniques, graded exercise, positive thinking, adaptive strategies, and other individualized supportive measures. Individuals with SSD can be difficult to treat and seem to receive the most benefit from supportive measures of caring and coping to deal with somatic complaints and bodily distress that is real to them.[67]

Conversion disorder can be difficult to treat due to the inability of the individual to understand the psychological cause of the physical symptoms. It often results in increased health care utilization and decreased work productivity.[3] The occupational therapy assessment should include formulating a comprehensive list of symptoms reported by the individual, evaluating ADL performance and use of adaptations and aids, documenting time use, routines, and habits, identifying psychological and physical barriers to rehabilitation, and assessing the individual's understanding of the diagnosis of conversion disorder.[69] Developing a strong therapeutic relationship with the individual is essential. Early attempts to explain the disorder should be avoided; instead, providing reassurance and validation that the symptoms are real to the person are important in building trust. Providing common examples of diseases that are well known to be stress-related and examples of stress-related symptoms can lead to a discussion of personal stress and conflict as related to the symptoms being experienced. Explaining the lack of an organic cause for the symptoms and encouraging the individual to accept that the symptoms are a manifestation of psychological conflict and stress can help the individual begin to accept the diagnosis and focus on specific goals for symptom management and recovery.[68]

Despite the occurrence of conversion disorder, there has been a lack of literature supporting the role of occupational therapy in its treatment. One study[44] has presented a review of the disorder and highlighted the importance and role of occupational therapy in the assessment and treatment of conversion disorder. An occupational therapist's dual training in physical health and mental health, and focus on ADLs rather than on the diagnosis, make them uniquely placed to provide valuable interventions for FND patients, a disorder that is at the interface between neurology and psychiatry.[44]

Although the use of aids and assistive devices are an integral part of occupational therapy services, current treatment approaches recommend active rehabilitation, with minimal emphasis on aids and adaptations, because they can encourage compensatory movement patterns instead of a return to the individual's normal movement patterns. Grading purposeful everyday activities to increase occupational performance is the focus of treatment, and strategies to motivate engagement are emphasized. If the individual is unable to engage in physical occupation as part of active rehabilitation, initiating a contract and/or a self-management program throughout treatment may be helpful. Gradually decreasing the frequency of sessions, with more responsibility directed toward the individual with a home program, may be beneficial. However, some individuals, despite provision of psychotherapeutic and rehabilitation services, do not improve.[69]

FDs can also be difficult to treat due to the resistance of the individual to recognize and acknowledge the psychological cause of the disorder. An interprofessional team-based approach led by the primary care doctor is the recommended approach for managing FD.[73] With all somatic symptom and related disorders, increased psychotherapeutic approaches such as CBT can be used to address the psychological conflicts that are at the root of the physical symptoms, and medication can be used to treat depression and anxiety if needed.[68]

SUMMARY

Other disorders included in the DSM-5[6] but not covered in this text include the categories of neurodevelopmental disorders, sleep-wake disorders, elimination disorders, sexual dysfunction, gender dysphoria, paraphilic disorders, and disruptive impulse control, and conduct disorders. Additionally, there is a category for specified or unspecified mental disorders, with or without another medical condition, and a category for medication-induced disorders.

"Neurodevelopmental disorders are a group of heterogeneous conditions characterized by a delay or disturbance in the acquisition of skills in a variety of developmental domains, including motor, social, language, and cognition."[79] These disorders develop during childhood as a result of abnormal brain maturation.[79] The category of neurodevelopmental disorders includes intellectual disabilities, global developmental delay, communication disorders, autism spectrum disorder, attention-deficit/hyperactivity disorder, specific learning disorders, developmental coordination disorders, stereotypical movement disorders, tic disorders, and Tourette syndrome.[6] Children diagnosed with neurodevelopmental disorders present with a variety of difficulties, including cognitive, social, and behavioral issues that impede typical development. They benefit from occupational therapy treatment and may receive services in pediatric treatment settings such as clinics and schools, as well as in the home.[80] Occupational therapists working in pediatrics will also likely treat children and teenagers with disruptive, impulse control, and conduct disorders. This category includes oppositional defiant disorder, intermittent explosive disorder, conduct disorder, antisocial personality disorder, pyromania, and kleptomania. These disorders usually develop during childhood or adolescence and may co-occur with neurodevelopmental or other disorders. Evidence-based behavioral management strategies and an interprofessional team approach are needed for successful treatment of these disorders.

Sleep-wake disorders include insomnia disorder, hypersomnolence disorder, and narcolepsy and subcategories of breathing-related sleep disorders and parasomnias. Breathing-related sleep disorders include four different diagnoses—obstructive sleep apnea hypopnea, central sleep apnea, sleep-related hypoventilation, and circadian rhythm sleep-wake disorders. Parasomnias are sleep disorders that involve abnormal movements, behaviors, emotions, perceptions, and dreams that occur while falling asleep, sleeping, between sleep stages, or during arousal from sleep. These includes disorders such as sleepwalking, sleep terrors, nightmare disorder, rapid eye movement sleep behavior disorder, and restless legs syndrome.[6]

Rest and sleep are occupations addressed in the OTPF.[63] Healthy sleep behavior is necessary for optimal occupational performance, participation, and engagement in daily life.[81] "Occupational therapists use knowledge of sleep physiology, sleep disorders, and evidence-based sleep promotion practices to evaluate and address the ramifications of sleep insufficiency or sleep disorders on occupational performance and participation."[81]

Elimination disorders, sexual dysfunction, gender dysphoria, and paraphilic disorders (e.g., voyeuristic disorder and exhibitionistic disorder) are other mental disorders not covered in this text. Although these disorders may be less likely to present in occupational therapy treatment, occupational therapists should be prepared to assess the impact on occupational performance if presented with a client with one of these disorders.

SUGGESTED LEARNING ACTIVITIES

1. Watch the Netflix original movie "To the Bone," which focuses on a 20-year-old woman's journey to recovery from anorexia nervosa in an inpatient group home for eating disorders. With therapy, she learns how to cope with her dysfunctional family and find self-acceptance. How does therapy help patients who are suffering from eating disorders?

2. Take an online self-assessment for eating disorders (https://eatingdisorder.org/eating-disorder-information/online-self-assessment). How helpful do you think self-assessment is for someone who may have an eating disorder?

3. Identify the common features for each personality disorder cluster (A, B, C). At what point do personality characteristics become a personality disorder?

4. View the following vignette on borderline personality disorder (BPD; https://www. youtube.com/watch?v=5tvwhqfGezQ). What are your impressions of BPD?

5. Explore mental health worksheets on dialectic behavioral therapy (DBT; https://www. therapistaid.com/therapy-worksheets/dbt/none).

6. View the movie "Love You to Death," about Dee Blanchard, who was alleged to have Munchausen syndrome by proxy and had been presenting her daughter, Gypsy Rose Blanchard, as disabled and chronically ill for many years. This is an extreme case and, despite some suspicions, Gypsy Rose was not removed from the care of her mother. Why do you think there was a lack of intervention from health care professionals or others?

7. Explore the self-help website managed by Dr. Jon Stone, a neurologist, for individuals with functional or dissociative neurologic symptoms (https://www.neurosymptoms.org). How helpful do you think this is for individuals with functional neurologic disorders?

8. Keep a personal sleep diary, and evaluate your sleep routine and sleep quality. Try one of the apps from the American Sleep Association (https://www.sleepassociation.org/sleep-treatments/sleep-apps). How can occupational therapy practitioners best work with clients with difficulties with rest and sleep?

REFLECTION QUESTIONS

1. Reflect on the role of occupational therapy in treating eating disorders. What does occupational therapy offer that is unique in the treatment of this population?

2. What is the impact of social media on eating disorders? How is social media use helpful, and how can it be harmful?

3. Considering the features of various personality disorders, are there individuals you know that you suspect may have a personality disorder? What difficulties have you observed with social relationships and occupational functioning?

4. Have you ever experienced dissociation? If yes, describe how it felt. How can occupational therapy practitioners best treat individuals with dissociative disorders?

5. How would you manage an individual with a somatic symptom and related disorder? Consider the differences between somatic symptom disorder, illness anxiety disorder, conversion disorder, and factitious disorder. What are the unique challenges of each disorder?

REFERENCES

1. National Institute of Mental Health. *Eating disorders*. 2017. Available at: https://www.nimh.nih.gov/health/statistics/eating-disorders.shtml.
2. Hudson JI, Hiripi E, Pope HG, Kessler RC. The prevalence and correlates of eating disorders in the national comorbidity survey replication. *Biol Psychiatry*. 2007;61(3):348-358.
3. Le Grange D, Swanson SA, Crow SJ, Merikangas KR. Eating disorder not otherwise specified presentation in the US population. *Int J Eat Disord*. 2012;45(5):711-718.
4. Smink FE, van Hoeken D, Hoek HW. Epidemiology of eating disorders: incidence, prevalence and mortality rates. *Curr Psychiatry Rep*. 2012;14(4):406-414.
5. Arcelus J, Mitchel AJ, Wales J, Nielson S. Mortality rates in patients with anorexia nervosa and other eating disorders. *Arch Gen Psychiatry*. 2011;68(7):724-731.
6. American Psychiatric Association. *Diagnostic and Statistical Manual of Mental Disorders*. 5th ed. Washington, DC; American Psychiatric Association; 2013.
7. Ulfvebrand S, Birgegard A, Norring C, Hogdahl L, von Hausswolff-Juhlin Y. Psychiatric comorbidity in women and men with eating disorders results from a large clinical database. *Psychiatry Res*. 2015;230(2):294-299.
8. National Eating Disorders Association. *Treatment*. 2018. Available at: https://www.nationaleatingdisorders.org/treatment.
9. Stip E, Lungu OV. Salience network and olanzapine in schizophrenia: implications for treatment in anorexia nervosa. *Can J Psychiatry*. 2015;60(suppl 2):35-39.
10. Dold M, Aigner M, Klabunde M, et al. Second-generation antipsychotic drugs in anorexia nervosa: a meta-analysis of randomized controlled trials. Psychother Psychosom. 2015;84(2):110-116.
11. Berg KC, Wonderlich SA. Emerging psychological treatments in the field of eating disorders. *Curr Psychiatry Rep*. 2013;15(407).
12. Roberts ME, Treasure J, Stahl D, Southgate L, Treasure J. A systematic review and meta-analysis of set-shifting ability in eating disorders. *Psychol Med*. 2007;37:1075-1084.
13. Tchanturia K, Davies H, Campbell IC. Cognitive remediation therapy for patients with anorexia nervosa: preliminary findings. *Ann Gen Psychiatry*. 2007;6:14.
14. Agras WS, Telch CF. The effects of caloric deprivation and negative affect on binge eating in obese binge-eating disordered women. *Behav Ther*. 1998;29:491-503.
15. Crosby RD, Wonderlich SA, Engel SG, Simmonich H, Smyth J, Mitchell JE. Daily mood patterns and bulimic behaviors in the natural environment. *Behav Res Ther*. 2009;47:181-188.
16. Smyth JM, Wonderlich SA, Heron KE, Sliwinski MJ, Crosby RD, Mitchell JE, et al. Daily and momentary mood and stress are associated with binge eating and vomiting in bulimia nervosa patients in the natural environment. *J Consult Clin Psychol*. 2007;75:629-638.
17. Hayes SC, Strosahl KD, Wilson KG. *Acceptance and Commitment Therapy: An Experiential Approach to Behavior Change*. New York: Guilford Press; 1999.
18. Manlick CF, Cochran SV, Koon J. Acceptance and commitment therapy for eating disorders: rationale and literature review. *J Contemp Psychother*. 2013;43:115-122.
19. Rosenfeld SM. *DBT in the treatment of eating disorders*. 2016. Available at: https://www.mirror-mirror.org/dbt-eating-disorder-treatment.htm.
20. Fassino S, Piero A, Gramaglia C, Abbate-Daga G. Clinical, psychopathological and personality correlates of interoceptive awareness in anorexia nervoa, bulimia nervosa, and obesity. *Psychopathology*. 2004;37:168-174.
21. Wanden-Berghe RG, Sanz-Valero J, Wanden-Berghe C. The application of mindfulness to eating disorders treatment: a systematic review. *Eat Disord*. 2011;19:34-48.
22. Safer DL, Robinson AH, Jo B. Outcome from a randomized controlled trial of group therapy for binge eating disorder: comparing dialectical behavior therapy adapted for binge eating to an active comparison group therapy. *Behav Ther*. 2010;41:106-120.
23. Telch CF, Agras WS, Linehan MM. Dialectical behavior therapy for binge eating disorder. *J Consult Clin Psychol*. 2001;69:1061-1065.
24. Koskina A, Campbell IC, Schmidt U. Exposure therapy in eating disorders revisited. *Neurosci Biobehav Rev*. 2013;37:193-208.
25. Carter FA, Bulik CM. Exposure treatments for bulimia nervosa: procedure, efficacy, and mechanisms. *Adv Behav Res Ther*. 1994;16:77-129.
26. McIntosh VVW, Carter FA, Bulik CM, Frampton CMA, Joyce PR. Five-year outcome of cognitive behavioral therapy and exposure with response prevention for bulimia nervosa. *Psychol Med*. 2011;41:1061-1071.
27. Glasofer DR, Albano AM, Simpson HB, Steinglass JE. Overcoming fear of eating: a case study of a novel use of exposure and response prevention. *Psychotherapy*. 2016;53(2):223-231.
28. Steinglass JE, Albano AM, Simpson HB, et al. Confronting fear using exposure and response prevention for anorexia nervosa: a randomized controlled pilot study. *Int J Eat Disord*. 2014;47(2):174-180.
29. Hildebrandt T, Loeb K, Troupe S, Delinsky S. Adjunctive mirror exposure for eating disorders: a randomized controlled pilot study. *Behav Res Ther*. 2012;50:797-804.
30. Key A, George CL, Beattie D, Stammers K, Lacey H, Waller G. Body image treatment within an inpatient program for anorexia nervosa: the role of mirror exposure in the desensitization process. *Int J Eat Disord*. 2002;31:185-190.
31. Cassin SE, von Ranson KM, Heng K, Brar J, Wojtowiez AE. Adapted motivational interviewing for women with binge eating disorder: a randomized controlled trial. *Psychol Addict Behav*. 2008;22:417-425.
32. Geller J, Brown KE, Srikameswaran S. The efficacy of a brief motivational intervention for individuals with eating disorders: a randomized control trial. *Int J Eat Disord*. 2011;44:497-505.
33. Geller J, Dunn EC. Integrating motivational interviewing and cognitive behavioral therapy in the treatment of eating disorders: tailoring interventions to patient readiness for change. *Cogn Behav Pract*. 2011;18:5-15.
34. Dray J, Wade TD. Is the transtheoretical model and motivational interviewing approach applicable to the treatment of eating disorders? A review. *Clin Psychol Rev*. 2012;32:558-565.

35. Macdonald P, Hibbs R, Corfield F, Treasure J. The use of motivational interviewing in eating disorders: a systematic review. *Psychiatry Res.* 2012;200:1-11.

36. Fairburn CG. *Cognitive Behavior Therapy and Eating Disorders.* New York: Guilford Press; 2008.

37. Wonderlich SA, Peterson CB, Crosby RD, Smith TL, Klein MH, Mitchell JE, et al. A randomized controlled comparison of integrative cognitive-affective therapy (ICAT) and enhanced cognitive behavioral therapy (CBT-E) for bulimia nervosa. *Psychol Med.* 2014;44(3):543-553.

38. Strober M, Freeman R, Morrell W. The long-term course of severe anorexia nervosa in adolescents: survival analysis of recovery, relapse, and outcome predictors over 10–15 years in a prospective study. *Int J Eat Disord.* 1997;22:339-360.

39. Lock J, Le Grange D. Family-based treatment of eating disorders. *Int J Eat Disord.* 2005;37:S64-S67.

40. Lock J, Le Grange D, Agras WS, Moye A, Bryson SW, Jo B. Randomized control trial comparing family-based treatment with adolescent-focused individual therapy for adolescents with anorexia nervosa. *Arch Gen Psychiatry.* 2010;67:1025-1032.

41. Costa DM. Eating disorders: occupational therapy's role. *Occup Ther Pract.* 2009;14(11):13-16.

42. Clark M, Nayar S. Recovery from eating disorders: a role for occupational therapy. *N Z J Occup Ther.* 2012;59(1):13-17.

43. National Eating Disorders Association. *Warning signs and symptoms.* 2018. Available at: https://www.nationaleatingdisorders.org/warning-signs-and-symptoms.

44. Gardiner C, Brown N. Is there a role for occupational therapy within a specialist child and adolescent mental health eating disorder service? *Br J Occup Ther.* 2010;73(1):38-43.

45. Livingston M, Reimann K, Coffey E, Thayer S, Hampton K, Gibson C. *The role of occupational therapy in the treatment of eating disorders.* Available at: https://www.motafunctionfirst.org/assets/2017-Conference-Presentation/3D%20-%20OT%20and%20Eating%20Disorders.pdf.

46. Newbridge Treatment for Eating Disorders. *Occupational therapy.* 2019. Available at: https://www.newbridge-health.org.uk/the-newbridge-treatment-model/therapies/occupational-therapy.

47. The Center for Eating Disorders. *Occupational therapy at the Center for Eating Disorders.* 2015. Available at: https://www.eatingdisorder.org/treatment-and-support/therapeutic-modalities/occupational-therapy.

48. Berghuis H, Kamphuis JH, Verheul R. Core features of personality disorder: differentiating general personality dysfunctioning from personality traits. *J Pers Disord.* 2012;26:704-716.

49. American Psychiatric Association. *What are personality disorders?* 2018. Available at: https://www.psychiatry.org/patients-families/personality-disorders/what-are-personality-disorders.

50. Hoermann S, Zupanick CE, Dombeck M. *DSM-5:* The ten personality disorders: cluster A. Available at: https://www.mentalhelp.net/articles/dsm-5-the-ten-personality-disorders-cluster-a.

51. Bressert S. *Schizotypal personality disorder.* 2017. Available at: https://psychcentral.com/disorders/schizotypal-personality-disorder/.

52. Hoermann S, Zupanick CE, Dombeck M. *DSM-5:* The ten personality disorders: cluster B. Available at: https://www.mentalhelp.net/articles/dsm-5-the-ten-personality-disorders-cluster-b.

53. Hoermann S, Zupanick CE, Dombeck M. *DSM-5:* The ten personality disorders: cluster. Available at: https://www.mentalhelp.net/articles/dsm-5-the-ten-personality-disorders-cluster-c.

54. Volkert J, Gablonski T, Rabung S. Prevalence of personality disorders in the general adult population in Western countries: systematic review and meta-analysis. *Br J Psychiatry.* 2018;213:709-715.

55. Gask L, Evans M, Kessler E. Personality disorder. *BMJ.* 2013;347(f5276):1-7.

56. Evershed S. Treatment of personality disorder: skills-based therapies. *Adv Psychiatr Treat.* 2011;17:206-213.

57. Ripoll LH, Triebwasser J, Siever LJ. Evidence-based pharmacotherapy for personality disorders. *Int J Neuropsychopharmacol.* 2011;14:1257-1288.

58. May JM, Richardi TM, Barth KS. Dialectical behavior therapy as treatment for borderline personality disorder. *Ment Health Clin.* 2016;6(2):62-67.

59. Kendall T, Pilling S, Tyrer P, Duggan C, Burbeck R, Meader N, et al. Borderline and antisocial personality disorders: summary of NICE guidance. *BMJ.* 2009;338:293-295.

60. Larivière N, Desrosiers J, Tousignant M, Boyer R. Exploring social participation of people with Cluster B Personality Disorders. *Occup Ther Ment Health.* 2010;26:4: 375-386.

61. Falklöf I, Haglund L. Daily occupations and adaptation to daily life described by women suffering from Borderline Personality Disorder. *Occup Ther Ment Health.* 2010;26(4): 354-374.

62. Lee S, Harris M. The development of an effective occupational therapy assessment and treatment pathway for women with a diagnosis of borderline personality disorder in an inpatient setting: implementing the Model of Human Occupation. *Br J Occup Ther.* 2010;73(11): 559-563.

63. American Occupational Therapy Association. Occupational therapy practice framework: domain and process, 3rd ed. *Am J Occup Ther.* 2014;68(suppl 1):S1-S51.

64. TraumaDissociation.com. *Dissociative disorders.* 2018. Available at: http://traumadissociation.com/dissociative.

65. American Psychiatric Association. *Diagnostic and Statistical Manual of Mental Disorders.* 3rd ed. Washington, DC: American Psychiatric Association; 1980.

66. American Psychiatric Association. What are dissociative disorders? 2018. Available at: https://www.psychiatry.org/patients-families/dissociative-disorders/what-are-dissociative-disorders.

67. Henningsen P. Management of somatic symptom disorder. *Dialogues Clin Neurosci.* 2018;20(1):23-30.

68. Ali S, Jabeen S, Pate RJ, et al. Conversion disorder—mind versus body: a review. *Innov Clin Neurosci.* 2015;12(5-6): 27-33.

69. Gardiner P, MacGregor L, Carson A, Stone J. Occupational therapy for functional neurological disorders: a scoping

review and agenda for research. *CNS Spectr.* 2018;23: 205-212.

70. Stone J, Carson A, Duncan R, Roberts R, Warlow C, Hibberd C, et al. Who is referred to neurology clinics? The diagnoses made in 3781 new patients. *Clin Neurol Neurosurg.* 2010;112(9):747-751.

71. Stone J, Warlow C, Sharpe M. The symptom of functional weakness: a controlled study of 107 patients. *Brain.* 2010;133(Pt 5):1537-1551.

72. Yates GP, Feldman MD. Factitious disorder: a systematic review of 455 cases in the professional literature. *Gen Hosp Psychiatry.* 2016;41:20-28.

73. Bass C, Halligan P. Factitious disorders and malingering: challenges for clinical assessment and management. *Lancet.* 2014;383:1422-1432.

74. Tyrer P, Seivewright N, Seivewright H. Long-term outcome of hypochondriacal personality disorder. *J Psychosom Res.* 1999;46:177-185.

75. Bass C, Jones D. Psychopathology of perpetrators of fabricated or induced illness in children: case series. *Br J Psychiatry.* 2011; 199:113-118.

76. Asher R. Munchausen's syndrome. *Lancet.* 1951;1(6650); 339-341.

77. Turner J, Reid S. Munchausen's syndrome. *Lancet.* 2002;359(9303):346-349.

78. Meadow R. Munchausen syndrome by proxy: the hinterland of child abuse. *Lancet.* 1977;2(8033):343-345.

79. Jeste SS. Neurodevelopmental behavioral and cognitive disorders. *Continuum (Minneap Minn).* 2015;21(3):690-714.

80. Ahn S, Hwang S. Cognitive rehabilitation of adaptive behavior in children with neurodevelopmental disorders: a meta-analysis. *Occup Ther Int.* 2018;5029571:1-7.

81. American Occupational Therapy Association. *Occupational therapy's role in sleep.* 2017. Available at: https://www.aota .org/~/media/Corporate/Files/AboutOT/ Professionals/ WhatIsOT/HW/Facts/Sleep-fact-sheet.pdf.

15

Emotional Impact of Physical Illness or Injury

Joy Crawford

LEARNING OBJECTIVES

1. Identify and discuss the psychosocial implications related to various physical pathologies.
2. Articulate the importance of engagement in occupations, roles, and routines and how engagement may affect health and wellness.
3. Describe various therapeutic interventions that may be used to promote independence, health, and wellness for clients with psychosocial impairments resulting from physical illness or injury.
4. Discuss the role of the occupational therapy practitioner with the client with psychosocial impairments related to physical illness or injury.

INTRODUCTION

Physical illness or injury may affect an individual's mental health, as well as the body part or systems affected. As a result, disruptions to one's life balance may occur. These disruptions may lead to changes in one's mental health.

The degree to which one experiences a disruption, and mental health changes, may vary. Mental health stability may change over time in those with illness or injury because mental health and well-being are known to be a dynamic state of being.[1] According to the World Health Organization (WHO), mental health is a state of well-being in which an individual is able to cope, adapt, and engage in their life productively.[2] The experience and response to disease and injury is a personal one; however, the inability to engage in one's chosen life occupations is effectively likely to occur on some level due to illness or injury.

Individuals with illness and/or injury may experience a plethora of emotions. Despair, anger, panic, apathy, fear, uncertainty, loneliness, frustration, and feelings of being out of control may surface as the individual is faced with the physical changes. Self-efficacy, which has to do with the individual's perception of personal competence, may be directly affected.[3] As a person's perception of personal competence changes, behaviors, personal adaptation, goal setting, goal achievement, and overall engagement in occupations may decline.[3] Occupations may become impoverished or disengagement may occur. As noted in the *Occupational Therapy Practice Framework* (OTPF), one's overall sense of well-being and health is sustained through engagement.[4] Considering this, challenges with coping strategies and potential mental health changes should be anticipated.

Clients may experience changes in performance patterns and performance skills as a result of physical illness or injury. Roles may shift or be abandoned and routines may be interrupted or halted. Rituals and habits that are typically a part of the individual's daily life may no longer hold the same importance or may be neglected. Skills that were used to engage in occupations of choice may be impaired, and the level of independence may change. As this occurs, changes in attitudes, expectations, and self-esteem may be anticipated. Motivation and initiation to participate in occupations that were previously meaningful may be diminished. Impairment or impoverishment in any of

219

the occupational therapy domains, including occupations, client factors, performance skills, performance patterns, contexts, and environments, may be affected as a result of physical illness or injury and are of concern to the occupational therapy practitioner.[4]

The role of the occupational therapy practitioner is to provide client-centered therapy.[4] The process begins with the completion of an occupational profile and the determination of what occupations and roles the client wants and needs to engage in. An analysis of occupational performance is completed, and the practitioner collaborates with the client, family, and/or caregivers to determine goals. The treatment plan is then established, and treatment implementation is initiated.[4] The collaborative dynamic therapeutic process that follows should progress the client toward productive and balanced life engagement.

This chapter is organized into 12 sections by illness or injury. Each section provides a review of the potential effect on the psychosocial well-being of the individual as a result of the condition. Occupational therapy implications for each are included, with examples of occupational therapy approaches to support psychosocial functioning and occupational performance.

AMPUTATIONS

Amputations may occur due to planned surgical interventions or trauma. The type and causes of amputation, severity, location, and prior level of mental health and well-being will affect an individual's response to an amputation.[5] Individuals may feel emotions that are typically experienced in times of loss. Disbelief, grief, fear, bargaining, guilt, anger, and feelings of uncertainty may surface. However, in many cases, with time and success with engagement in occupations, adjustment to the amputation will occur.[5]

Following an amputation, changes may occur in varied occupations, performance skills, and performance patterns. Self-image, self-esteem, and body image may be significantly affected as a result of the loss, resulting in impairments in social and sexual relationships. Among individuals who have experienced an amputation, concerns regarding their ability to engage socially and be financially productive have been found to be of paramount concern.[6] Other factors that have been identified as being significant to this population are a sense of uncertainty and feeling powerless.[6] Anxiety, depression, and posttraumatic stress disorder (PTSD) may result in those who are unable to develop adequate coping strategies.[5]

Occupational Therapy Implications

Dependent on the needs, interests, and goals of the client, the occupational therapy practitioner may choose to use occupation-based interventions, therapeutic activity, or preparatory methods during the treatment process.

Clients may be educated in the use of relaxation techniques to address stress, anxiety, pain, and sleep disruption. Cognitive behavioral therapy strategies, coping strategies, and positive self-talk may be beneficial in the process of the acceptance of the new self and for overall goal achievement. Leisure and vocation interest checklists, along with discussion, may be meaningful for the client who values engagement in social and work activities. Activities that offer opportunities for self-expression and mindfulness may be beneficial for addressing anger, stress, fear, and grief.

When planning therapy sessions, the clinician should consider activities with the potential for built-in successes, and opportunity for choices to improve the client's self-efficacy, self-worth, self-esteem, and sense of empowerment. As identified in the OTPF, occupational engagement is essential to one's perception of competence and sense of self.[4] Keeping this in mind, the goal of the practitioner is to provide opportunities for engagement that address the wide range of occupations that one may choose to embrace.

BURNS

The mechanism of a burn injury and the location and degree of the burn will affect the physical and mental health well-being of a client. Clients who have experienced burns may experience mental health disorders such as PTSD, affective disorder, substance abuse disorder, or adjustment disorder.[7] The prevalence of PTSD among burn patients is relativity high.[7] Reports have indicated that PTSD in adults ranges from 31% to 45.2% compared with the rate of 9% to 30% in the general population.[7] These psychosocial affects may be lifelong.

Various area of occupation may be affected as a result of burn injuries. In addition to the psychological effects of burn injuries, clients may experience significant physical issues such as pain, itching, loss of mobility, decreased strength, and decreased range of motion, which may limit engagement in occupations. Roles, routines, habits, and the context in which these engagements occur may be disrupted, which may further limit the client's ability to participate in activities of daily living. These limitations may lead to frustration, anger, and fear.

Clients may experience changes with self-esteem, self-image, and body image as a result of burn injuries. As a result, disengagement may occur in the social realm. Sexual and romantic relationships may suffer due to the individual's perceptions of any existing disfigurement. Perceptions of self-efficacy and self-worth may also affect the client's engagement in occupations and with personal relationships.

Occupational Therapy Implications

The role of occupational therapy with the client with a burn injury is to address the various domains of occupation to return the client to a productive meaningful life, and foster a sense of competency.[4] Interventions may vary and should be prioritized based on the client's personal goals and needs. The occupational therapy practitioner will consider the significant psychosocial effects that the burn injury may have on the individual. Issues related to disfigurement, pain, and impaired performance are paramount and are addressed throughout the occupational therapy process.

To promote healthy coping skills the occupational therapy practitioner may engage the client in relaxation techniques, stress management strategies, imagery, sensory modulation, and anger management. Once learned, these strategies may be applied throughout the client's recovery.

The use of therapeutic activities such as arts and crafts may be beneficial for developing a sense of competency. This may also be used as a method of self-expression or it may be used as a means of distraction from stressors or pain. Engagement in the described therapeutic activities may prove to be a wonderful outlet for the individual who is unable to voice feelings or is reluctant to share them.

Positive self-talk, cognitive behavior therapy, role playing, and self-esteem building activities may be beneficial in preparing the client for social interactions and in resuming healthy relationships. Acceptance of the new self and increased confidence may be a product of these therapeutic interventions.

Participation in basic activities of daily living (BADLs) and instrumental activities of daily living (IADLs) provides the client with the opportunity to engage in their occupations of choice. This participation may develop self-efficacy and promote a sense of control and personal achievement. The effect of "doing" and acting on the environment is powerful and may be motivating, stimulating, and rewarding to the client who is able to engage.

Ultimately, there are a multitude of activities and interventions that may be beneficial for the client who has experienced a burn injury. Addressing the psychosocial needs of the client includes addressing the effects of the physical limitations on their overall mental health and well-being. The client-centered clinician will match the client's interests with the most effective and beneficial interventions to foster health, wellness, and independence.

CANCER

The effects of cancer on one's physical and mental health may vary dependent on the type of cancer, stage of cancer, and treatment method used.[8] Client skill levels and the ability to engage in chosen occupations will affect the client's life satisfaction, sense of well-being, and mental health.

Research studies have indicated that the rate of decreased mental health in individuals with cancer is higher than in the general population.[8] As a result, the occupational therapy practitioner may anticipate the need to address related mental health issues. Clients who have received a diagnosis of cancer may experience feelings of fear, uncertainty, loss of control, anxiety, denial, anger, and depression. Impairments in BADLs, IADLs, work, leisure, socialization, sleep, and educational pursuits may occur. Self-image, self-esteem, and self-efficacy may be affected as the client moves through the disease process and treatment. Roles, routines, habits, rituals, and relationships may change due to disengagement and skill loss. Complications from treatments, and the disease itself, may limit engagement in life occupations.

Occupational Therapy Implications

The goal of occupational therapy with the client with cancer is to provide client-centered interventions that move the client toward personal goal achievement. The therapist should be mindful of the unique presentations of each client and how their performance may be affected by the type and stage of cancer with which they have been diagnosed. As the disease progresses, or the client improves, the clinician should anticipate that the individual's mental health needs may change as well. Based on client responses and needs, the occupational therapy practitioner will modify treatment sessions and goals accordingly. Occupations that are meaningful to the client should be the focus of occupational therapy treatment session. Goals, set in collaboration with the client, may be achieved through skill development, adaptations, modifications, and use of various strategies.

The occupational therapy practitioner may recommend adaptive strategies and techniques or make recommendations for home modifications to facilitate engagement in varied BADLs and IADLs. In some cases, the therapist may suggest task delegation to minimize client stress and fatigue and allow the client to be more productive in areas that are deemed more important. Stress management techniques, anger management strategies, visualization and imagery, deep breathing, progressive muscle relaxation, sensory modulation techniques, and journaling may be recommended to promote optimal coping skills and a sense of peace and wellness. The occupational therapy practitioner may use varied activities and strategies for self-esteem building. Programs that focus on "feeling and looking good" may be recommended to improve self-esteem and provide a sense of normalcy. Arts and crafts may be used to promote self-expression or as a healthy means of distraction.

Spirituality and faith may be of concern to some clients. In these cases, meditation, prayer, listening to music or nature sounds, or reading materials related to one's beliefs may be encouraged to promote a sense of peace, hope, and being grounded. If indicated, the therapist may assist the client with finding adaptive strategies that will allow them to engage in their spiritual practices as they move through the disease process.

Dependent on the disease progression, end-of-life preparation may be addressed to facilitate a sense of control. The therapist may assist the client in organizing personal items of importance, preparing letters or videos for loved ones, and/or tying up loose ends to promote a sense of control and closure.

Yoga, tai chi, leisure exploration, sleep preparation strategies, and positive self-talk may all be used to address varied psychosocial and physical needs and to promote a more balanced, healthy, and fulfilled life.

CARDIOPULMONARY CONDITIONS

Psychosocial conditions are common among clients with a diagnosis of cardiopulmonary illnesses.[9] It has been reported that individuals with chronic obstructive pulmonary disease (COPD) and congestive heart failure (CHF) are two to five times more likely to experience anxiety and depressive disorders than the general population.[9] PTSD is also not uncommon, because clients with cardiopulmonary conditions may have experienced health-related events that were traumatic.

Clients who are diagnosed with cardiopulmonary conditions may experience feelings of fear, panic, disbelief, anger, frustration, and lack of control. Physiologic symptoms associated with the conditions may affect the client's ability to engage in chosen occupation and life roles. Impairments in areas of occupations may further exacerbate existing psychosocial issues related to the existing conditions. Coping skills may be maladaptive or nonexistent. Self-efficacy and self-esteem may be negatively affected as a result of impoverished engagement. Fear of exacerbation of physical symptoms or death may prevent the client from engaging in their lives fully. The overall quality of life of the client may be negatively affected as a result of the physical and psychosocial effects of the conditions.

Occupational Therapy Implications

Occupational therapy practitioners may use a variety of interventions with the client with cardiopulmonary conditions. Close collaboration with other health care providers may be indicated due to the physiologic nature of the conditions.

Coping skills may be a significant area of focus due to the rate of anxiety among this population. Relaxation techniques may be a helpful strategy to address this issue. The occupational therapy practitioner may encourage the client to engage in visualization, progressive muscle relaxation, pursed-lip breathing, meditation, or prayer. Modified yoga or tai chi may be beneficial for managing stress and anxiety and for its physical health benefits.

Offering opportunities for self-expression may be beneficial for addressing issues of anger, fear, frustration, and lack of control. Art, crafts, and woodworking are methods that may be useful in achieving goals related to coping and may be goods tool to distract the client from unwarranted worries.

Lifestyle modifications, work simplification, and energy conservation may reduce stress and anxiety and increase self-efficacy because the client may be able to increase engagement in occupations of choice and gain a sense of control by adopting the strategies. The occupational therapy practitioner is keenly aware that the ability to be an active participant in one's life is beneficial physically, mentally, and spiritually. Using their unique skill set, therapists determine the methods that are best based on each client's unique needs, which then moves the client forward to resuming engagement in life at the optimal level.

CEREBROVASCULAR ACCIDENT

The physical, cognitive, perceptual, and behavioral presentations due to a cerebrovascular accident will vary from client to client, depending on the area of the brain in which blood flow was interrupted. The resulting impairment and their effects on the client's ability to engage in chosen occupations will likely affect the client's state of mental health. Depression, mania, anxiety, PTSD, and psychosis are not uncommon with this diagnosis.[10] Depression is cited in 20% to 50% of individuals who have experienced a stroke and often is associated with anxiety; PTSD is present in 3% to 37% of the population.[10]

Following a cerebrovascular accident, clients may experience a wide range of emotions. Disbelief, fear, grief, anger, frustration, uncertainty, a sense of loss, and decreased self-worth are common. The resulting physical manifestations of the event, loss of skill, ability to engage in preferred occupations, and changes in roles and routines may be devastating for the client. Due to the frequency of depression with this population, it is crucial to have the client engage in chosen occupations, at some level, to prevent disengagement because this may have a lasting effect on outcomes and recovery.

Occupational Therapy Implications

Occupational therapy practitioners may choose to use a variety of therapeutic interventions for skill development and acquisition. Occupation-based interventions, therapeutic activity, or preparatory methods may be used to meet the client's needs, interests, and goals.

The clinician should consider activities with the potential for built-in success and opportunity for choices to improve the client's self-efficacy, self-worth, self-esteem, and sense of empowerment. Coping strategies may be taught to address anger, fear, anxiety, and frustration. Depending on the client's cognitive status, the clinician may educate and demonstrate relaxation techniques, stress management strategies, and sensory modulation techniques.

Offering opportunities for engagement in activities such as arts and crafts may be beneficial for both psychosocial and physical impairments. Matching the client's skill level to the activity is of the utmost importance to avoid frustration and further loss of self-efficacy. The experience of engagement in the presented tasks may provide an opportunity for the client to get lost in the act of doing, which in and of itself is therapeutic. Producing an end product may also create a sense of accomplishment that may be lacking and also provides an opportunity for self-expression.

Exploration of former or new leisure interests may be of benefit for the client who values or could benefit from leisure pursuits. This may be done during casual conversation or with the use of structured leisure checklists. In some cases, the clinician may determine that it is beneficial to offer opportunities to engage in new leisure pursuits as a part of treatment sessions.

As the clinician engages the client who has experienced a cerebrovascular accident, they need to consider both the psychosocial and physical needs of the client and how they are affecting the client's ability to engage in a healthy fulfilled life safely, effectively, and meaningfully.

CHRONIC DISEASES

Chronic disease may be defined as a condition that is long-lasting and that may be managed but not cured.[11] Individuals with chronic diseases may experience depression, anxiety, and adjustment disorders. Research has indicated that chronic disease affects mental health, and impairments in mental health complicate the treatment of chronic disease.[12] Approximately 50% of individuals with chronic illnesses experience depression. Depression may disrupt the individual's ability to cope and engage in life occupations fully.[13]

Individuals who live with chronic disease are challenged with managing and coping with their condition. The results of dealing with the daily health issues may prove to be physically and mentally exhausting. Changes in the way occupations are done, or the inability to engage in meaningful activities, may affect the client's perceptions of themselves, their abilities, and their quality of life. Feelings of anger, fear, shame, guilt, and frustration may surface as a result of the ongoing management of the disease and the limitations incurred due to the nature of the disease. Family members, caregivers, and health care providers are encouraged to be mindful of the effect of their unique role, and the nature of chronic conditions, as they engage with and provide care to the individual who is dealing with a chronic condition.

Occupational Therapy Implications

When addressing the needs of the client with chronic disease, the occupational therapy practitioner will consider the nature of the disease as well as performance skills, patterns, client factors, and occupations relevant to the client. Various therapeutic interventions may be used to address performance skills and related occupations, as well as emotional responses. Of particular relevance with this population is the ability to self-manage the disease. Empowering the client to do so will promote a sense of control and self-efficacy, which will inevitably affect the quality of life and overall mental wellness. Education in lifestyle modification, self-monitoring, and adaptations and modifications for tasks can facilitate improved health, wellness, and independence. Facilitating and acknowledging successes and assisting the client in setting realistic goals may encourage the frustrated client to think positively and attain a focus on tasks that are of the most important for their life satisfaction. Based on the client's needs and presentations, the occupational therapy practitioner, in collaboration with the client, will identify coping skills most beneficial for their unique life experience.

CHRONIC PAIN

Chronic pain may be defined as pain that persists beyond 3 months.[14] The cause of chronic pain may be as a result of injury, surgery, or disease. According to the National Institutes of Health (NIH), more than 76 million American live with chronic pain.[14] In individuals with chronic pain, major depression occurred in 2% to 61% of the population, and the prevalence of substance abuse among those with chronic pain ranges from 27% to 87%.[15] Anxiety disorders among those with chronic pain ranges from 1% to 65%, and suicidal ideations in those with chronic pain occurred, with 28% to 48% of those individuals seeking treatment.[15]

Pain can result in preoccupation with pain and pain relief and can affect social engagement, relationships, self-image, and physical functioning.[16] Individuals who experience chronic pain may develop a sense of helplessness and hopelessness. Disengagement and avoidance of various daily life tasks may occur due to the anticipation of pain.

Skill loss may accompany disengagement, further complicating the sequela.

Occupational Therapy Implications

Occupational therapy interventions for the client who is dealing with chronic pain may vary from client to client because each person's response to pain is unique to their experience. Individuals will vary in their tolerance to pain, perceptions of pain, and expectations of potential outcomes.

In addition to recommendations for adaptive strategies and techniques to increase engagement in occupations, the occupational therapy practitioner may make recommendations for medication management, sleep preparation, stress management, and relaxation techniques. Tai chi, yoga, qi gong, prayer, and meditation may be suggested and demonstrated to reduce stress, redirect negative thinking, and improve overall health and wellness.

DEGENERATIVE DISEASES OF THE CENTRAL NERVOUS SYSTEM

The very nature of progressive degenerative disease requires that the client, family members, and health care providers consider the ever-changing needs of the client. The unique characteristics, symptoms, and progression of various degenerative diseases affect the client's personal experience.[17] The decline of the client's physical and/or cognitive abilities will vary and is dependent on the nature of the disease, complications related to the disease, and access to and compliance with health care recommendations.

As the disease progresses, the client's ability to engage in meaningful life occupations, roles, and routines fully and effectively will decrease. These changes and loss of autonomy and independence can significantly affect the individual's mental health, well-being, and quality of life.[18] Clients may experience feelings of fear, uncertainty, loss of control, anxiety, denial, anger, and depression. They may feel guilt and worry about the demands placed on their family and caregivers as their needs increase. Financial worries may further compound the client's feelings of anxiety.

Occupational Therapy Implications

The occupational therapy practitioner will collaborate with the client, family, and caregivers to identify goals and address needs and wants. Various strategies for engagement in daily life tasks may be addressed to maintain the ability to participate in valued occupations and foster a sense of autonomy and control.

Clients may be encouraged to prioritize, plan, pace, and simplify. Treatment sessions may include education in effective coping strategies, stress management strategies, relaxation techniques, and anger management. Grounding activities, positive affirmations, listening to nature sounds, encouraging commentaries, and journaling are some effective coping techniques that may be recommended to address the emotional challenges that accompany the disease process.

HAND INJURIES

Hands are the tools of the human with which they may engage in doing, creating, expressing, and loving.[19] As a result of this, injury to the hand may have significant effects psychosocially. This is often overlooked by health care professionals, the client, and society.

An individual's response to a hand injury is as unique as individuals themselves. The extent of the injury, cause of injury, appearance of the injury, and client's perception of those factors will inevitably affect the way they respond to and cope with the injury.

The ability to engage in occupations following a hand injury may be affected due to changes in range of motion, sensation, coordination, strength, pain, fear, or even medical restrictions. This alone may result in changes in one's mental health and wellness. Disfigurement or scarring of the hand may further add to the client's negative perception of themselves. The client may experience a wide range of emotions, including embarrassment, shame, disbelief, fear, or even anger. Self-efficacy, self-worth, and self-esteem may be affected. The client may avoid looking in the mirror, touching, or being touched. Social interaction and sexual activity may be negatively affected.

It is imperative that the occupational therapy practitioner be sensitive to the client's subtle and overt responses to the injury because clients may be reluctant to acknowledge or address their emotional needs. A knowledgeable, client-centered therapist will address the client's needs from a holistic perspective, moving the client toward success, wellness, and goal achievement.

Occupational Therapy Implications

As with all physical and psychosocial impairments, the clinician will address performance skills, patterns, client factors, and occupations that are important to the client. Issues related to range of motion, pain, sensation, coordination, and scar management should be addressed to promote skill development, goal achievement, and an increased sense of well-being. Creating an environment in which the client feels that they can freely and safely share their feelings and concerns is important.

Encouraging the client to touch and view the injured extremity during therapy sessions may be helpful in minimizing dread and fear and may also be helpful in coming to terms with the results of the injury. The therapist may encourage the use of visualization as a method to prepare the client for interactions with which they are concerned and promote successful outcomes in those interactions. Positive self-talk, stress management, and relaxation may be warranted to improve coping skills and increase the quality of life.

ORTHOPEDIC CONDITIONS AND TRAUMAS

Orthopedic conditions and physical traumas of the upper and lower extremities and spine may have a significant effect on the client's ability to engage in daily routines and tasks safely and effectively. Pain, fear, immobility, and physical limitations may affect the individual's self-efficacy. Depression, anxiety, and impaired coping skills may result and may affect the client's overall mental health and functional outcomes.[20]

In some cases, orthopedic surgeries are necessary due to preexisting degenerative conditions, or trauma. In the case of preexisting degenerative conditions such as arthritis, the effects of long-term disability or pain may have resulted in disengagement and maladaptive coping skills. In these cases, clients may be more reluctant or fearful to attempt to engage in life once again. Clients who are postsurgical may be especially fearful of mobility and may worry that they will be unable to care for themselves. Concerns may arise regarding the care of others or pets, return to work, or financial responsibilities. The inability to effectively engage in varied occupations and concerns regarding potential outcomes may magnify already existing anxieties.

Occupational Therapy Implications

The occupational therapy practitioner may focus on the reestablishment of routines and roles because these factors are key elements in increasing the client's sense of self-efficacy and control. Opportunities for engagement in BADLs, IADLs, and leisure activities, and built-in successes in those tasks, will increase confidence, decrease fear and worry, and empower the client. Assisting the client with setting realistic and achievable personal goals may provide the client with the necessary focus for embracing meaningful occupations that may have been neglected. Adaptive strategies may be used to promote independence and reduce fear and pain that may have previously been associated with activity. The therapist may provide the client with education on techniques for pain reduction, stress management, and relaxation to promote sleep and rest, healing, and an overall sense of well-being. Establishing rapport and building a relationship of mutual respect and trust are essential for participation and goal achievement.

SPINAL CORD INJURY

Individuals who experience spinal cord injuries (SCIs) will be faced with physical and emotional challenges. Adjustment to spinal cord injuries may be dependent on a variety of factors, including the severity of the injury, social support, and the client's premorbid mental health.[21] Clients may experience feelings of disbelief, hopelessness, anger, grief, and frustration. Depression and anxiety are common among this population and will have a negative effect on the individual's quality of life and overall sense of well-being.[21]

The inevitable changes in areas of occupations, roles, and routines may cause the client to experience decreased self-esteem, motivation, and self-efficacy. The client's perception of their body image and the potential to love and be loved may be altered. Adjustments to a new way of living life and changes in the ability to live their lives with autonomy may affect the individual's overall experience and perception of quality of life.[21] Healthy coping skills are essential as the client deals with both the physical and emotional challenges that have occurred as a result of the injury.

Occupational Therapy Implications

When treating the client with an SCI, the occupational therapy practitioner should consider the importance of engagement in occupation as a means of achieving a sense of well-being. Engaging the client in activities using adaptive strategies and techniques will move them toward independence and increase their sense of control and self-worth. The clinician may encourage the client to engage in activities previously enjoyed or explore new activities to promote skill development and participation. With each successful encounter, motivation, hope, and self-efficacy will increase.

Coping strategies may be used throughout the client's life as they encounter unique situations and stressors and adjust to their new normal. Stress management, relaxation techniques, and anger management may be addressed. Positive self-talk, reflection, and support groups may be suggested to address issues of self-worth and to increase quality of life.

TRAUMATIC OR ACQUIRED BRAIN INJURY

Mental health issues among those with traumatic brain injury (TBI) or acquired brain injury (ABI) are typical. The rate of depression following a TBI or ABI is reported to be 18.5% to 61%.[22] Anxiety disorders were found to be present in 41.2% of the population.[22] Other mental health issues, such as PTSD, aggressive behavior, psychosis, affective lability, apathy, mania, and obsessive-compulsive disorder, may occur, but were cited at lower rates.[22]

Following a TBI or ABI, the client may experience minimal or significant changes in their physical and cognitive abilities and ability to manage their emotions. The ability to communicate, socially engage, and participate in routine occupations effectively may prove to be frustrating and overwhelming. Outbursts of anger and tearfulness are not uncommon in the early stage of recovery and may cause feelings of embarrassment and guilt. Relationships may change, roles may shift, and new routines may need to be developed. The client may feel out of control, uncertain, and fearful. The world they once knew may now be unfamiliar.

The effective client-centered therapist will acknowledge the unique presentation and needs of each client. Establishment of rapport and building a sense of trust is of extreme importance to promote participation and progress the client toward goal achievement.

Occupational Therapy Implications

When planning treatment interventions, the occupational therapy practitioner will need to determine the client's level of functioning based on the Ranchos Los Amigos Scale.[23] Methods and strategies used will vary according to the client's cognitive and physical abilities.

Engagement in varied occupations may promote skill development and a sense of self-efficacy and well-being. Activities may be used to empower, redirect, and promote successful engagement. Coping strategies may be used to improve the client's quality of life and increase appropriate social interactions. The therapist may choose to use discussion, role playing, and modeling as preparatory methods for planned real-life engagements and build the client's self-esteem. Encouragement, empathy, and understanding are needed as the client engages in the journey toward physical and mental wellness.

SUMMARY

When addressing the psychosocial needs of the client with a physical illness or injury, the occupational therapy practitioner should take a client-centered, collaborative, holistic approach. Varied frames of reference and models of practice may be considered as the therapist plans therapeutic interventions. Existing performance skills, performance patterns, and context in which the client engages in chosen occupations are considered during the evaluation, implementation, and outcomes process. The insightful therapist is mindful that limitations in the ability to engage in an occupation of choice will negatively affect the client's mental health and well-being, and that the client's mental health and well-being will affect the client's engagement in occupations. As a result, the occupational therapy practitioner will choose therapeutic interventions that provide the appropriate challenge and opportunity for success, self-expression, and skill development. Engagement in an occupation-based activity, therapeutic activity, or preparatory method need not be exclusive of one another but may be used in conjunction with each other for goal achievement. The results of effective, client-centered therapeutic interventions are clients who are, once again, able to engage in their daily lives to the fullest.

CASE STUDY 15.1   Jim

Client Profile and Occupational Performance Analysis

Jim is a 60-year-old man who lives in a single-story home with his wife. He has two grown children and grandchildren and works full time as a sales manager for a pharmaceutical company. Jim reports that he takes care of the lawn, assists with some housekeeping chores, and prepares most of the meals because he likes to cook. He enjoys fishing, playing golf, and playing poker with his friends. He reports that he engages in leisure activities as much as time allows.

Jim recently experienced an above-knee amputation as a result of complications from diabetes mellitus. He received inpatient rehabilitation and was just discharged to home. His physician ordered occupational therapy to ensure safety and independence in the home environment. During the evaluation process, the occupational therapist learns that Jim was independent with all aspects of BADLs and IADLs prior to admission to the hospital. Currently, he is modified independent with BADLs. Jim reports that his wife is taking care of the home management and household tasks at this time. He stated that he was too tired to worry about taking care of things at home and was having difficulty sleeping. He reports that he has not invited his friends over for a game of poker since the surgery because he is too tired, and he really doesn't want to see anyone. Jim shared that he and his wife frequently argue about his lack of activity and anger outbursts. He voiced concerns that his wife might not want to "hang around to see how life pans out with a grumpy man with one leg." He is certain that he will have to make major life changes and doubts that he will be able to return to work, leisure, or social activities.

CASE STUDY 15.1 Jim—cont'd

Collaboration and Interventions

After completing the evaluation process, the occupational therapist discussed with Jim the areas of occupation, roles, routines, skills, contexts, and environments that were affected by the recent physical and psychosocial changes he was experiencing. During the conversation, she highlighted the fact that the way one feels about themselves, and a situation, have a significant effect on the individual's engagement and success. She encouraged Jim to list and reflect on his positive attributes, abilities, relationships, and opportunities in his life.

With the therapist's guidance, Jim identified and prioritized occupations that were most meaningful to him. Goals were set collaboratively, and treatments were planned. Jim and the therapist determined that meal preparation would be on the top of the list of occupations in which to engage. Jim's occupational therapist understood that approaching treatment from a client-centered perspective is key in client engagement and successful therapy outcomes. She is also aware that having Jim engage in meal preparation (using occupation as a means and end) would address issues related to self-efficacy, self-esteem, and productivity, as well as the development of performance skills for physical engagement. Engaging Jim in his role of chef would likely change his perceptions of his ability to contribute to the family and would provide a sense of accomplishment. The opportunity to become immersed in the activity and the natural rhythm of the task may be calming and redirecting for Jim as well.

Sleep hygiene was addressed, and recommendations were made at the time of evaluation as the therapist has insights into the effects of sleep on health and wellness. The therapist also assisted Jim in identifying the triggers that facilitate anger outbursts. Appropriate responses to anger were discussed, as well as anger management strategies. Timely interventions in this area of concern were relevant to Jim's mental wellness and relationships with family members.

With the therapist's encouragement, Jim has agreed to make phone contact with a few of his friends in the next week. Jim's therapist acknowledges that this method may be a safe way for Jim to reinitiate the relationships that have been avoided.

The therapist and Jim have discussed future sessions, which will include putting golf balls in the backyard and exploration of wheelchair-accessible sites for fishing. Because Jim's therapist engages in evidence-based practice, she is aware of the strong correlation to wellness and life balance as it is related to leisure engagement. The occupational therapist anticipates that Jim's relationships will become healthier and more balanced as he is able to resume his life roles and engagement in occupations of choice. With that in mind, occupation-based interventions are a focus of his treatment sessions.

Jim is considering using journaling as a means of expressing his thoughts and feelings, as recommended by his therapist. He and the occupational therapist agree that this strategy may be an effective means of coping with thoughts and feelings that are negatively affecting his overall sense of well-being. Plans to educate Jim in the benefits of stress management techniques, positive self-talk, and affirmations are included in the treatment plan. These strategies will be used during future treatment sessions, and Jim will be encouraged to use them as needed within the context of each unique occupation.

Jim and his occupational therapist are planning a community re-entry activity prior to discharge. At this point in his recovery, Jim is beginning to believe that he may be able to take the risk and go out into the community once again. With each success and each goal met, Jim senses that life is becoming more balanced, and attaining wellness is on the horizon.

CASE STUDY 15.2 Julie

Client Profile and Occupational Performance Analysis

Julie, a 23-year-old dance instructor, is receiving outpatient occupational therapy due to a laceration injury to her dominant hand. Julie lives alone in a small condo near her work. She has a busy work and social life and is known for being gregarious and outgoing. She recently began dating a man she met through mutual friends and is hopeful that the relationship will continue to develop. Prior to the injury, Julie was independent with all aspects of BADLs and IADLs. She engaged in a variety of outdoor leisure activities, including hiking, kayaking, and swimming.

On evaluation, Julie's presented with decreased active range of motion, strength, and fine motor skills in her right dominant hand. Moderate edema and hypertrophic scarring were noted, as well as mild atrophy of the thenar

Continued

CASE STUDY 15.2   **Julie—cont'd**

and hypothenar eminences. During the evaluation process, Julie was noted to be guarded and uncomfortable with other clients who were sharing the clinic area. Julie reported that she is able to complete basic daily life tasks on her own, with minimal to moderate difficulty using her nondominant hand. She reported that she has the most difficulty with cutting foods, putting on jewelry, and putting on her bra. She reported that she has had few social interactions since the accident, preferring to stay at home. She stated that she had been working her regular schedule at the dance studio until recently, when the surgeon insisted that she stop wearing the previously provided splint. Since then, she reports she has "had to call out a few times."

Collaboration and Interventions

During the evaluation process, the occupational therapist provided opportunities for Julie to share her concerns and personal goals. Using therapeutic use of self, the occupational therapist established rapport and began the process of trust building. Julie was encouraged to identify occupations that were most relevant to her, roles that were most significantly affected, and skills with which she was most concerned. Approaching the client's care using a holistic approach, the occupational therapist chose to administer the Canadian Occupational Performance Measure (COPM) to assist with identifying the client's perception of her occupational performance and the Wheel of Life satisfaction tool to determine her sense of well-being. As the session unfolded, Julie revealed that although she felt inept with some of her daily tasks and was fearful of further injury, the disfigurement of her hand was more of a concern. She acknowledged that she had deliberately withdrawn from social interactions and work activities due to her perceived disfigurement. Julie went on to explain that her hands were an important tool in dance and, in its current condition, her right hand was "too horrendous to show in public." She admits that she has had limited interactions with her new boyfriend due to her embarrassment and stated that she is unsure as to how long she can keep him at arm's length.

Julie's occupational therapist acknowledged the importance of addressing Julie's physical and psychosocial needs. As she and Julie collaborated on a treatment plan and goals, the therapist explained to Julie the effects that her injury, physical limitations, and physical presentations are having on her engagement in her life roles, work, relationships, daily life activities, and mental health and wellness. The therapist suggested to Julie that addressing issues related to her physical and mental wellness are of equal importance and should be considered during therapy sessions.

During the initial therapy session, the therapist addressed using modalities to decrease edema and scar management techniques to reduce scarring. The client was provided with an edema glove and educated on its application and wear schedule. Scar management techniques were taught, and Julie was able to demonstrate the techniques independently. Adaptive strategies were demonstrated and discussed for engagement in chosen occupations. The occupational therapist is aware that although the techniques and strategies used will directly affect Julie's physical impairments and presentations, they will also serve as tools of empowerment because Julie will be able to be involved in her own care and outcomes. Self-efficacy and an increased sense of self-worth are anticipated to improve as Julie assumes more control over her current situation and as engagement and healing occur.

As the sessions continued, the occupational therapist encouraged Julie to practice dance moves in front of a mirror at home to increase visual exposure to her injured hand and engage in positive self-talk during the exercise. The therapist suggested that Julie consider using visualization techniques and instructed her in the process. Julie envisioned herself participating in varied social encounters and personal and work relationships with confidence, poise, and success. The therapist anticipates that Julie will increase her self-confidence, coping skills, and self-esteem as she applies the techniques and experiences successes.

Future therapy sessions will include a combination of occupation-based interventions, therapeutic activities, exercises, and modalities to increase the functional use of Julie's hand. The therapist acknowledges the effect that "doing" has on an individual's emotional health and wellness. As she addresses issues of scar management, strengthening, and range of motion, the therapist will be mindful of the effects these interventions will have not only on Julie's function, but on her perception of herself as well. She understands, as a therapist who engages in evidence- based practice, that as the physical presentation of Julie's hand changes, the joy of doing, expressing, creating, and loving will emerge once again.[4] Elements of built-in success will be incorporated into the sessions; appropriate challenging measures will be provided to ensure that Julie continues to develop confidence and skills. Julie's occupational therapist will continue to assess her

CASE STUDY 15.2 Julie—cont'd

physical and psychosocial needs and will respond accordingly. Stress management and relaxation techniques will be explored as tools for coping during times of increased stress. The therapist anticipates that Julie will be able to use the provided coping strategies effectively as she moves through the process of healing, both physically and mentally.

Approaching Julie's care through the holistic lens of occupational therapy will ensure the best possible outcomes and will be key in helping her return to the life she loves.

SUGGESTED LEARNING ACTIVITIES

1. Attend a support group in your community for individuals with physical illness or disease. Consider the stated and implied effects that the illness or disease is having on the participant's life balance and well-being.
2. Search the web for blog sites written by individuals with a particular physical health issue. Identify trends or themes that were noted regarding the effects of the disease on the individual's perception of quality of life, locus of control, and emotional well-being. Reflect on the effect of those perceptions on one's overall mental and physical health (e.g., https://www.msconnection.org/Blog).
3. Ask a friend, family member, or acquaintance with a physical impairment to complete a life satisfaction survey. Review the results and consider how the physical impairment is affecting the individual's level of stress, ability to cope, satisfaction with life roles, relationships, spirituality, and perception of life balance. Think about methods that an occupational therapist may use to address impoverishment or imbalance in these areas (e.g., https://qli.org.uic.edu/index.htm, or http://minerva.stkate.edu/LBI.nsf).

REFLECTION QUESTIONS

1. When addressing mental health and wellness with the client with physical impairments, what methods can the occupational therapy practitioner incorporate into treatment sessions to address both the physical and mental health needs of the client? Is it necessary to view and address the two areas of need independently of one another? Why or why not?
2. Clients may be reluctant to acknowledge or address mental health needs that may have arisen as a result of a physical illness or injury. If this is the case, how should the therapist address this issue? What concerns may arise? What should the therapist anticipate?
3. Illness or injury may disrupt one's life balance. Considering this, how may the occupational therapy practitioner facilitate life balance? Is it possible for the therapist to approach life balance from a preventative perspective? If so, what methods could the therapist use? What outcomes are likely to occur?

REFERENCES

1. Barry M, Jenkins R. *Implementing Mental Health Promotion.* Edinburgh, Scotland: Churchill Livingstone/Elsevier; 2007.
2. World Health Organization. Mental Health: A state of well-being. 2014. Available at: http://www.who.int/features/factfiles/mental_health/en.
3. Bandura A. *Self-Efficacy: The Exercise of Control.* New York: Freeman; 1997.
4. American Occupational Therapy Association. Occupational Therapy Practice Framework: Domain and Process. 3rd ed. 2014. Available at: https://ajot.aota.org/article.aspx? articleid=1860439.
5. Belon HP, Vigoda DF. Emotional adaptation to limb loss. *Phys Med Rehabil Clin N Am.* 2014;25(1):53-74.
6. Levy N, Gillibrand W, Kola-Palmer S. Minor amputation and quality of life: is it time to give the patient a voice? *Diabet Foot J.* 2017;20(4):228-234.
7. Gardner PJ, Knittel-Keren D, Gomez M. The Posttraumatic Stress Disorder Checklist as a screening measure for posttraumatic stress disorder in rehabilitation after burn injuries. *Arch Phys Med Rehabil.* 2012;93(4):623-628.
8. Boer H, Elving W, Seydel E. Psychosocial factors and mental health in cancer patients: opportunities for health promotion. *Psychol Health Med.* 2007;3:71-79.

9. Ratcliff CG, Barrera TL, Petersen NJ, Sansgiry S, Kauth MR, Kunik ME, et al. Recognition of anxiety, depression, and PTSD in patients with COPD and CHF: who gets missed? *Gen Hosp Psychiatry*. 2017;47:61-67.

10. Sutter M, Olabarrieta Landa L, Calderón Chagualá A, Chacón Peralta H, Vergara Torres G, Perrin PB, et al. Comparing the course of mental health over the first year after stroke with healthy controls in Colombia, South America. *PM R*. 2017;9:8-14.

11. Center for Managing Chronic Disease. About chronic disease. 2018. Available at: http://cmcd.sph.umich.edu/about/about-chronic-disease.

12. Chapman DP, Perry GS, Strine TW. The vital link between chronic disease and depressive disorders. *Prev Chronic Dis*. 2005;2(1):A14.

13. Di Benedetto M, Lindner H, Aucote H, Churcher J, McKenzie S, Croning N, et al. Co-morbid depression and chronic illness related to coping and physical and mental health status. *Psychol Health Med*. 2014;19(3):253-262.

14. National Institutes of Health, Medline Plus. Safely managing chronic pain. 2011. Available at: https://medlineplus.gov/magazine/issues/spring11/articles/spring11pg4.html.

15. Hooten M. Chronic pain and mental health disorder: shared neural mechanisms, epidemiology and treatment. *Mayo Clin Proc*. 2016;91(7):955-970.

16. Ansara A. Psychosocial aspects of pain management: a mind-body-hand treatment approach. *American Occupational Therapy Association*, 2013;36(4).

17. Kern RZ, Brown AD. Disease adaptation may have decreased quality-of-life responsiveness in patients with chronic progressive neurological disorders. *J Clin Epidemiol*. 2004;57(10):1033-1039.

18. Kratz A, Ehde D, Hanley M, Jensen M, Osborne T, Kraft G. Cross-sectional examination of the associations between symptoms, community integration, and mental health in multiple sclerosis. *Arch Phys Med Rehabil*. 2016;97:386-394.

19. Lohman H, Royeen C. Posttraumatic stress disorder and traumatic hand injuries: a neuro-occupational view. *Am J Occupational Therapy*. 2002;56(5):527-537.

20. Ayers DC, Franklin PD, Ring DC. The role of emotional health in functional outcomes after orthopaedic surgery: extending the biopsychosocial model to orthopaedics. *J Bone Joint Surg Am*. 2013;95(21):e165.

21. Arango-Lasprilla J, Nicholls E, Olivera S, Perdomo J, Arango J. Health-related quality of life in individuals with spinal cord injury in Colombia, South America. *Neurorehabilitation*. 2010;27(4):313-319.

22. Schwarzbold M, Diaz A, Martins ET, et al. Psychiatric disorders and traumatic brain injury. *Neuropsychiatr Dis Treat*. 2008;4(4):797-816.

23. Rancho Los Amigos National Rehabilitation Center. (1 March 2011). The Rancho Levels of Cognitive Functioning. Retrieved from https://web.archive.org/web/20110514024558/http://rancho.org/Research_RanchoLevels.aspx

Pediatric Mental Health

Monica Keen

INTRODUCTION

Occupational therapy practitioners provide services to children ranging in age from birth through adolescence. Addressing the mental health needs of the child as part of the overall treatment approach is essential. In the United States, 14% to 15% of children between the ages of 2 to 8 years have a mental, behavioral, or developmental disorder as reported by the child's parent in a national survey.[1] For children 13 to 18 years old, 20%, or over 17 million young people, have or will have a serious mental illness.[2,3] Mental health disorders are the most common health issues for school-age children in the United States.[2] Worldwide, 10% to 20% of children and adolescents are diagnosed with a mental disorder, and neuropsychiatric conditions are the leading cause of disability in this age group across all geographic areas.[4] Half of all lifetime cases of mental illness start by the age of 14 years.[3,4] Health care professionals working with children should be prepared to address the mental health needs of these children. Occupational therapy practitioners are trained to recognize and address mental health concerns through the occupational profile and provision of occupation-based treatment. Additional training may be needed for advanced or specialized clinical skills.

Addressing the mental health needs of an infant is a more recent concept that may not be well understood by the health care team. When the words "mental illness" are spoken, images of a baby or even young children do not come to mind. However, at these young ages, mental illness can develop. Even when in the womb, stress and depression can influence a newborn's ability to tolerate and respond to external stimulation.[5] Environmental, biological, developmental, and social factors affect a child's mental health, whether individually or as a whole.

The environment in which a child is raised, as well as the interactions that they have during the course of growing up, can influence their mental health. Exposing a child to a stable and protective environment where they are nurtured and are in healthy consistent relationships lays the groundwork for good mental health.[5] Babies born prematurely or medically fragile also need to feel protected and secure. Additionally, it is paramount that children have consistent relationships with caretakers. This is important for healthy mental health development throughout childhood, from birth through the teenage years.

As a child transitions into school, the need for a stable and protective environment remains. By the year 2020, it is anticipated that mental health–related problems will increase by over 50%, with 80% of these disorders emerging during childhood or adolescence.[6] These statistics are staggering. School is the environment where a child spends most of their waking hours for more than 12 years of their life. Consequently, this environment needs to be well equipped to address the mental health needs of the students. Sadly, that is not always the case. In one survey of school workers in Canada, 80% of the respondents stated that there are mental health needs in schools that go unaddressed.[6] The rise in school shootings is an example of students dealing with mental health issues that have not been identified, resolved, or met by the school or any other mental health facility.

Occupational therapy can and does play a role in the mental health of children. Being a holistic practice, occupational therapy is concerned with the entire individual, which includes mind, body, and spirit. Occupational therapy practitioners are an invaluable resource for supporting healthy mental development in the neonatal intensive care unit, home, clinic, and school setting. This chapter focuses on two areas of pediatric mental health, infant mental health as an emerging area of practice and school-based mental health, because many occupational therapy practitioners are employed in school systems and have the opportunity to address behavioral concerns as part of the intervention process.

INFANT MENTAL HEALTH

This section examines typical and atypical infant mental health and the many factors that influence infant mental health. A discussion of the importance of family and its role in developing both positive and negative mental health of an infant is provided. The aspects of the typical developing infant versus the infant with special needs will be explored, and the influence on the mental health of the infant, parents, and extended family will be discussed. The role of occupational therapy in delivering infant, family, and therapist-oriented services will be addressed.[7]

Infant mental health is defined as "the developing capacity of the child from birth to three to: experience, regulate, and express emotions; form close interpersonal relationships; and explore environment and learn—-all in the context of family, community, and cultural expectations for young children."[5] From the moment a baby is born, their mental health is being shaped as a result of the numerous experiences and relationships introduced to them in a myriad of contexts on a daily basis. Evidence supporting the influence of early experiences and relationships on the development of an infant's mental health has resulted in more research to increase knowledge on how to support these early experiences and relationships positively.[5]

Factors

There are numerous factors that can influence infant mental health. This section examines the biological, developmental, environmental, and social factors that can make an impact in the development and growth, both positive and negative, on an infant's mental health.

Biological Influences

Physical health, physical attributes, personality, and genetic influences can play a role in affecting the mental health of infants from birth to 3 years.[5] It is important to note that the brain develops the most during the third trimester of pregnancy through the second year of life. However, development is dissected into structural and functional modules. In utero, structural development is completed over the gestation period, but functional development occurs after birth and is a cropping of sorts of the neuronal synapses that occurs secondary to prenatal and postnatal experiences. The physical health of the infant plays a role in determining what type of care they need, as well as how the infant's caregivers are going to respond to that need. In turn, the response(s) of the caregivers play a part in the process of the baby's mental evolution and development. This closely compares with the child's temperament. However, physical attributes, as well as the personality of the baby, can control the caregiver's desire to engage in or walk away from interactions and overall support of the child. Consider the children who do not like to be held or coddled as opposed to the one who loves human contact. These characteristics of the child can affect, positively and/or negatively, the parental interaction with the developing baby. Another example could include how physical disfigurement and medical fragility can cause a parent to shy away from interacting with the child. These experiences, positive and negative, play a significant role in the mental health of the infant.

Developmental Influences

The first 3 years of life is the time when the most rapid development occurs in the life span of a human.[5,8] Developmental challenges can affect an infant's mental health. Even at a sensory level, newborns are adept in identifying the ones who are caring for them. In the first few months of the child's existence, they are learning ways to make their wants and needs known. It is how these wants and needs are being met, if at all, that play a role in molding the child's mental well-being. Studies have found that babies who are exposed to violence, trauma, or numerous medical procedures may experience developmental delays and developmental challenges. They have an increased risk of having "abnormal patterns in the expression of emotion; unusual or deviant behaviors including increased motor activity; distractibility and inattention; disruptions in feeding and sleeping patterns; and/or development delays in motor and language skills."[5]

Environmental Influences

Environmental influences such as family, culture, and ethnicity play a significant role in the development of a baby's mental health. As varied as families, cultures, and ethnicities are, so are parenting beliefs and behaviors. One child may be raised in a home where there is a mom and dad while another grows up in a single-parent home. Another child may have parents who have high expectations for their children to succeed, yet other parents cannot provide the opportunities or resources to reach such goals. Still others may be raised in a biracial home where there is a difference in ethnicity as well as culture. Consider the child raised in foster care or even in an orphanage and how their experience differs exponentially from the child raised in a home with biological or adoptive parents. However, there are some ideals that have no boundaries, including keeping a child healthy, ensuring their safety, and the hope that the child will be a self-sufficient and good citizen in society.[5]

Social Influences

The infant–caregiver relationship is one that makes a deep impression on the life of a child. Events occurring in this relationship play a significant role in influencing emotions.[5] This relationship is a conduit from which the child starts to develop self-concepts, such as competence and self-worth, as well as how to interact with other people.[5] Factors such as environmental and intrinsic risks also shape the infant–caregiver relationship. What is key is not necessarily what the child experiences, but how the child experiences the environment. For example, a child can be raised in poverty, but if the child experiences support and love, the experience of the environment does not have such a negative impact. However, if the infant is in an environment where there is domestic abuse or mental illness, the impact can be problematic. The temperament of a challenging infant is another way in which the best parents can be disheartened; however, if the child experiences a relationship with the parent that is consistently stable and responsive, it is possible that the temperament of the child can be molded. Finally, the infant–caregiver relationships that are secure during the first year of life are the ones that typically yield confident relationships for the child in the future. In contrast, the infant–caregiver relationships that may involve issues such as maternal depression, domestic violence, drug abuse, or unresolved grief can shape a child who will be anxious and insecure in future relationships.

As stated above, it is more important how a child experiences the environment than what the child experiences. The same concept goes for relationships. It is not the individual who makes the relationship; rather, it is the quality of the relationship that results in the most secure attachment. For the child, this relationship requires more than being fed, clothed, diapered, and housed. This relationship also requires the feelings and emotional expectations that are afforded by this attachment. However, the child is able to make more than one attachment to a caregiver.

The relationship that is the most nurturing, responsive, and consistent is the one that the child experiences as the most secure. This is referred to as "relationship-specific."[5] Overall, the most important aspect of infant mental health is derived from the parent–infant relationship; however, it is vital that the relationships with other caregivers and service providers are positive as well.

Disorders in Infant Mental Health

The parent–infant relationship is a powerful existence. It has the capability of shaping the emotional well-being or lack thereof in a child.[8] The first year of life is a vital one, and even during this early period, abnormal behaviors, emotional responses, and even emotional problems can form. This is sometimes the result when the parent–infant relationship is compromised secondary to the state of the relationship being changed or if the relationship is strained.

There are numerous reasons that a child displays patterns of behaviors or demonstrates poor social-emotional functioning. Some behaviors are seen as atypical or even maladaptive in children ranging in age from birth to 3 years. Children having difficulty in these areas are considered as being at risk.[5] When assessing these children, it is paramount that their life experiences be taken into account. Abuse, neglect, mental illness of the significant caregiver, institutionalization, and significant trauma can all play a role in altering the child's ability to possess appropriate social and emotional skills. Consequently, when assessing these children, due diligence must be afforded to the individual experiences of the infant and caregiver. In doing so, it can bring clarity to understanding the child's behavior.

The goal of any treatment session is to improve the relationship between the caregiver and child, both from an individual as well as from a dual perspective.[5] In the case of the infant, one has to be trained in specialized practices to complete a comprehensive assessment. There is continual research being conducted to deepen the understanding of how the developmental processes influence how mental disorders are manifested, how they are diagnosed and classified, and what interventions are effective. To summarize, principles of infant mental health include the following[5]:

- Infant mental health is synonymous with healthy social and emotional development.
- Consistent relationships that are nurturing, protective, stable, and consistent are fundamental building blocks for infant mental health.
- Behavioral markers of infant mental health include emotion regulation, the ability to communicate feelings to the caregivers, and active exploration of the environment.
- Any factors that affect the relationship between the infant and caregiver have the potential to affect the infant's mental health.

- Programs that address infant mental health must focus on relationships, be based on current developmental knowledge, and be supportive of the family.
- Families need to be involved in the planning and delivery of infant mental health services.
- Values, including personal, family, ethnic, cultural, professional, and organizational, affect every aspect of infant mental health.

Positive and Negative Impact of Maternal Relationship

The bond between a mother and child is very unique, and the relationship that is formed through interactions between the two are significant.[9] This is the first relationship that the infant forms when in utero, and the choices that are made by the mother will significantly affect her developing baby. A child's emotional well-being can be shaped from the child's genetic, biological, and/or psychosocial factors, and if the relationship between the parent and child is not properly fashioned, the outcomes can be detrimental.[9]

There are numerous factors that can affect the relationship between the mother and child. "During the transition to motherhood, a woman experiences a shift in psychological and bodily processes that may have consequences for roles, mood states, and social interactions."[7] Some examples would be "acute or chronic illness of the child, parental psychopathology, mother's preoccupation with her worries because of life adversities, or poor parenting."[9] During the first 3 years of the child's life, the events that occur are crucial to emotional well-being. Developmental changes are occurring rapidly during this time, and the foundation for emotional stability, even at this early age, is being fashioned.[9] By the end of a child's first year of life, the child is able to gauge events and is even capable of "evaluating...the emotional responses of others."[9] Both the infant and mother have responsibilities in the dyadic relationship, and each influences the behavior of the other.[10] For example, the mother should be responsive to the child's needs, both emotional and physical. Engaging the child in joint attention, having moments of sharing smiles and laughter, and the mutual reciprocity of interaction is vital to a healthy connection between the mother and child. Unfortunately, there are psychiatric components that may affect the parent–child relationship. Mothers who are dealing with postpartum depression, living in environments that are of low socioeconomic status, or those living in volatile conditions run a significant risk of having the inability to interact appropriately with their infant.

More research is needed regarding the mother–child relationship. Specifically, research on early mother–infant interactions in the community, as well as any associations with maternal psychopathology, is needed.[9] Depression and anxiety are the most common subclinical forms of psychopathology that prevail in the community, with differences being shown in mother–child relationships in the low socioeconomic class versus upper- and middle-class mothers.[9] More research will provide a better understanding regarding the mother–child relationship. This will help in designing interventions used to train mothers dealing with these issues to be better equipped to interact with their babies.

Impacts of Typical Versus Nontypical Infant Development

Throughout this section, two concepts have been emphasized. One regards the importance of the relationship between the caregiver and infant and how it shapes the baby's emotional well-being. The other concept emphasizes how the environment plays a substantial role in shaping the emotional well-being of the child. It would stand to reason that an uncomplicated birth that results in a typical healthy child would provide the foundation for a solid start to life and emotional stability. Continue to consider that this child will be brought home to a house that has electricity and running water. In this home, the child will be provided with a place to sleep and will have a mother who is there to feed, clothe, and diaper the child, as well as a father who will do the same. This child is held, swaddled, communicated and sung to, and is comforted whenever they cry. The child will be loved. Now, consider the infant boy who is born prematurely via emergency cesarean section and suffers a brain bleed shortly after birth. He cannot breathe on his own and undergoes numerous attempts to be intubated. Consider that he is stuck with needles to start IVs, one of which is in his head. Furthermore, he is in an incubator and is hooked up to numerous machines that are beeping constantly. Additionally, he has a nasogastric (NG) tube placed. He has not been held by anyone; instead, when touched for diapering or positioning, it is painful. Who do you think has the more positive start in life? Who has a more secure environment? Which baby do you think will have the best relationship with the caregiver?

The experiences that a baby goes through affect the child's behavior in future relationships.[10] There are four theories regarding the mother–child relationship and how it is formed. They are described in Box 16.1.

So, what does all of this mean? The data truly reflects on the importance of the infant–caregiver relationship and how these relationships can become disordered due to external factors, environmental factors, and factors regarding infants with special medical needs. Consequently, there needs to be an intervention for the baby, caregiver, and family unit that will develop secure relationships among all

BOX 17.1 Theories of Mother-Child Relationship

Bowlby J (1958, 1969, 1973, 1980)—according to Bowlby, the affectionate bond between the mother and child "is biologically rooted in a behavioral system that promotes the survival of the species through protecting its infants from harm."[11-14]

Ainsworth MDS (1979)—Ainsworth had a theory that the infant–caregiver relationship develops through a process of interactive negotiations that revolve around a series of issues, with the earliest ones being sleep, wakefulness, and feeding. These later develop into more complex issues, such as intentions, feeling, and expressions.[15] Sander's theory supports the idea that the behavior of both the baby and mother dually affect the interaction between the two.

Sander IW (1964)—Sander has noted that it is the nature of the highly individualized and patterned caregiver interactions rather than the frequency of the specific behaviors that determines the quality of the attachment relationship.[16]

Sroufe AL & Fleeson J (1986)[17]—Sroufe and Fleeson have proposed that each participant in the relationship, the mother and child, come to the relationship as individuals, bringing their own unique characteristics. They have further noted that outside this interaction, there is minimal significance.

the members of that system. This is called the "family system" and is indeed an interactive one. The Fraiberg model describes one model for intervention.[10] This proposes that in the child's first year of life, its role is to forge the emotional relationship with its caregiver, and the caregiver's role is to provide physical and emotional support, as well as protection. This is accomplished by providing home-based services to mothers and infants from the time of pregnancy until the age of 3 years. The Fraiberg model uses a multidisciplinary team approach with team members including but not limited to education, social work, nursing, and psychology. The goals of the Fraiberg model include emotional support to the caregivers, access to resources, directions on developmental expectations, psychotherapy for the caregiver and infant to address emotional walls that may be hindering healthy attachments, and advocacy to build up communication between the family and community support system.[10]

Occupational Therapy and Infant Mental Health

"The goal of …occupational therapy, like the goal of infant mental health practice, is to assist the client to achieve satisfactory function socially, emotionally, and psychologically in a natural environment."[18] Changes have been occurring in the area of infant mental health and occupational therapy. Occupational therapy must look beyond just the child as the only client and recognize that the family is a vital piece to the child's well-being, physical and mental. Dual sets of occupations must be addressed. For the infant, their occupations include eating, sleeping, exploring, growing, and starting to develop a sense of individuality. The caregivers now have the new occupation of parenting and have all the responsibilities that come with it. Occupational therapy can assist them in this new role by teaching the importance of the parent–child relationship.[19] Should the child be born with special needs, the parents may

experience additional stressors, as well as dealing with intense feelings of guilt, self-blame, anger, and sadness.[19] Occupational therapy practitioners have the skills to help parents process through these emotions and provide them with guidance on how to strengthen the parent–child bond through holding, feeding, touching, and communicating with the baby through talking and singing. Additionally, occupational therapy practitioners can teach parents how to maintain their individuality and provide insights into the importance of maintaining a balance in their daily, including intentionally taking the time to engage in preferred activities of leisure.

Occupational therapy is just one member of the team that works with infants whose lives begin in the neonatal intensive care unit (NICU).[10] In working within the model of family-centered care, occupational therapy has three areas to address: infant-oriented services, family-oriented services, and therapist-oriented services.[10] Infant-oriented services involve the activities that are going to be provided directly to the child to achieve full potential and can include client-centered tasks such as positioning, handling, feeding, splinting, and environmental modulation.[10] Family-oriented services assist the family in helping the infant achieve maximal development. Occupational therapy practitioners call on their knowledge regarding neurodevelopment, understanding the medical interventions for the fragile infant and being aware of the occupational tasks involved with parenting.[10] Therapist-oriented services require a plan to avoid burnout and imply an understanding of the parallel processes that are at work during the relationship building.[10]

Occupational therapy strives to be client-centered; the goal is to re-engage the client in the occupations that bring them satisfaction and purpose. How can that be done from a family-centered approach? How involved an occupational therapy practitioner becomes with the family may depend on other professionals, how available they are to deliver services, and the nature of the parental issues.[19] For example, it is essential to work interprofessionally and coordinate services when working with families in rural areas to provide the most comprehensive care. Additionally, the occupational therapy practitioner needs to understand when to make referrals to other medical professionals because the nature and severity of the situation is beyond the scope of the occupational therapy practitioner. Using a family–centered approach ensures that all family members are getting the appropriate intervention and are being supported.[19] The family-centered approach requires advocating for all family members, including the child. An example of advocating for the child may be on the parent's behalf because of feeling intimidated by not only what is happening to their child, but being unable to understand the process that their child is going through. We may be able to explain the plan of care to the parents and siblings. Occupational therapists may also encourage the parents to step out for some fresh air because they have been awake for over 24 hours sitting by their child's crib in the NICU.

In conclusion, this section has discussed the numerous factors that affect infant mental health. Even while in utero, events can happen that shape the emotional well-being of the infant. Once born, additional factors such as the mother–child relationship, environment, culture, and socioeconomic status can affect the child's mental health. Other considerations are the quality of the environment and the quality of the relationships among the child, parent(s), and other caregivers. Is the environment where the child is being raised free from violence and drugs? Are the caregivers providing stability, reliability, and consistency in regard to meeting the physical and emotional needs of the child? It is important to remember that it is not the quantity of the interactions, but the quality of the interactions that build relationships, that promote good mental health.

Family-centered care is the focus of occupational therapy as it relates to infant mental health. Occupational therapy practitioners focus on the family to teach them how to best care for the needs of the child, especially babies born with special needs. Occupational therapy practitioners are able to provide the individual care needed for the client (baby) and his or her needs, but are also sensitive to the parents regarding their emotional well-being in their occupation as parent and caregiver. Occupational therapy practitioners combine the two units, look at it from the family perspective, and work to provide interventions that will fortify the bond of the family while preserving the individuality of each family member. Occupational therapy's aim is "achieving health, well-being, and participation in life through engagement in occupation, no matter the age."[20]

CASE STUDY 16.1

Meg and Bryce are expecting their first child in the summer, with a due date of August 31. However, in early April, Meg goes into labor and delivers a baby girl, named Molly, weighing 1 pound, 5 ounces. Molly is not able to breathe on her own and is placed on a respirator. Additionally, she suffers a brain bleed and is demonstrating right-sided weakness.

Working within the context of family-centered care in the NICU, Meg and Bryce are introduced to a team of practitioners that will be caring for Molly in the days and weeks to come. The team leader, Dr. Smith, spends some time with the parents to discuss Molly's case, as well as explain to them about other team members who will be working with not only Molly, but also with them, the parents.

Marcy, the occupational therapist, comes by later in the afternoon to do her evaluation of Molly. As she is working with her, she takes the time to get to know Meg and Bryce. She is careful to explain what she is doing in her evaluation and educates the parents on her findings. She also takes the time to talk about the importance of building emotional and physical bonds with Molly during this time of hospitalization. Marcy describes how the kangaroo technique is done, and assures them that this will be a very important sensory part of both theirs and Molly's day. Marcy shows Meg and Bryce some positioning techniques and also discusses the importance of controlling the sounds, sights, and movements in Molly's room to create and maintain a soft sensory environment.

Marcy continues to work with Molly and her parents throughout the course of her hospital stay. During the weeks before discharge, Marcy plans with the parents to have Molly enrolled in BabyNet on discharge. (BabyNet is a developmental program that helps an infant or toddler with special needs move toward his or her full potential.) Marcy continues to educate Meg and Bryce regarding the importance of keeping up with occupational therapy, physical therapy, and speech therapy and provides the parents with the names of therapists who are contracted with the BabyNet agency. She also provides Meg and Bryce with contact information that will be needed for future resources as they continue to raise Molly.

SCHOOL-BASED MENTAL HEALTH

Mental health is defined as "a state of well-being in which an individual realizes his or her own abilities, can cope with the normal stresses of life, can work productively and is able to make a contribution to his or community."[21] The consequences for children with mental health issues, their families, and the schools that educate them are substantial.[21] "Children with emotional disturbance often struggle with interpersonal relationships, exhibit inappropriate behavior and express feelings of general pervasive unhappiness or depression."[17] Mental illness in children and youth has become a significant issue in this country and worldwide. The statistics are concerning. As many as 20% of school-age youth have a diagnosable mental illness, and up to 75% of them are not receiving treatment and/or not getting adequate intervention.[21,23] In Canada, approximately 1.2 million children have mental illness to the degree that their occupational performance is affected.[6] With early detection, evaluation, and intervention, about 70% of childhood mental illnesses can be ameliorated and, in doing so, the child has a better opportunity to engage in and contribute to society, as well as experience an improved quality of life.[6] Many mental health issues can be identified at a young age and, if treated successfully, the child can experience increased success in education, employment, and family roles.[21]

Many children do not have the resources they need or the necessary skills to address the emotional needs they experience.[24] The most common mental health issues in school-age children are depression, anxiety, substance abuse, and having a hard time in social relationships, with depression and anxiety being the most common.[6] Overall, it is estimated that 10 million children would benefit from engaging in professional mental health services from the time they enter school in kindergarten until they graduate from high school.[25] It is during this time of life that these youth are engaging in the occupation of being a student. As a student, they are spending more time in school than anywhere else during the course of their day. It would therefore be common sense that this would be an appropriate environment to have mental health services available to those who need them. Occupational therapists have emphasized that "the need for preventative and responsive school-based mental health services is growing at an alarming rate."[25] However, there are not enough resources in our schools on a worldwide basis that would help address the mental health needs of students.[6] There is a global shortage of mental health workers, and it is estimated that this will continue to increase.[25]

Research has also shown that how well a student is doing emotionally and socially directly affects their academic performance and success in the school.[23] Statistically, students who are dealing with mental health issues demonstrate deficits in their academic performance and, sadly, are less likely to graduate.[23] Moreover, these same students can also affect the learning outcomes of other students, as well as the overall school environment.[23] There are classrooms around the country that are being emptied during instruction time for the safety of students while one of their classmates is engaging in destructive and aggressive behavior because they do not know how to express their frustration and anger properly and safely. There are numerous examples of children being bullied, physically accosted, and emotionally abused while at school, with no recourse for the offender and no emotional or mental health support for the offended. Unfortunately, the mental health needs of students are forced to take a back seat because school districts are pushing to have higher academic standards met.[25]

Some schools are doing what they can to help these students in their times of need. However, most schools are using the traditional method of calling on personnel such as school psychologists, counselors, and social workers to deal with the students who are in crisis. Although these professionals do have a mental health background, they also have other responsibilities, resulting in high caseloads and leaving them with little time to address the needs of the students efficiently.[25] Their high caseloads are directly related to the shortage of highly qualified school personnel who are better equipped to work with this population.[25] "There is a need for a highly trained workforce with knowledge and skills related to evidence-based practices and programs to effectively work with children and their families."[25] In some cases, the most common service used to meet the mental health needs of the student is meeting with an educator in an individual setting who has no formal mental health training.[6]

Occupational Therapy and School-Based Mental Health

Occupational therapy's roots originated working in the field of mental health. Occupational therapy is concerned with the totality of the individual including the mind, body, and spirit. Further, engagement in occupation assists the individual in obtaining optimal health and well-being. According to the Occupational Therapy Framework Domain and Process,[20] "Practitioners [occupational therapists] use their knowledge of the transactional relationship among the person, his or her engagement in valuable occupations, and the context to design occupation-based intervention plans that facilitate change or growth in client factors and skills needed for successful participation." Occupational therapy is occupation-based, contextual, and client-centered, incorporating evidence-based practice to guide assessment and intervention of the client.[20]

School officials do not always understand the role of occupational therapy in addressing the mental health needs of students.[25] However, occupational therapists have much to offer the team and student to promote optimal engagement in the classroom. Through collaboration with other school personnel, a solid, interprofessional mental health service delivery plan is obtainable.[25] There is a growing support for the collaborative model, which incorporates mental health workers and schools to meet the needs of the child.[23] Together, this interprofessional team works collaboratively to provide intervention and support to those youth whose emotional well-being is impaired.[23]

One of the barriers that impedes occupational therapists from taking an active role in school-based mental health is the lack of understanding regarding occupational therapy's role in addressing mental health. "Defining the role of occupational therapy practitioners in school mental health and educating other team members about the value of occupational therapy [is crucial] in establishing the foothold for occupational therapy in school-based mental health services."[25] The lack of understanding regarding the role of occupational therapy in mental health could be a reason for the loss of occupational therapists in this field.[25] So, how can education regarding the value of occupational therapy in school based mental health be accomplished? Some websites offer information regarding this topic. For example, occupational therapist Susan Bazyck has created a program called "Every Moment Counts," which is "a mental health promotion initiative developed to help all children and youth become mentally healthy to succeed in school, at home and in the community."[26] On the program's website, a variety of model programs, tool kits, and building capacity materials can be found. Another resource can be found on the American Occupational Therapy Association's website. The School Mental Health Tool Kit[27] includes a variety of articles on how to promote positive mental health in the school setting.

Articles include issues such as bullying prevention, childhood trauma, anxiety disorders, and creating a positive environment in the cafeteria.[27] In educating others, occupational therapy's distinct value will be recognized by school administrators, such as principals and assistant principals, who can support occupation-based interventions for mental health to be initiated by occupational therapy practitioners. By educating the administration about the unique skill set that occupational therapy can bring to the table in the area of mental health, barriers such as budget, time, and space in the building for such programming can be eliminated.[21]

The number of children diagnosed with mental illness or dealing with mental health issues has been increasing.[28] Today, the number of youth in the United States who are dealing with unaddressed mental health issues is a critical social issue.[21] Our schools are being pushed to be academically superior at the expense of putting students who are emotionally unstable into the proverbial waiting room. Occupational therapy is concerned with the well-being of the entire human being, meaning mind, soul, and spirit. Occupational therapy's beginnings were rooted in mental health, and occupational therapy has much to offer those who are in need of mental health intervention. In the school setting, traditional personnel are currently being used to address the mental health needs of the school. However, due to high caseloads of the "traditional team" and a shortage or even lack of highly qualified personnel, these emotionally charged youth are receiving minimal, if any, assistance at all. Education about occupational therapy's role in mental health is necessary so that its full potential in the school setting can be realized. Occupational therapy has a tremendous responsibility to present evidence-based practice to make our presence and valuable contributions to this area of need known. In doing so, the profession can help bridge the gap to better mental health for all children in school settings.

CASE STUDY 16.2

Mike is a school-based occupational therapist that works for South Lexington School District. This is his fifth year as a school-based practitioner. The Title One school that he serves is located in the rural part of the county, where farming is prevalent. Many of the students who attend this school are children of sharecroppers, and they come from very humble backgrounds. Quite a few do not have running water, and electricity in the homes is sparse. Additionally, many of the sharecropping children do not have enough to eat; consequently, they receive most of their nutrition in the school setting. These families are also known to move often, with the changing of the seasons. The school houses grades K to 5, and Mike is at the school 5 days a week.

Mike sees children with many needs in his school. During his work week, Mike is able to serve all his students who have occupational therapy on their Individualized Education Program (IEP) on Monday, Tuesday, and Thursday. On Wednesday, he runs a variety of groups that promote simple life skills, such as preparing simple meals and snacks, improving hygiene, and bettering oral care.

CASE STUDY 16.2—cont'd

Another group he implements is the "How are you feeling" group. This group is designed for the students referred by the guidance counselor who are having trouble forming and maintaining relationships, who are being bullied or bullying, and/or those dealing with traumatic events that are occurring outside the school setting. This group works on social skills and addresses how to deal with and handle anger, sadness, and frustration appropriately.

He also incorporates school-wide mental health activities recommended by Every Moment Counts. Some of these programs include Creating a Comfortable Cafeteria,

Refreshing Recess, and After School Leisure Coaching. All these programs promote good mental health and the overall happiness of the students in the school. He works closely with the school's guidance counselor and has open office hours to work with students in crisis, as well as provide a safe environment for the students to talk. On Fridays, Mike coordinates and implements Backpack Buddies, which is a program that supplies nonperishable food items discreetly placed in the backpacks of students whose families will not have enough food to feed their families over the weekend.

SUGGESTED LEARNING ACTIVITIES

1. Familiarize yourself with NICU and the types of sensory stimulation present. What sensory information could be too much? What sensory information could be lacking?
2. What are some techniques that can be used to help introduce the newborn to the sensory experiences they have in the NICU?
3. Familiarize yourself with information regarding behavior and emotional red flags that can be observed in children who move often.
4. Familiarize yourself with state and federal initiatives that promote good nutrition in schools.

REFLECTION QUESTIONS

1. Why is occupational therapy's presence in the NICU valuable?
2. How will you go about educating child caregivers regarding an infant's unique needs?
3. What can you do to assist the caretaker during this time of transition? What are the most important issues to address first?
4. How could you incorporate therapeutic use of self in a situation such as this?
5. What are some group activities that occupational therapists can lead for students who move often and are having difficulty making friends and experiencing feelings of belonging?
6. What are some group activities that occupational therapists can lead for the stationary students to assist them in forming friendships with the transient student population?
7. What can be done beyond BackPack Buddies to address the lack of food in the homes of these students?
8. How can occupational therapy work with the school administration in meeting the academic needs of these students?

REFERENCES

1. Centers for Disease Control. *Children's Mental Health*. 2018. Available at: https://www.cdc.gov/childrensmentalhealth/data.html.
2. Child Mind Institute. 2016 Children's Mental Health Report. 2016. Available at: https://childmind.org/report/2016-childrens-mental-health-report/.
3. National Alliance of Mental Illness. Mental Health Facts: Children and Teens. 2018. Available at: https://www.nami.org/NAMI/media/NAMI-Media/Infographics/Children-MH-Facts-NAMI.pdf.
4. World Health Organization. Child and Adolescent Mental Health. 2018. Available at: http://www.who.int/mental_health/maternal-child/child_adolescent/en/.

5. Zeanah PD, Stafford BS, Nagle GA, Rice T. Addressing social-emotional development and infant mental health in early childhood systems. Available at: https://files.eric.ed.gov/fulltext/ED496853.pdf.

6. Chan C, Dennis D, Kim SJ, Jankowski J. An integrative review of school-based mental health interventions for elementary students: implications for occupational therapy. *Occup Ther Mental Health*. 2017;33(1):81-101.

7. Pizur-Barnekow K. Maternal health after the birth of a medically complex infant: setting the context for evaluation of co-occupational performance. *Am J Occup Ther*. 2010;64:642-649.

8. Clinton J, Feller AF, Williams RC. The importance of infant mental health. *Pediatr Child Health*. 2016;21(5):239-241.

9. Singhal M, Sinha UK. Quality of mother-infant interactions in maternal emotional disturbance: a pilot study. *J Indian Assoc Child Adolesc Mental Health*. 2012;8(4):78-104.

10. Olson JA, Baltman K. Infant mental health in occupational therapy practice in the neonatal intensive care unit. *Am J Occupational Therapy*. 1994;48(6):499-505.

11. Bowlby J. The nature of a child's tie to his mother. *Int J Psychoanal*. 1958;39:350-373.

12. Bowlby J. *Attachment and Loss*. 2nd ed. Vol 1. *Attachment*. London: Hogarth; 1982.

13. Bowlby J. *Attachment and Loss*. Vol 2. *Separation: Anxiety and Anger*. London: Hogarth; 1973.

14. Bowlby J. *Attachment and Loss*, Vol 3. *Loss: Sadness and Depression*. London: Hogarth; 1980.

15. Ainsworth MDS. Attachment as related to mother-infant interaction. In: Rosenblatt JS, Hinde RA, Beer C, Busnel M, eds. *Advances in the Study of Behavior*. New York: Academic Press; 1979:9.

16. Sander IW. Adaptive relationships in early mother-child interaction. *J Am Acad Child Psychiatry*. 1964;3:231-264.

17. Sroufe A L, Fleeson J. Attachment and the construction of relationships. In: Hartup WW, Rubin Z, eds. *Relationships and Development*. Hillsdale, NJ: Erlbaum; 1986:51-71.

18. Krohn WS, Cara E. Occupational therapy in early intervention: applying concepts from infant mental health. *Am J Occup Ther*. 2000;54(5), 550-554.

19. Anderson J, Hinojosa J. Parents and therapists in a professional partnership. *Am J Occup Ther*. 1984;3(7):452-461.

20. American Occupational Therapy Association (AOTA). Occupational Therapy Practice Framework: Domain And Process. 3rd ed. *Am J Occup Ther*. 2014;68:S1-S48.

21. Blackman KF, Powers JD, Edwards JD, Wegmann KM, Lechner E, Swick DC. Closing the gap: principal perspective on an innovative school-based mental health intervention. *Urban Rev*. 2016;48:245-263.

22. Smith CJ, Archer L. School-based services for students with emotional disturbance: findings and recommendations. *OT Pract*. 2008;1:17-21.

23. Capp G. Our community, our schools: A case study of program design for school-based mental health services. *Child Sch*. 2015;37(4) 241-248.

24. Maas C, Mason R, Candler C. When I get mad. *OT Practice*. 2008;19:9-14.

25. Cahill SM, Egan BE. Perceptions of occupational therapy involvement in school mental health: a pilot study. Available at: https://scholarworks.wmich.edu/ojot/vol5/iss1/5.

26. Every Moment Counts. Welcome to Every Moment Counts! Available at: http://www.everymomentcounts.org/.

27. American Occupational Therapy Association (AOTA). School Mental Health Tool Kit. 2018. Available at: https://www.aota.org/Practice/Children-Youth/Mental%20Health/School-Mental-Health.aspx.

28. Twenge JM. Time period and birth cohort differences in depressive symptoms in the U.S., 1982-2013. *Soc Indic Res*. 2015;121:437-454.

17

Trauma-Informed Care

Tina Champagne

LEARNING OBJECTIVES

1. Define trauma-informed care.
2. Examine the impact of trauma on the developmental process.
3. Contrast a trauma-informed versus a non–trauma-informed approach.
4. Identify at least three to five ways that occupational therapy practitioners engage in trauma-informed care.
5. Recognize the importance of trauma-informed care across all areas of occupational therapy practice.

INTRODUCTION

In 2003, the trauma-informed care (TIC) initiative was launched across the United States in response to the President's New Freedom Commission,[1] which included TIC as part of its federal mandates to all mental health organizations. TIC is a model of care requiring that everyone working with persons with mental illness recognize the high prevalence of trauma in this population and understand the pervasive neurophysiological, social, and emotional impact of trauma.[2-4] TIC also requires that the care provided to people with mental illness is collaborative, individualized, and addresses each individual's trauma-related needs and goals. Similar to how the definition of the term *trauma* has evolved radically over the past 2 decades, TIC has also evolved as a construct and in the therapeutic guidelines promoted for practical application. This chapter provides an overview of trauma, TIC, trauma-informed approaches, and a review of some of the ways occupational therapy practitioners support the TIC initiative and often take a leadership role in its implementation.

TRAUMA

To become trauma-informed, it is necessary to understand what trauma is and how it affects the ability to participate safely and functionally in meaningful life roles, routines, and occupations. It is widely documented in the scientific literature that abuse and violence often lead to the development of trauma-related and other mental health and medical symptoms and diagnoses.[5-7]

Trauma is an experience, not an event. Trauma is anything that you experience that overwhelms your ability to cope, integrate your experience, and continue to function in your daily life roles, routines, and occupations. Some examples of experiences or events that can be traumatic in nature include but are not limited to the following:

- Abuse (physical, sexual, emotional, verbal): assault, witnessing, or neglect
- Poverty
- Homelessness and frequent moves
- Displacement (refugee status, relocation)
- War and combat exposure
- Sexual slavery, human trafficking, exploitation
- Exposure to death, dying, or grotesque situations or work experiences
- Being disenfranchised due to ethnicity, religion, other types of minority status
- Incarceration
- Human rights violations
- Witnessing or experiencing acts of terrorism

The Substance Abuse Mental Health Services Administration[8] published an update to its working definition of trauma as being an experience that stems from an event, series of events, or set of circumstances perceived as being physically or emotionally harmful or life-threatening and that has lasting adverse effects on the person's functioning and emotional, social, mental, physical, and/or spiritual well-being. Furthermore, there are different types of trauma—acute, chronic, complex, and neglect. Acute trauma is a single event that is relatively brief or time-limited. Chronic trauma typically involves multiple events that occur over a relatively long period of time. Complex trauma occurs when there are multiple cumulative traumatic experiences starting early in life, with much of the trauma inflicted by one's primary caregiver(s).[9]

The way trauma affects individuals is very subjective and complex, which is part of the reason why it is difficult to define concretely. Two people may encounter the exact same event and yet each may go on to have similar or even very different perceptions of the experience and outcomes. This difference in effect occurs because trauma is the outcome of one's perception of what happened, and not solely due to the event(s) or experience(s) encountered or witnessed. Not all trauma experiences are remembered—for example, when trauma occurs in utero or infancy.

Although one's natural responses to perceived threat or danger are protective and adaptive responses of self-preservation, which are critical to survival, once the threat or danger is no longer present, the triggering of these neurophysiologic and psychological processes typically subsides. For those with trauma histories, these protective responses often misfire or continue in intensity for long periods of time. This is because the nervous system becomes shaped in a manner that perceives danger and more extreme fear in the face of stressors, or at times misperceives stress, benign situations (e.g., minor corrections on a paper or test), or even what others may view as positive experiences as threatening or dangerous (e.g., fear or paranoia increases when forming a close relationship). Imagine the effect of being continuously fearful, hypervigilant, and/or paranoid on the ability to engage in everyday roles, activities, and relationships as one's protective response continues to be triggered intensely and repeatedly, and when perceptions may be distorted due to past trauma experiences.

Neurophysiology and Traumatic Experiences

Occupational therapy practitioners (OTPs) are well versed in the role of the central nervous system on the ability to function and participate in meaningful life roles, routines, and activities, given the academic preparation they have received in anatomy, physiology, neuroscience, mental health, and other courses. Few other professions receive this type of entry level preparation; therefore, OTPs are well positioned to support the TIC initiative and provide direct care services to those experiencing trauma or with trauma histories, given the understanding of the complexity of the mind-body connection, the central role of attachment and the therapeutic relationship, and the correlations with occupational participation.

One of the ways that trauma (traumatic stress) influences the development of the brain and body (central nervous system, which includes the sensory and motor systems), and hormonal systems (hypothalamic-pituitary-adrenal [HPA] axis) is through the triggering of the stress response.[10,11] When the stress response is triggered, one of the systems of the central nervous system that plays a primary role is the autonomic nervous system (ANS), which is comprised of the sympathetic (SNS) and parasympathetic (PNS) nervous systems. The SNS is often known for triggering the mobilization of the brain and bodily systems to support the fight-or-flight response during times of threat or danger. The PNS triggers the rest-and-digest mode when in a calm mode and not triggered by stress and supports the social engagement capacities to attune and interact socially. When the SNS response is not sufficient in diffusing the threat, however, the PNS goes into a different mode known as the "freeze response," supported largely by the vagus nerve, in the attempt to self-protect.[12-14] When a person has repeated or chronic traumatic stress and goes into the mobilized, externalized, fight-or-flight mode, this pattern of response may become the predominant response of the nervous system.[9] When the PNS response goes into the immobilized, internalized freeze mode, this pattern may become the predominant response of the nervous system.[9,14] It is also common for people to have a more complex presentation, where the person may present with either of these modes of response, sometimes in rapid succession.

When a person experiences trauma (including neglect) while these neurophysiologic structures and systems are still forming, especially when trauma occurs in a repeated or chronic manner, these experiences affect the development of brain structures in a use-dependent and sequential manner due in part to neurogenesis, neuroplasticity, synaptic migration, and/or pruning during the different stages of development.[10] There are also sensitive periods of development when the nervous system is apt to be even more sensitive and, therefore, significantly influenced by one's experiences. One example of an area of the brain that has evidence supporting the negative affect of early childhood trauma is the amygdala. The amygdala is a part of the brain that processes emotional information (e.g., fear) at a preconscious level of awareness. Due to the continued triggering of the traumatic stress response, the amygdala becomes highly sensitive and overresponsive to social and emotional input (e.g., seeing an upset or angry facial expression) to the degree that the nervous system is "primed" for threat detection and hypervigilance.[15-21] Research has also revealed that there is reduced thickness in the structures of the brain involved in the emotional processing of social information, called the "ventromedial prefrontal cortex."[16,22,23] Many studies have demonstrated a variety of different types of sensory processing patterns and relational and occupational influences due to traumatic experience.[24-27] For example, recent research using neuroimaging on the effects of trauma on the vestibular system and cerebellum has revealed the links among posttraumatic stress disorder (PTSD), dissociation, body awareness, and balance.[28,29]

Although it is not the purpose of this chapter to provide an extensive review of the effect of trauma on the brain and development, a brief review of some of the research is provided to support the understanding of the pervasive effect of trauma. These neurophysiologic systems are some of the key structures whose development supports functional outcomes, such as a positive and safe sense of self and others and the developmental capacities supporting occupational participation. The *Diagnostic and Statistical Manual of Mental Disorders* (DSM-5)[9] also states that the variability of one's response to stress and trauma is remarkable, and that fear and anxiety are at the core of many of the trauma-related symptoms experienced.[9] Although there is much more research needed to establish a strong evidence base on the effect of trauma on overall development, a growing body of literature has validated that traumatic experiences are complex and provides a window into that complexity.

All of this knowledge is important to take into account when working with people with trauma histories. Having an understanding of how trauma affects neurophysiological, social, emotional, behavioral, and occupational capacities helps OTPs engage with clients collaboratively and compassionately and informs the clinical reasoning process that supports ideas related to the OT evaluation and intervention planning and implementation processes.

Trauma's Affect: Occupational Participation

Everyone is unique, and therefore it is common for people with trauma histories, or those experiencing ongoing forms of trauma, to have difficulty engaging in different aspects of occupational participation. Although this is not an all-inclusive list, the following are examples of how trauma-related symptoms may affect occupational performance skills and participation:

- Cognition (executive functioning): difficulty with cognitive flexibility (planning and problem solving), paying attention and focusing on task, screening out distractions and triggers from the environment; difficulty with dissociation and

not feeling bodily grounded, which may interfere with safe or efficient participation in daily occupations (e.g., not being fully aware when at school or at work, when shopping, cooking, safety when driving).
- Emotional: anxiety, depression, fear, paranoia, or panic to the degree that negatively affects the ability to participate in daily routines and activities (e.g., home care, school or work participation, child care, pet care, leisure participation).
- Neurophysiological: high levels of ANS arousal, difficulty with body awareness, hypersensitivities to sensation(s) (e.g., touch, sounds, smells), difficulty with self-regulation and inhibitory control, balance and spatial awareness, fine motor skills, and/or praxis skills (e.g., difficulty with dressing; the ability to focus, read, or complete other tasks at school or at work; the ability to drive).
- Relational: difficulty with forming close, trusting, intimate relationships (attachment formation); difficulty with being paranoid, anxious, and/or insecure in relationships limiting social and leisure opportunities, work, and school participation.
- Occupational: difficulty falling asleep, staying asleep, and/or poor quality of sleep, difficulty with completion of work and school tasks, self-care, home care, and social and leisure engagement.

Diagnostic Classifications

The quest continues for an all-encompassing definition of trauma, a more comprehensive taxonomy of trauma-related disorders, and a broader understanding that takes into account the many variables that affect how trauma-related sequela manifest in individuals, including the following:

- Age(s) of exposure
- The type of relationship the person has with the perpetrator(s)
- Types and degrees of trauma experienced or witnessed
- Socioeconomic and cultural variables
- Other risk and protective factors

In the meantime, the DSM-5 provides the taxonomy and diagnostic information used by doctors and practitioners for diagnostic, educational, and research purposes to date.[9] Given the recent surge in the research on stress and trauma, the DSM-5 created an entirely new diagnostic category called *trauma- and stressor-related disorders*, which includes the following diagnoses:

- Reactive attachment disorder
- Disinhibited social engagement disorder
- Posttraumatic stress disorder
- Acute stress disorder
- Adjustment disorders

- Other specified trauma- and stressor-related disorders
- Unspecified trauma- and stressor-related disorders

Dissociation is another symptom often experienced by those with trauma histories. Dissociation is a state of mind that can be experienced at different degrees of severity and may be accompanied by the loss of awareness of perceptual cues from the physical and/or social environment, loss of spatial awareness, time, balance, the ability to process auditory input, decreased facial expression, and decreased body and pain awareness.[9] Dissociation is often considered as being on a continuum, ranging from its least to most severe symptoms. Everyone has experienced a minor form of dissociation when daydreaming or "spacing out," but the more moderate or severe forms of dissociation can involve feeling numb, having out-of-body experiences, loss of memory, and even multiple personalities.[9] The DSM-5 has added dissociation to some of the different trauma-related disorder diagnostic criteria, as well as continuing to give it an entire category of its own called "dissociative disorders." For more information on the diagnostic criteria of trauma and stress-related disorders, refer to Chapter 10; for dissociative disorders, refer to Chapter 14.

It is clear that there is still a long way to go to create a unified taxonomy of trauma-related disorders and, without such a taxonomy it is difficult to engage in high-quality research and develop evidence-based practice guidelines and public policy. Still, efforts continue in researching trauma-related areas in need of further attention, such as developmental trauma, complex trauma, and adverse childhood experiences. Research in the area of TIC and its application in physical medicine and rehabilitation services have also begun, but these efforts are in the early stages.

Developmental Trauma

Many professionals advocating for the increased focus on trauma over the past two decades also promoted the importance of the inclusion of developmental trauma as a diagnostic category in the DMS-5. There has been extensive research and publishing on the effect on a child's neurophysiological and relational foundations of development when trauma occurs before the age of 5 years, particularly when repeated, severe, prolonged, or inflicted by a caregiver.[30-34] According to van der Kolk,[30] developmental trauma helps to describe better:

> …the complex disruptions of affect regulation, the disturbed attachment patterns, the rapid behavioral regressions and shifts in emotional states, the loss of autonomous strivings, the aggressive behavior against self and others, the failure to achieve developmental competencies; the loss of bodily regulation in the areas

> of sleep, food and self-care; the altered schemas of the world; the anticipatory behavior and traumatic expectations; the multiple somatic problems, from gastrointestinal distress to headaches; the apparent lack of awareness of danger and resulting self-endangering behaviors; the self-hatred and self-blame and the chronic feelings of ineffectiveness.

There has also been a heightened focus on the effects of variables that may occur in utero or soon after birth that negatively affect neurodevelopment and attachment formation, such as exposure to viruses or toxins, lack of oxygen to the brain, prematurity, maternal substance abuse while in utero, muscular and other disorders (e.g., cerebral palsy), invasive medical procedures, and extended hospital stays in infancy.

Although developmental trauma did not get accepted into the DSM-5 as a diagnostic category, the term continues to be used in the research and literature on the subject. The extensive research completed on developmental trauma, however, has contributed to the addition of new criteria for diagnosing PTSD in children younger than 6 years.[9] Although the addition of the new PTSD criteria is a significant stride, it continues to lack the degree of sensitivity and specificity indicating the extent of the effect of early childhood trauma and attachment disruption. Research efforts continue to identify more comprehensive research methodologies and diagnostic criteria related to the effect of childhood trauma, which ultimately informs the clinical reasoning related to individualized therapeutic interventions. A recent pilot study using occupational therapy assessment tools (in addition to other trauma-related tools) has revealed that children with developmental trauma appear to have sensory processing challenges across many areas of praxis (e.g., postural, constructional, oral, sequencing, and praxis on verbal command), graphesthesia, design copy, and standing walking balance.[35] Correlations with trauma, dissociation, and occupation were also explored, although more research is necessary to establish an evidence base and demonstrate occupational therapy's distinct value in working with people with trauma histories. Some general examples of the effect of developmental trauma on occupational participation are outlined in Table 17.1 (note that this list is not all-inclusive).

Adverse Childhood Experiences

The adverse childhood experiences (ACE) study has provided ground-breaking research that has brought a significant shift in the understanding of what happens to individuals neuropsychologically, behaviorally, and medically when the person has unaddressed trauma.[5,7] The original ACE study included over 17,000 participants and was

TABLE 17.1 Examples of Occupational Barriers Due to Trauma

Areas of Occupation	Occupational Barriers
Activities of daily living	Sleep problems: difficulty falling asleep, staying asleep, and with nightmares Difficulty, avoidance or refusal of performing dressing, bathing, and/or grooming tasks due to: • Fearful or anxious due to trauma triggers • Sensory over-responsivies • Fine motor control • Body, self-awareness • Dyspraxia • Dissociation
School performance	Difficulty with: • Staying focused in class • Maintaining safe behaviors • Problem solving • Being in a loud or chaotic cafeteria or physical environment • Participating in gym class • Forming and/or maintaining social relationships • Engaging in cooperative projects or groups • Lack of self-esteem • Lack of self-identity or identification of subjects they are skilled in • Feeling like a failure or triggered when corrected by adults and teachers
Play and leisure participation	Difficulty with: • Safe use of playground, play, or sports equipment • Social and communication skills • Lack of trust with others • Self-regulation • Impulse control • Dyspraxia • Sensory overresponsivity • Hypervigilance • Staying focused and engaged during play or leisure activities • Tolerating turn taking, lack of skill with games or sports, not winning • Lack of self-identity, identification of likes and dislikes with play and leisure participation

conducted by physicians at Kaiser Permanente.[7] The results of the ACE study have demonstrated the pervasive nature of ACEs and expanded the knowledge of the types of experiences and situations that may be considered traumatic when encountered before the age of 18 years. Thus, the ACE study expanded the scope of the definition of trauma and age-related considerations.[7] The ACE study identified the following experiences as traumatic and, therefore, have come to be known as ACEs[7]:

- Abuse
  - Physical, sexual, or verbal abuse
  - Physical and emotional neglect
- Household challenges
  - Having a household family member with depression, mental illness, or attempted suicide
  - Having a family member who is incarcerated
  - Witnessing intimate partner (domestic) violence
  - Household family member with problems with substance abuse
  - Parental separation, divorce, or other reasons related to parental loss

The ACE score is identified by adding up the number of ACEs that the person experiences before the age of 18 (scores range from 0–10 ACEs). The higher the ACE score, the higher the risk of the following:

- Chronic health conditions (e.g., heart disease, autoimmune disorders, asthma)
- Health risk behaviors (e.g., substance abuse, self-injury)
- Trauma-related symptoms (e.g., depression, suicidality)
- Disrupted neurodevelopment
- Difficulty reaching one's full potential (e.g., social participation, graduation rate, difficulty maintaining a job, low academic achievement)
- Early death (in some situations)

The ACE pyramid is a widely published visual representation of the mechanisms identified in the ACE study.[36] The ACE pyramid is shown in Fig. 17.1.

The US Department of Health and Human Services[37] has revealed that ACEs continue to be very common in children. In 2015, child protective services reported approximately 4 million referrals, involving 7.2 million children for maltreatment.[37] The number of confirmed child maltreatment and fatality rates have risen significantly from 2011 to 2015 in the United States.[37] The ACE study has been supported by other research that shows that childhood abuse and neglect cause pervasive developmental, health, and societal effects that persist into adulthood if left unaddressed.[5,7,38-40] In addition, when children are removed from those inflicting maltreatment, they are often placed with other relatives or in foster care. At times in these placements, further experiences of separation, loss, and further victimization may occur. Taking into account

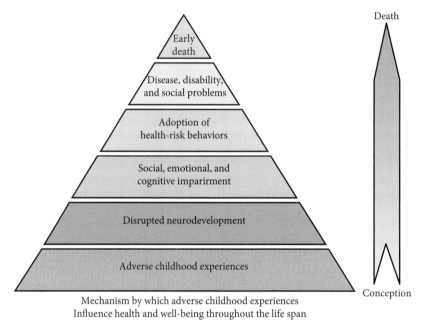

Fig. 17.1 Adverse childhood experiences: mechanisms influencing health and well-being. (From Centers for Disease Control and Prevention. The ACE pyramid. 2016. Available at: https://www.cdc.gov/violenceprevention/acestudy/about.html.)

all of these experiences that children entering into the child welfare system may face, it is easier to understand how children facing higher levels of adversity tend to require more mental health services than those who have not experienced maltreatment.[41,42]

Complex Trauma and Disorders of Extreme Stress Not Otherwise Specified

Similar to the initiative with developmental trauma, the diagnostic criteria in the DSM-5 for trauma-related disorders that are more complex, severe, prolonged, or repeated in nature and go beyond early childhood is not sufficiently represented in the DSM-5.[43-45] In fact, it is possible to go through childhood without experiencing ACEs but in adulthood experience chronic and severe trauma (e.g., active combat, abduction, prisoners of war).

The categories and descriptions of trauma reviewed in this section are supplemental to those categorized in the DSM-5. The ongoing explosion of information and research on this subject continues to challenge and shape our evolving understanding of the definition, prevalence, and pervasive effects of trauma as it occurs across the life span. This information is critical to identifying ways to prevent maltreatment and trauma and developing and engaging in innovative and evidence-based practices with those who have experienced trauma.

Although the field has come a long way in its understanding of trauma, there are still many areas in need of exploration. Some of the areas in need of more research include the impact of invasive medical procedures, pain, and rehabilitation services that are perceived as experiences of traumatic stress. Research into study trauma related to other types of adverse experiences, such as living with mental illness, developmental or learning disabilities, traumatic or progressive brain injuries or disorders, and neurodegenerative diseases is also needed.

Protective and Risk Factors: Building Resilience

Although diagnostic classifications are useful in describing patterns of trauma-related symptoms and behaviors to support a better understanding of what individuals are experiencing, when actually working with people with trauma histories, it is important to use a strength-based, collaborative, individualized, and TIC approach that fosters empowerment, resilience, and occupational participation.[46-48] Resilience refers to the inherent ability of each person to recover and thrive in the face of adversity; it is a capacity that all people have to varying degrees, and this capacity may change over time. Some of the variables that support resilience include one's neurophysiology, temperament, sense of self-identity and self-efficacy, one's belief system prior to the trauma experience(s), supportive relationships, and ability to experience positive emotions.[49-52] Situational and contextual factors, as well as the degree of support that the individual believes he or she has, significantly influences resilience and the recovery process (e.g., socioeconomic, cultural).

Similar to the literature on resilience, factors having a significant influence on whether a person has a higher or lower vulnerability of victimization, perpetration, or maltreatment are referred to as "protective and risk factors."[53,54] Risk factors are the variables that contribute to a person having a higher probability of maltreatment and trauma; protective factors are variables that reduce this risk.[53,54] Protective and risk factors are often divided into the following categories: individual, familial, peer and social, community and societal.[53,54] Table 17.2 provides examples of protective and risk factors. It is important to note that the factors contributing to resilience are similar to those in the protective factor category, and those listed as risk factors are similar to those identified as ACEs.

OTPs work collaboratively with clients, parents, caregivers, staff, and communities to help identify and use protective

TABLE 17.2 Protective and Risk Factors

Group	Protective	Risk
Individual	Internal locus of control Good overall health and adequate development Hobbies and interests Good peer relationships Positive temperament, disposition, and social orientation Minimal to no childhood trauma Highly developed skills in the following areas—social skills and competence, executive functioning and realistic planning skills, emotional intelligence, above-average cognitive intelligence Balance between help seeking and autonomy High aspirations for academic achievement and levels of academic achievement Positivity in attitudes and beliefs Lack of exposure to violence or significant conflict in the family system Spirituality or religiosity	External locus of control Premature birth, birth anomalies, low birth weight, exposure to toxins in utero Lack of hobbies and interests Temperament: slow or hard to warm up to Childhood trauma History of high emotional distress, poor impulse control, low frustration tolerance, lack of trust, aggressive behaviors, difficulty with behavioral control, treatment for emotional problems Attention deficits, hyperactivity, learning disorders, or low IQ Antisocial attitudes and beliefs Involvement with alcohol, drugs, or tobacco Exposure to violence or significant conflict in the family system
Parental, familial	Secure and stable attachment relationship(s); supportive, warm and positive parent-child relationship Supportive family environment Extended family support and involvement Familial expectation of prosocial behaviors Consistent presence of parent(s) or primary caregiver(s) during at least one of the following: when waking up, getting home from school, evening mealtime, going to bed Connectedness to family or adults outside the family Consistent parental employment Frequent engagement in shared and social activities Ability to discuss problems with parents Parent and family use of constructive coping mechanisms Positive adult role models outside of the family High parental education	Insecure attachment relationship(s) Authoritarian style parenting Harsh, inconsistent, or lax disciplinary practices Low or neglectful emotional attachment to or involvement with parents or primary caregivers High parental conflict, domestic violence, separation, divorce Poor overall family functioning; high stress Parental unemployment; homelessness Parental psychopathology Parental substance abuse or criminal behavior Low parental income Low parental education Inaccurate expectations or knowledge about child development

Continued

TABLE 17.2 Protective and Risk Factors—cont'd

Group	Protective	Risk
Peer and social	Positive social relationships with those at school that are prosocial, close, and strong Invested in, committed to, and doing well in school Close relationships with nondeviant peers Membership in peer groups with strong prosocial values and that engage in prosocial activities Exposure to schools that have: • Trauma-informed approach • Intensive supervision • Clear rules for behavior • Engagement of parents and teachers • Consistent and appropriate reinforcements for positive behaviors versus aggression	Social rejection from peers Stressful life events Low commitment to school, school failure, or poor academic performance Social isolation; bullying Exposure to racism, discrimination Associating with delinquent peers Lack of exposure to schools that have: • Trauma-informed approach • Intensive supervision • Clear rules for behavior • Engagement of parents and teachers • Consistent and appropriate reinforcements for positive behaviors versus aggression
Community and societal	Middle to high socioeconomic status Access to health care and social services Adequate housing High concentration of residents with mid to high socioeconomic status Active community engagement Supportive neighborhoods Low, minimal community violence	Low socioeconomic status Lack of access to health care and social services Inadequate housing or homelessness High concentration of neighborhood residents with low incomes Low community participation Socially disorganized neighborhoods High level of transiency Dangerous, violent neighborhood Community violence

Adapted from Centers for Disease Control and Prevention. Youth violence: risk and protective factors. 2017. Available at: https://www.cdc.gov/violenceprevention/youthviolence/riskprotectivefactors.html; Child Welfare Information Gateway. Risk and protective factors for child abuse and neglect. 2004. Available at: https://www.childwelfare.gov/pubPDFs/riskprotectivefactors.pdf.

factors for prevention and intervention purposes. Additionally, OTPs help to prevent and counter the effects of risk factors, such as trauma and the lack of positive attachment relationships, while also supporting safety, stability, self-organization, positive relational engagement, and occupational participation. Helping clients build occupational performance skills, identify and access the supports and resources necessary to build prosocial experiences, and enhance self-awareness, self-esteem, self-identity, resilience, and recovery are just some of the many ways OTPs work with clients from a trauma-informed approach.

TRAUMA-INFORMED CARE

Given the radical culture change required by organizations to meet this charge, TIC continues to be a national and international initiative, and due to the complexity involved, most mental health organizations are still working to achieve this goal. The term *universal precautions* has

been adopted to emphasize that to be trauma-informed it is necessary to assume that whether or not the client acknowledges it, trauma is likely to have been part of each person's experience. This is important because[52]:

> …the characteristics of the trauma and the subsequent traumatic stress reactions can dramatically influence how individuals respond to their environment, relationships, interventions, and treatment services and those same characteristics can also shape assumptions that clients/consumers make about their world (e.g., their view of others, sense of safety), their future (e.g., hopefulness, fear of a foreshortened future), and themselves (e.g., feeling resilient, feeling incompetent in regulating emotions).

For this reason, a trauma-informed culture is one that infuses trauma informed knowledge, skills, and the resources necessary to implement and sustain trauma informed principles and practices.

According to the Substance Abuse Mental Health Services Administration (SAMHSA),[48] trauma-informed principles include the following:

1. Safety and stability: across each practice setting all clients, caregivers, and staff feel safe.
2. Trustworthiness and transparency: organizational operations and decisions are transparent, compassionate, and work toward an overall goal of building and maintaining trust among staff, clients, and caregivers.
3. Peer support and mutual self-help: both are integral to the organizational and service delivery approach and are understood as a key vehicle for establishing safety, trust building, and empowerment.
4. Collaboration and mutuality: the organization recognizes that everyone has a central role to play in the therapeutic process; therefore, the leveling of power differences is recognized as a way to share decision making, empower, and build the trusting relationships necessary for healing and recovery.
5. Empowerment, voice, and choice: a strength-based approach is used across all aspects of care. The organization strives to build on client, caregiver, and staff strengths, and views choice and an individualized approach as essential to TIC. It is also a core belief that all persons, organizations, and communities are able to heal and recover.
6. Cultural, historical, and gender responsivity: the organization removes cultural biases and stereotypes and strives to implement cultural sensitivity and competence, leveraging cultural opportunities that support the healing process. The organization offers gender-responsive services and recognizes and addresses historical and intergenerational trauma.

TIC must be part of occupational therapy practice given that a significant number of clients who seek out occupational therapy services after an accident, injury, or invasive medical procedure or due to mental health, developmental, learning, intellectual, or physical challenges affecting occupational participation. Although not all clients will experience symptoms warranting a trauma-related diagnosis, many will have minimally had adverse experiences and may continue to struggle with pain, fear, depression, anxiety, grief, or loss as a direct result of the challenges they experienced prior to engagement in occupational therapy services. In addition, many clients may or may not be aware that they have a high number of ACEs or traumatic experiences prior to the event or injury that leads them to occupational therapy services. TIC is part of what OTPs must be aware of and intentionally incorporate into their practices in addition to supporting its incorporation on an organizational scale from their respective positions (e.g., consultant, committee member, administrator, advocate, team member, educator).

Trauma-Informed Approaches

Although TIC continues to be a requirement of mental health organizations, the model has transformed to also include *trauma-informed approaches* (TIAs). The SAMHSA[55] has stated that a TIA "can be implemented in any type of service setting or organization and is distinct from trauma-specific interventions or treatments that are designed specifically to address the consequences of trauma and to facilitate healing." TIAs came about after it became clear that there are different disciplines that do not have the skill set necessary to provide direct therapeutic services to people with trauma-related needs and goals, yet are part of the broader community of services necessary to support safety, education, and other community-based supports. All individuals interfacing with those experiencing trauma or with trauma histories must understand the prevalence and effects of trauma, TIC principles, and how not to retraumatize people with trauma histories (e.g., school personnel, emergency services personnel, prison guards). TIAs also promote the universal precautions approach to help society recognize and understand the effects of trauma and necessity of TIAs. To become a trauma-informed society, a variety of interventions and approaches at the client, provider, organizational, community, state, federal, and policy levels are necessary.

Occupational Therapy: Organizational and Community-Based Models

When OTPs work with programs, organizations, and communities to achieve goals related to TIC and the culture change, it is important to know about the evidence-based models and promising strategies that support this initiative.[56] One of the primary evidence-based models for helping to implement trauma-informed organizational culture change is the Six Core Strategies.[2,57]

Six Core Strategies

In addition to the TIC guiding principles, the Six Core Strategies for TIC and restraint and seclusion reduction is an evidence-based practice used by organizations to create a trauma-informed strategic plan.[2,57,58] Starting at the level of the organization's vision, mission, and strategic planning process, strong leadership support and full engagement are critical to the ability to become trauma-informed because TIC requires culture change and leadership support to achieve and sustain progress over time. The Six Core Strategies include the following:

1. Leadership toward organizational change
2. Use of data to inform practice
3. Workforce development
4. Use of seclusion and restraint prevention tools
5. Consumer roles
6. Debriefing

TABLE 17.3	Six Core Strategies and the Occupational Therapy Practitioner (OTP) Role
Core Strategies	**OTP Role Examples**
1. Leadership toward organizational change	Work with administrators, committees, and/or team members to co-create and implement the trauma-informed care (TIC) strategic plan.
	Work with leadership to identify resources that help support the implementation of the TIC strategic plan.
2. Use of data to inform practice	Work with administrators, committees, and/or team members to create and track outcomes related to the TIC initiative.
3. Workforce development	Provide trainings to staff on the effects of trauma, TIC, the Six Core Strategies, specific TIC-related interventions related to TIC, and the occupational therapy (OT) role as part of the treatment team.
	Provide training on the therapeutic approaches used by the agency (e.g., Attachment, Regulation and Competency [ARC], Dialectical Behavior Therapy [DBT], Neurosequential Model of Therapeutics [NMT]).
	Support staff in understanding how to individualize therapeutic interventions.
	Provide in-services on any TIC-related trainings attended outside the agency.
4. Use of seclusion and restraint prevention tools	Assist in assessing the client's trauma and attachment history, triggers, warning signs, and helpful strategies.
	Help the client create and/or team enhance the client's list of helpful strategies based on client's OT assessment results.
5. Consumer roles	Support client's and caregivers in client-centered and guided therapeutic services.
	Model how to provide services in a client-centered and trauma informed manner.
6. Debriefing	Support staff in the process of debriefing when incidents, seclusion and/or restraint events occur (in a nonpunitive manner) to identify ways to change the outcome in the future.
	Help modify client's individualized plans based on any information obtained throughout the debriefing process.

A brief summary of the Six Core Strategies and examples of ways that OTPs participate in each strategy is provided in Table 17.3.

There are clear indicators as to whether an organization is trauma-informed or not. One of the first distinctions is the shift in all staff attitudes toward persons served, such as the change to considering what happened to the person rather than focusing on what is wrong with them. An individualized approach, rather than one focused exclusively on rules and behavioral techniques, that values a therapeutic relationship-based focus, as well as evidence-based and promising TIC practices, is essential. Table 17.4 demonstrates practical examples of some differences between trauma-informed and non–trauma-informed attitudes, practices, and behaviors.[2,4] Although, initially, providers may think changing to a TIC approach is merely a change in semantics, reviewing some of the differences from a nonjudgmental stance will help demonstrate that knowledge and culture change are necessary to becoming trauma-informed.

Since TIC was initially introduced, the SAMHSA and National Association for State Mental Health Program Directors (NASMHPD) have and continue to provide a wide variety of training and technical assistance supports (including direct consultation) to mental health agencies and providers to help them obtain the consultation and training resources often necessary to create and implement trauma-informed strategic plans across many different types of mental health, educational, and forensic organizations. The Six Core Strategies is now an internationally recognized organizational guideline for TIC and seclusion and restraint reduction and is implemented by mental health, forensic, school-based, and other organization types with guidelines available specific to organizations' strategic planning.[3,4] OTPs often assist administrators in developing and implementing a TIC strategic plan as part of a TIC committee or member of the treatment team. Additionally, OTPs practicing in administrative or consultation roles help lead or coach organizations in achieving the goal of becoming trauma-informed. For more information on the Six Core Strategies, refer to the online resource section at the end of the chapter.

Building Bridges

The Building Bridges Initiative (BBI) was created to help child and adolescent residential and community-based

TABLE 17.4 Trauma-Informed Versus Non–Trauma-Informed Approaches

Trauma-Informed	Non–Trauma-Informed
Universal precautions approach (assumes that all clients have trauma history)	Does not use a universal precautions approach
Lack of training on trauma and trauma-informed care (TIC)	Lack of training on trauma and TIC
Client is expert on their own experiences and the change agent in their care and recovery process	Professional viewed as the expert and perceived as the change agent in the client's care and recovery process
Collaborative service provision that holds the client's voice and choice as central to the service provision	Minimally includes the client's voice and choice throughout service provision
Assesses for trauma history and symptoms	Does not assess, minimally considers trauma history and symptoms
Uses the information gathered in the assessment for intervention planning	Does not use information gathered in the assessment for intervention planning
Helps client identify individualized triggers, warning signs and helpful strategies	Does not help client identify individualized triggers, warning signs, and helpful strategies
Focuses on "what happened to you"	Focuses on "what is wrong with you"
Language—respectful, neutral, nonjudgmental	Language—disrespectful and judgmental (e.g., manipulative, needy)
Avoids shaming, blaming, humiliating	Use of shaming, blaming, humiliating, and views as therapeutic
Power and control dynamics minimized; staff collaborative and compassionate	Staff viewed as rule enforcers, in charge versus collaborative and compassionate
Recognizes and strives to minimize organizational culture, practices that retraumatize	Overreliance on physical interventions (seclusion, restraint)
Minimizes the use of physical interventions (seclusion, restraint)	Development and use of therapeutic relationship not seen as a primary intervention
Development and use of therapeutic relationships viewed as a primary intervention	Does not value or provide nurturing and healing therapeutic and environmental options
Values and provides nurturing and healing therapeutic and environmental options	Leadership not passionate about or dedicated to the TIC initiative
Leadership passionate about and dedicated to the TIC initiative	

Adapted from National Association for State Mental Health Program Directors (NASMHPD). *Trauma-Informed Care Module*. Alexandria, VA: NASMHPD, National Technical Assistance Center for State Mental Health Planning; 2003; and National Association for State Mental Health Program Directors (NASMHPD). *Trauma-Informed Care Module*. 9th ed. Alexandria, VA: NASMHPD, National Technical Assistance Center for State Mental Health Planning; 2009.

mental health programs not only meet but exceed the expectations and outcomes of TIC.[59] The BBI values and core principles that promote high-quality care and positive outcomes include the following:
- Youth-guided and family-driven care
  - Individualized and strengths-based
  - Collaborative and coordinated
  - Comprehensive, integrated, and flexible
- Trauma-informed care
- Preventing seclusion and restraint
- Cultural and linguistic competence
- Linking residential with community
- Working with youth in transition
- Promising and best practices in medication
- Evidence-based and practice-informed
- Sustained positive outcomes

Building on each of the Six Core Strategies, BBI promotes the following seven essential elements as areas for organizations and therapeutic teams to focus on to change short-term residential services to become not only trauma-informed and client-centered (central to and involved in the process) but also client-directed (leading the process with support)[59]:
- Effective leadership
- Family and youth engagement and inclusion
- Workforce development
- Practice strategies and tools
- Using data to inform practice
- Quality improvement
- Fiscal strategies

Both the Six Core Strategies and BBI models demonstrate that organizational culture change requires strong leadership, and the entire organization must be part of the process. It is common for OTPs to feel overwhelmed when trying to integrate TIC into their own practice, particularly if the organization for which they work is not actively engaging in the aforementioned culture change process as well. Both the Six Core Strategies and BBI principles and their respective core strategies and elements are synchronous with occupational therapy values, ethics, and strength-based approaches. When adding the knowledge of TIC organizational change processes to the OTP repertoire, OTPs become uniquely positioned to assist organizations in the mission to become trauma-informed.

Self-Healing Communities Model

There are many resources available to assist communities in becoming more trauma-informed, such as the self-healing communities model (SHCM). The SHCM promotes the widespread application of TIAs and provides guidelines to help communities implement TIAs. One of the primary ways that the SHCM fosters a TIA is by not only helping communities become more aware of TIC and TIAs and strengthen how they understand and provide services from a trauma-informed perspective, but also by emphasizing and supporting the centrality of clients and caregivers in the overall initiative and empowering them as primary agents of the trauma-informed culture change.[60] Expanding community capacity is another component of the SHCM, where groups of people in a community get together and form relationships and identify and create community-based awareness and supports that foster collective action toward health and social equality, thereby decreasing stigma and incidents of ACEs over time.[61] In one research study using the SHCM in Washington state, it was found to reduce the rates of seven different major social problems affecting ACEs over the course of 8 years.[62] Involving local community leaders, emergency services, judicial and other legal personnel, and the general public supports the widespread implementation. With the rates of maltreatment and other forms of trauma on the rise across much of the United States, it is critical for OTPs to provide TIC across all areas and types of OT practice and to become involved in community-based TIC efforts.

Occupational Therapy: Individual and Group Services

It is well established that the profession of occupational therapy first began in mental health care institutions and, according to the American Occupational Therapy Association,[63] OTPs are qualified mental health practitioners. OTPs must include TIC as part of the occupational therapy (OT) process, which requires an understanding of TIC and the national initiatives, research, promising, and evidence-based practices associated with TIC.[64] OTPs have the educational background necessary to promote mental health, wellness, resiliency, and recovery from traumatic experiences.[64-68]

Applying the totality of the OT process when working with people with trauma histories is essential to providing skilled OT services and promising evidence-based interventions. Through the OT assessment process, a person's strengths, trauma history, protective and risk factors, and how each affects the individual are identified and integrated into the OT profile (e.g., identify trauma-related symptoms, developmental skill levels across the areas of occupational performance and participation; effects on occupations [sleep, self-care, school or work performance]). Such a comprehensive approach is critical to the OT process and the client, involved caregivers, and the treatment team to identify areas of strengths and needs and guide the ability to target each client's interventions at the appropriate challenge level. Identifying where the client is performing from a developmental perspective is just one example of the critical information that OTPs provide to the client and therapeutic team. For example, the identification of developmental capacities is important when working with children and adolescents with trauma histories because they tend to have developmental skill levels (in some areas) that are below chronologic age expectations, hindering participation, wellness, and the recovery process. For example, if it is expected that a child should be participating in groups but is only at the developmental stage of parallel play, this information is critical to the treatment planning and intervention processes. An example with an adult client may involve the expectation that the client completes a bathing and dressing routine independently, but if the person is highly tactile overresponsive (hypersensitive) and has difficulty sequencing through the steps of the activity, prompts and individualized supports are needed to help cue the client to complete the self-care tasks successfully and manage the sensory overresponsivity. Understanding the client's trauma history provides another layer of understanding. For instance, it is possible that the client's trauma occurred (in part or totally) during self-care routines. In such cases, client education about tactile overresponsivity and the correlations with the traumatic experience is often helpful to increase self-awareness and identify ways to cope with or work to change the sensory processing pattern, if that is part of the client's wishes. This is just one way that the evaluation process is essential to identifying the client's strengths and areas of need collaboratively, and how OT services support the overall therapeutic process with each client.

OTPs also work with clients and caregivers to provide education and training on the interrelatedness of the mind-body connection, (e.g., sensory and motor patterns) and other potential areas of need to help determine individualized goals, stress reduction techniques, and coping strategies (e.g., yoga, mindfulness, sensory-based modalities), and increase occupational participation.[69-71] These are just some examples of how an OTP may work with a client with a trauma history on an individual level.

Wellness and Recovery Initiatives

Research identifying the significant degree of health disparities among people with substance abuse and mental health disorders and the general public has revealed staggering results. The SAMHSA[72] created the wellness initiative to support increased awareness of this issue and promote tools that can be used to help foster healthy lifestyles supporting wellness, quality of life, and recovery. The eight dimensions of wellness[72] are promoted as areas of focus that help lead to a lifestyle that will support positive health and well-being:

1. Emotional
2. Environmental
3. Financial
4. Intellectual
5. Occupational
6. Physical
7. Social
8. Spiritual

Each of the eight dimensions of wellness is complex and can be broken down further into examples of positive health and wellness strategies. OTPs provide therapeutic services that target health, wellness, and quality of life and work collaboratively with people with mental health and substance abuse disorders to help identify, prioritize, and meet preferred goals related to these eight dimensions.

The *recovery initiative* was introduced in 2003; the most recent working definition of recovery is "a process of change through which individuals improve their health and wellness, live self-directed lives, and strive to reach their full potential."[73,74] The SAMHSA[74] promotes the four major dimensions of recovery, identified as primary areas to support persons actively engaged in the recovery process:

1. Health: helping address the person's overall health
2. Home: obtaining and sustaining a stable and safe home environment
3. Purpose: identifying and engaging in meaningful roles and occupations, including income and the means for occupational participation in society
4. Community: assisting the person in developing sense of purpose, belonging, hope, and connectedness in relationships

In addition to the four major dimensions of recovery, the 10 guiding principles of recovery include person-driven, hope, respect, strengths, and responsibility and address trauma, holistic pathways, peer support, and relational and cultural factors.[73] The wellness and recovery initiatives are both trauma-informed at the core and are often used in a collaborative and individualized way to support safety, stability, and resilience as part of the OT process.

Although the life experiences and challenges encountered that are related to mental health and substance abuse can be very taxing to the person and their relationships, one of the key areas supporting recovery is a sense of belonging and connection. People with mental health, substance abuse, and traumatic experiences often have attachment or relational challenges that, if not identified or addressed, may continue across the life span and negatively affect relationships (e.g., attachment disorders, codependency). Thus, it is imperative to support the client in developing these capacities and to obtain the resources necessary to embark on and sustain the recovery process, but part of this process is to create and engage in relationships in safe, stable, and supported ways. The wellness and recovery initiatives are similar in that both aim to support the health, wellness, and quality of life of clients with mental health and trauma-related needs and goals by fostering increased resilience throughout the recovery process. These and other TIC, wellness, and recovery-oriented models created by mental health agencies are meant to provide organizations and practitioners with resources to guide and support culture change and service provision. For more information on these initiatives, refer to the online resources section at the end of the chapter.

Occupational Therapy Process

OTPs use the OT process.[75] As part of this process, establishing the therapeutic relationship and completing a collaborative evaluation is the starting point through which the occupational therapist helps each client identify strengths, values, and areas of need, which then supports goal setting, intervention planning, and outcome monitoring.[75]

Evaluation. The OT evaluation process requires working collaboratively with each client to identify strengths and priorities for goal setting and intervention planning and is typically the starting point of OT services. When it is unclear as to whether skilled OT services are necessary, an initial screening process may be a first step to make this determination. The evaluation process may also be used to identify the appropriateness of services. It is important to conduct an evaluation or, minimally, a screening process to determine whether a more comprehensive evaluation would be beneficial. Chart review, interview, observation, and assessment tools are used to create an occupational profile. The collaborative identification of goals, intervention planning and implementation, and outcomes monitoring all stem from the evaluation process and the assessment results contained in the occupational profile.

To practice in a manner that is trauma-informed, it is necessary to assess whether the individual has had a trauma history and/or is currently experiencing trauma, any current trauma-related symptoms (regardless of whether they identify as having a trauma history), and any corresponding triggers, warning signs, and helpful strategies. A simple tool called the "safety tool" has been created, with samples available for use with child and adult populations, and is available as part of the publication titled *Resource Guide*.[64,76] (Refer to the online resources section at the end of this chapter for the Massachusetts Department of Mental Health website link to obtain these free resources.) Interdisciplinary staff, including occupational therapists, can use the safety tools or modify them as needed. Additionally, comprehensive lists of other trauma and attachment-related assessment and screening tools and tutorials are available through the National Center for Posttraumatic Stress Disorder and the National Child Traumatic Stress network (refer to the resource section at the end of the chapter for website information).

Due to the more recent identification of the impact of trauma on sensory processing and executive functioning skills, as well as other areas often affected by trauma, direct evaluation of all occupational performance areas should be included in the evaluation process (e.g., Quick Neurological Screening Tool, Clinical Observations of Motor Performance, School Function Assessment) and not solely limited to collecting subjective data from questionnaires (Sensory Profile, Sensory Processing Measure) as part of the OT process. Evaluation of the person's occupational performance values and goals, including areas of occupational strength and weakness, must also be part of the OT evaluation process to be trauma-informed (e.g., Canadian Occupational Performance Measure, Model Of Human Occupation [MOHO] tools).

Intervention. Trauma-informed intervention planning and implementation must be individualized and include focus on the client's strengths, preferences, and trauma-related needs and goals identified in the evaluation process. The occupational performance skills, patterns, and areas of occupation affected by trauma are part of what is targeted from a trauma-informed approach. There are several different models promoted by experts in working with people with trauma histories to help guide the intervention process. These models support OTPs as TIC is integrated into OT practice. The three-phase model of trauma treatment has been used for many years as a standard of practice by therapists working with people with trauma.[77] The three-phase model recommends focusing on stabilization before working on trauma processing (phase 2) or integration (phase 3). This is not a linear model and, therefore, it is possible to stay in one phase for a period of time or to see movement back and forth between the phases or work being done across areas. A components-based approach is also promoted for working with children, which focuses on safety, self-regulation, self-reflective information processing, identity formation, traumatic experiences integration, relational engagement, and positive affect enhancement.[78] These two approaches provide general guidelines that are supportive of the client's recovery process when used in a skilled manner as part of the OT process.

The dimensional model of childhood (DMC) experience proposes information that is helpful in terms of guiding clinical reasoning related to the type(s) of trauma that the individual has experienced. The DMC suggests that when one's traumatic experiences stem primarily from neglect, there tends to be a lack of development that would indicate the need for evaluation and intervention processes focused on identifying the specific areas affected and then targeting those areas with specific and graded interventions from more of a trauma-informed, developmental lens. A literature review of interventions for children with neurodevelopmental difficulties due to trauma has also suggested that it is beneficial to develop specific approaches for addressing each area of difficulty separately (e.g., building memory, attention, sensory processing, or language skills).[79] The DMC also notes that those primarily experiencing and/or witnessing threat or violence often benefit from evaluation and interventions focused on establishing safety, stabilization, and self-regulating and organizing interventions, building supportive and trusting relationships, and targeting other developmental and trauma-related challenges once the person feels more safe and stabilized. Certainly, there are a wide variety of traumatic and adverse childhood experiences that may not fit into these two broad categories, and situations where the client has had a variety of experiences over time, indicating the need for a combination of approaches.[16]

Perry's Neurosequential Model of Therapeutics (NMT) aims to match the interventions used with the specific brain regions, developmental stages and functional and relational problems identified in the NMT assessment process.[10,80] Interventions are relationship-based, experiential, and modified for developmental stage. Perry emphasizes the need for repetition, rhythmicity (drumming), sensory rich experiences (massage), consistency, routine, and respect throughout the intervention process. For example, if a person is presenting as unsafe and extremely dysregulated, interventions would be targeted at the brainstem level to support the ANS regulatory responses and feelings of safety. The NMT has different recommendations for interventions that are related to the different levels of brain organization (brainstem, diencephalon [cerebellum], limbic, and neocortex) and the corresponding skills and symptoms identified as being in need of support. (For more information on NMT, refer to the Child Trauma Academy link in the online resources at eh end of the chapter).

With child populations, OTPs work with children and families who have experienced trauma. It is important to help identify the strengths of the child (and caregivers), as well as the client's needs and goal areas using a trauma-informed lens as part of the OT process. Common areas that OTPs often target when working with children and families include supporting healthy attachment formation, self-awareness and regulation skills, self-esteem, self-identity, development of a variety of occupational performance skills as needed (e.g., sensory processing, executive functioning, motor performance), and occupational participation through preparatory, purposeful, and occupation-based interventions. Sleep-rest, self-care, school participation, play, social (family, friends) and community participation are some of the common areas of occupation that are often affected when children experience trauma. Difficulty with safety, emotion regulation, sensory processing, attention span, and impulse and behavior control are also areas that are typically affected. For some children, developmental challenges are more severe, and they may not function at their chronologic age level in some areas. The OT evaluation supports clients and interdisciplinary teams in understanding the child's developmental strengths and needs across performance skill areas and guides intervention planning to support safety, attachment, self-regulation, other targeted developmental skills, and occupational participation.[81]

When working with children and families, it is important to emphasize the necessity of fostering the child-caregiver attachment relationship.[82] It is common to see intergenerational trauma among families, and research has emphasized the role of safety and stability in families to support recovery.[83,84] Helping parent and child to feel safe, stabilized, and supported is always the first step when working with families. Activity participation that builds on the relational capacities of both the child and caregiver(s) increasingly to tolerate and enjoy safe and fun-filled, non-competitive experiences that support loving presence, attunement, and reciprocity (e.g., cook or bake together, go for a walk together, hold hands, read and tell stories) is recommended when the client and caregiver are ready for this step. Both the child and caregiver may have their own trauma-related needs and goals; therefore, the timing of the interventions is related to the healing journeys of all involved. Therapeutic interventions involving siblings may also be part of the process.

In addition to individual sessions targeting these areas, OTPs also offer group sessions. For some children, groups may be very difficult due to social, play, relational, and other developmental challenges. Modifications to the group expectations to match each child's individualized needs is necessary, such as incorporating movement that is at the right challenge level, making groups smaller, helping each child maintain personal physical boundaries in fun ways, using visuals to support executive functioning, and making groups geared toward the interests and goals of each child.[85]

OTPs also work with adult and older adult populations with trauma histories.[64,67,86] Adults may present with an array of mental health and medical symptoms and diagnoses if one's trauma history goes unidentified or unaddressed. An adult or older adult may not necessarily experience childhood trauma; instead, they may have experienced an acute or chronic traumatic experience later in life. When trauma is experienced in adulthood and not during childhood, the person has had a developmental advantage in that the nervous system and relational capacities have had the opportunity to develop without the effect of trauma. Nonetheless, the symptoms that emerge following traumatic experiences may affect few or many areas of occupational performance skills and participation. Relationships may be challenged, difficulty with sleep, self-care or home care, work performance, leisure, and social and community engagement are some of the areas that trauma may affect in adults and older adults. Groups may also be used with adults and older adults as part of the therapeutic intervention process.

Preparatory and occupation-based approaches. Preparatory and occupation-based interventions are used with people with trauma-related needs and goals. Preparatory interventions are typically used when a client is having difficulty with safety and stabilization. Preparatory interventions are used to support the person to and successfully engage in meaningful roles, routines, and activities safely.[75] Occupation-based interventions are typically infused as the person feels more able to branch out, explore, and safely participate. Occupation-based interventions are also used to help a person feel more stabilized, provided that the interventions are safe and modified at the appropriate challenge level. Stabilization is often difficult for people with trauma histories, and OTPs are often asked to begin working with people to help them begin to feel safer and more stabilized. The level of care and safety protocols in place also affect the types of interventions that may be used as part of OT practice.

The increased recognition of the necessity of including body-oriented approaches with people with trauma histories has put sensory-based and complementary approaches used by OTPs for decades into the spotlight. Sensory-based approaches are often viewed as preparatory interventions, but this depend on the person's perception. For example, engagement in exercise may be a preparatory intervention for one person experiencing severe dissociation and using exercise only to stabilize. However, it may be occupation-based for someone who engages in exercise regularly as a meaningful and purposeful activity as part of the daily routine and maybe also for stabilization. The more stabilized a person feels, the more they tend naturally to want to engage in meaningful life roles, routines, and occupations.

Ayres Sensory Integration[81,87] and other sensory-based approaches and frameworks are used with people with trauma histories as a primary intervention, secondary to another trauma-based intervention or in conjunction with other interventions.[64,67,86,88-91] The Sensory Modulation Program (SMP) was created to provide OTPs and interdisciplinary professionals with trauma-informed guidelines for implementing a range of sensory-based strategies that support safety, self-organization, and occupational participation in a skilled manner.[64,67] The SMP is often used as a supplement to trauma-focused and other mental health interventions, and it encompasses a variety of components that place an emphasis on sensory integration and processing and relational approaches: therapeutic use of self, evaluation through intervention implementation (individual and group sessions), sensorimotor activities and modalities, sensory diet (individualized daily routine inclusive of prevention and de-escalation interventions), environmental modifications and enhancements (e.g., sensory rooms), and client and caregiver education. Some interventions that may be used as part of an individualized SMP include the following:

- Animal-assisted therapies
- Expressive arts
- Playing an instrument
- Dance, gymnastics, acrobatics, yoga
- Biofeedback (neurofeedback, HeartMath)
- Sound therapy
- Weighted modalities
- Aromatherapy
- Creation and use of a sensory kit or cart
- Sensory supportive physical environments (e.g., sensory room, sensory garden)

The SMP guidelines offer a general structure and resources for training interdisciplinary staff. When used by OTPs, the SMP is a component of the overall OT process. For more information on the SMP and other sensory-based approaches, refer to Chapter 8.

In addition to direct care services, OTPs engage in mental health promotion, prevention, and intervention.[66,92] Many OTPs are leaders in the TIC initiative and play key roles in administration, academic, and public health policy promotion, advocating for the OTPs role in TIC.[2,4,76,88,93,94] One example of a program promoting positive mental health and participation in academic and nonacademic activities and through embedded supports in school and after school programs is Every Moment Counts (EMC).[65] The EMC model programs have been developed by OTPs but can be implemented and sustained by interdisciplinary staff, parents, and administrators. The following are the EMC model programs and examples of the embedded interventions:

- Creating a comfortable cafeteria
- Refreshing recess
- Embedded classroom strategies for mental health promotion
- After school leisure coaching

Evidence-based and evidence-supported approaches. There are a variety of evidence-based approaches promoted for working with people with trauma histories. Mindfulness and meditation practices are evidence-based interventions supporting trauma recovery and implemented with child, adult, and older adult populations.[69,95] Sensory-enhanced, trauma-informed yoga has been shown to have positive effects with military personnel experiencing combat stress,[71] as well as the use of high-intensity sports and other OT interventions with people with PTSD, depression, and combat stress.[70,96] Eye movement desensitization and reprocessing (EMDR) is another evidence-based modality used as part of trauma processing for people with trauma.[97]

In addition to trauma-informed interventions that have supporting evidence within the OT literature, there are a variety of evidence-based and evidence-supported trauma therapy models; with additional training, OTPs can use these methods as part of the OT process:

- Trauma-focused cognitive behavioral therapy (TF-CBT)[98]
- Neurosequential model of therapeutics[10]
- Attachment regulation and competence[99]
- Dialectic behavior therapy[100,101]
- Somatic experiencing[32]
- Sensorimotor psychotherapy[102]
- Circle of security[103]
- Theraplay[104]
- DIR Floortime[105]

SUMMARY

Trauma-informed care is a movement; its primary purpose has been to bring safe and skilled services, as well as compassion and a more humane approach, to working with people with trauma histories. Traumatic experiences are more common than previously thought, to the degree that a universal precautions approach to TIC is recommended. OTPs are qualified mental health practitioners who play a critical role as primary clinicians, as part of interdisciplinary teams, or as administrators, when working with people, organizations, and communities that experience trauma.[63,64,75] As the understanding of the prevalence of trauma among clients across most practice settings continues to rise, there will be a much larger scale adoption of TIC across the many areas of OT practice. This realization and broad-scale implementation will bring with it a significant need for more research, TIC promotion and trauma prevention efforts within and outside the OT profession, and more opportunities for OTPs to take a leadership role in the TIC initiative.

SUGGESTED LEARNING ACTIVITIES

Explore some of the resources listed below and identify three things that you have learned about trauma that supports occupational therapy's role in the TIC initiative.

REFLECTION QUESTIONS

1. How would you define trauma-informed care to someone who is not familiar with it?
2. What types of trauma are you most aware of in the clients you have observed or have worked with, and how has it affected their occupational performance?
3. Why is it important to understand the effects of trauma on clients receiving occupational therapy services?
4. What types of trauma-informed approaches are you most comfortable incorporating into practice?
5. What areas of occupational therapy practice still need to integrate more of a TIC approach, and how can the profession take steps toward recognizing and integrating it into those areas of practice?

ONLINE RESOURCES

- Adverse Childhood Experiences Study: http://www.acestudy.org
- American Occupation Therapy Association: www.aota.org
- Beacon House UK Resources: https://beaconhouse.org.uk/useful-resources
- Building Bridges Initiative: http://www.buildingbridges4youth.org/index.html
- Center for the Study of Traumatic Stress: www.centerforthestudyoftraumaticstress.org
- Child Trauma Academy: http://childtrauma.org
- Child Welfare Information Gateway: Evidence-based practice for child abuse prevention. https://www.childwelfare.gov/topics/preventing/evidence/?hasBeenRedirected=1
- Eight Dimensions of Wellness (video): https://www.youtube.com/watch?v=tDzQdRvLAfM&feature=youtube
- Essentials for Childhood: ttps://www.cdc.gov/violenceprevention/pdf/ essentials_for_childhood_framework.pdf
- Every Moment Counts: http://www.everymomentcounts.org
- International Society for the Study of Trauma and Dissociative Disorders: http://www.isst-d.org
- National Center for PTSD: http://www.ptsd.va.gov/
- National Center for Trauma-Informed Care: https://nasmhpd.org/content/national-center-trauma-informed-care-nctic-0http://www.nasmhpd.org/content/national-center-trauma-informed-care-nctic-0
- National Center on Family Homelessness: http://www.familyhomelessness.org/
- National Child Traumatic Stress Network: www.NCTSN.org
- National Institute for Trauma and Loss in Children: https://www.starr.org/training/tlc
- Massachusetts State Department of Mental Health Seclusion and Restraint Reduction Initiative: http://www.mass.gov/eohhs/gov/departments/dmh/restraintseclusionreduction-initiative.html
- OT Innovations: www.ot-innovations.com
- Substance Abuse Mental Health Services Administration (SAMHSA) Recovery Resources: https://www.samhsa.gov/recovery
- SAMHSA Trauma-Informed Care and Alternatives to Seclusion and Restraint: http://www.samhsa.gov/nctic/trauma-interventions
- Trauma Center: http://www.traumacenter.org
- US Health and Human Services Resilience Resources: https://www.hhs.gov/ash/oah/ adolescent-development/mental-health/positive-mental-health/index.html

REFERENCES

1. President's New Freedom Commission on Mental Health. Achieving the Promise: Transforming Mental Health Care in America. 2003. Available at: https://web. archive. org/ web/20050412233239/http://www. mentalhealthcommission .gov/reports/finalreport/ FullReport.htm.
2. National Association for State Mental Health Program Directors (NASMHPD). *Trauma-Informed Care Module.* Alexandria, VA: NASMHPD, National Technical Assistance Center for State Mental Health Planning; 2003.
3. National Association for State Mental Health Program Directors (NASMHPD). *Trauma-Informed Care (TIC) Planning Guidelines for Use in Developing an Organizational Action Plan: Transforming Cultures of Care Toward Recovery Oriented Services: Guidelines oward Creating a Trauma-Informed System of Care.* Alexandria, VA: NASMHPD; 2005.
4. National Association for State Mental Health Program Directors (NASMHPD). *Trauma-Informed Care Module.* 9th ed. Alexandria, VA: NASMHPD, National Technical Assistance Center for State Mental Health Planning; 2009.
5. Anda RF, Butchart A, Felitti VJ, Brown DW. Building a framework for global surveillance of the public health implications of adverse childhood experiences. *Am J Prev Med.* 2010;39:93-98.
6. Anda RF, Felitti VJ, Bremner JD, et al. The enduring effects of abuse and related adverse experiences of childhood. A convergence of evidence from neurobiology and epidemiology. *Eur Arch Psychiatry Clin Neurosci.* 2006; 256(3):174-186.
7. Felitti VJ, Anda RF, Nordenberg D, et al. Relationship of childhood abuse and household dysfunction to many of the leading causes of death in adults: the Adverse Childhood Experiences (ACE) study. *Am J Prev Med.* 1998;14:245-258.
8. Substance Abuse Mental Health Services Administration. Working Definition of Trauma. 2018. Available at: https:// www.samhsa.gov/trauma-violence.
9. American Psychiatric Association. *Diagnostic and Statistical Manual of Mental Health Disorders.* 5th ed. Washington, DC: Author; 2013.
10. Perry BD. Examining child maltreatment through a neurodevelopmental lens: clinical applications of the neurosequential model of therapeutics. *J Loss Trauma.* 2009;14:240-255.
11. Selye H. *Stress in Health and Disease.* Boston: Butterworth; 1976.
12. Porges SW. The polyvagal theory: phylogenetic substrates of a social nervous system. *Int J Psychophysiol.* 2001;42:123-146.
13. Porges SW. Social engagement and attachment: a phylogenetic perspective. Roots of mental illness in children. *Ann N Y Acad Sci.* 2003;1008:31-47.
14. Porges SW. The polyvagal perspective. *Biol Psychol.* 2007;72: 116-143.
15. McCrory EJ, De Brito SA, Sebastian CL, Mechelli A, Bird G, Kelly PA, et al. Heightened neural reactivity to threat in child victims of family violence. *Curr Biol.* 2011;21:R947-R948.
16. McLaughlin KA, Sheridan MA, Lambert HK. Childhood adversity and neural development: deprivation and threat as distinct dimensions of early experience. *Neurosci Biobehav Rev.* 2014;47:578-591.
17. McLean S. The Effect of Trauma on the Brain Development of Children: Evidence-based Principles for Supporting the Recovery of Children in Care. 2016. Available at: https://aifs .gov.au/cfca/publications/effect-trauma-brain-development-children.
18. Murrough JW, Huang Y, Hu J, et al. Reduced amygdala serotonin transporter binding in posttraumatic stress disorder. *Biol Psychiatry.* 2011;170:1033-1038.
19. Pollak SD, Klorman R, Thatcher JE, Cicchetti D. P3b reflects maltreated children's reactions to facial displays of emotion. *Psychophysiology.* 2001;38:267-274.
20. Pollak SD, Nelson CA, Schlaak MF, et al. Neurodevelopmental effects of early deprivation in post-institutionalized children. *Child Dev.* 2010;81:224-236
21. Pollak SD, Sinha P. Effects of early experience on children's recognition of facial displays of emotion. *Dev Psychopathol.* 2002;38:784-791.
22. De Brito SA, Viding E, Sebastian CL, Palmer AL, Mechelli A, Pingault JB, et al. Reduced orbitofrontal and temporal gray matter in a community sample of maltreated children. *J Child Psychol Psychiatry.* 2013;54:105-112.
23. Kelly PA, Viding E, Wallace GL, Schaer M, De Brito SA, Robustelli B, et al. Cortical thickness, surface area, and gyrification abnormalities in children exposed to maltreatment: neural markers of vulnerability? *Biol Psychiatry.* 2013;74:845-852.
24. Atchison B. Sensory modulation disorders among children with a history of trauma: a frame of reference for speech-language pathologists. *Lang, Speech, Hear Serv Sch.* 2007; 38:109-116.
25. Engel-Yeger B, Palgy-Levin D, Lev-Wiesel R. The relationship between posttraumatic stress disorder and sensory processing patterns. *Occup Ther Ment Health.* 2013;29:266-278.
26. Engel-Yeger B, Palgy-Levin D, Lev-Wiesel, R. Predicting fears of intimacy among individuals with post-traumatic stress symptoms by their sensory profile. *Br J Occup Ther.* 2015;78:51-57.
27. Meyer B, Ajchenbrenner M, Bowles DP. Sensory sensitivity, attachment experiences, and rejection responses among adults with borderline and avoidant features. *J Pers Disord.* 2005;19(6):641-658.
28. Rabellino D, Densmore M, Theberge J, McKinnon M, Lanius R. The cerebellum after trauma: resting-state functional connectivity of the cerebellum in posttraumatic stress disorder and its dissociative subtype. *Hum Brain Mapp.* 2018;1-21.
29. Sherain H, Nicholson A, Densmore M, Théberge J, McKinnon MC, Neufeld RWJ, et al. Sensory overload and imbalance: resting-state vestibular connectivity in PTSD and its dissociative subtype. *Neuropsychologia.* 2017;106:169-178.
30. Van der Kolk B, Rosh S, Pelcovitz D, Sunday S, Spinnazzola J. Disorders of extreme stress: The empirical foundation of a complex adaptation to trauma. *J Trauma Stress.* 2005;18(5): 389-399.
31. Van der Kolk B. Clinical implications of neuroscience research and PTSD. *Ann N Y Acad Sci.* 2006;1071:277-293.

32. Levine P. *Healing Trauma: A Pioneering Program for Restoring the Wisdom of Your Body*. Boulder, CO: Sounds True; 2005.

33. Perry BD, Szalavitz M. *The Boy Who Was Raised as a Dog: and Other Stories from a Child Psychiatrist's Notebook*. New York: Basic Books; 2017.

34. Schore A. Complex trauma in childhood and adolescence. Relational trauma, brain development, and dissociation. In: Ford JD, Courtois CA, eds. *Treating Complex Traumatic Stress Disorders in Children and Adolescents: Scientific Foundation and Therapeutic Models*. New York: Guilford Press; 2013:91-113

35. Champagne T, Saccomandi N. *Effects of Developmental Trauma on Sensory Processing and Participation*. Presented at the Massachusetts Occupational Therapy Association's Spring Conference, Boston; 2017.

36. Centers for Disease Control and Prevention. *The ACE Pyramid*. 2016. Available at: https://www.cdc.gov/violenceprevention/acestudy/about.html.

37. US Department of Health and Human Services. Child Welfare Outcomes: Report to Congress. 2015. Available at: https://www.acf.hhs.gov/sites/default/files/cb/cwo2015.pdf.

38. Krantz DS, Whittaker KS, Sheps DS. Psychosocial risk factors for coronary artery disease: pathophysiologic mechanisms. In: R. Allan and J. Fisher, eds., *Heart and Mind: Evolution of Cardiac Psychology*. Washington, DC: APA; 2011.

39. Miller GE, Chen E, Parker KJ. Psychological stress in childhood and susceptibility to the chronic diseases of aging: moving toward a model of behavioral and biological mechanisms. *Psychol Bull*. 2011;137:959-997.

40. Widom C, Czaja S, Bently T, Johnson M. A prospective investigation of health outcomes in abused and neglected children: new findings in a 30-year follow-up. *Am J Public Health*. 2012;102(6):1135-1144.

41. Bartlett J, Griffin J, Spinnazzola J, et al. The affect of state-wide trauma-informed care initiative in child welfare on the well-being of children and youth with complex trauma. *Child Youth Serv Rev*. 2018;84:110-117.

42. Yanos PT, Czaja SJ, Widom CS. A prospective examination of service use by abused and neglected children followed up into adulthood. *Psychiatric Serv*. 2010;61(8):796-802.

43. Luxenberg T, Spinazzola J, Hidalgo J, Hunt C, van der Kolk, B. Complex trauma and disorders of extreme stress (DESNOS) diagnosis, part two: treatment. *Dir Psychiatr*. 2001;21:373-392.

44. van der Kolk B. Developmental trauma disorder. *Psychiatric Ann*. 2005;35:401-408.

45. van der Kolk B. *The Body Keeps Score: Mind, Brain, and Body in the Healing of Trauma*. New York: Penguin Books; 2014.

46. LeBel J, Champagne T. Integrating sensory and trauma-informed interventions: a Massachusetts state initiative, part 2. *Mental Health Spec Interest Sect Q*. 2010;33(2):1-4.

47. Huckshorn KA, LeBel J. Trauma-informed care. In: Svendsen D, Yeager K, eds. *Textbook of Modern Community Mental Health Work: An Interdisciplinary Approach*. New York: Oxford University Press; 2013:62-83.

48. Substance Abuse Mental Health Services Administration. Guiding principles of trauma-informed care. *SAMHSA News*. 2014;22(2):1.

49. Bonanno G. Loss, trauma. And human resilience. *Am Psychol*. 2004;59:20-28.

50. Bonanno GA, Mancini AD. The human capacity to thrive in the face of extreme adversity. *Pediatrics*. 2008;121:369-375.

51. Feder Charney, Collins. Neurobiology of resilience. In: Southwick S, Litz B, Charney D, Friedman M, eds. *Resilience and Mental Health: Challenges Across the Lifespan*. Cambridge, MA: Cambridge University Press; 2011:1-15.

52. Substance Abuse Mental Health Services Administration. *Trauma-informed care in behavioral health services*. Rockville, MD: Author; 2014.

53. Centers for Disease Control and Prevention. Youth violence: risk and protective factors. 2017. Available at: https://www.cdc.gov/violenceprevention/youthviolence/riskprotectivefactors.html.

54. Child Welfare Information Gateway. Risk and Protective Factors for Child Abuse and Neglect. 2004. Available at: https://www.childwelfare.gov/pubPDFs/risk protectivefactors.pdf.

55. Substance Abuse Mental Health Services Administration. Trauma-Informed Approach. 2018. Available at: https://www.samhsa.gov/nctic/trauma-interventions.

56. World Health Organization and International Society for Prevention of Child Abuse and Neglect. *Preventing Child Maltreatment: A Guide to Taking Action and Generating Evidence*. Geneva (Switzerland): World Health Organization; 2006.

57. National Association for State Mental Health Program Directors. *National Executive Training Institute Curriculum for the Creation of Violence-free and Coercion-free Treatment Settings and the Reduction of Seclusion and Restraint*. 11th ed. Alexandria, VA: Author; 2013.

58. Substance Abuse Mental Health Service Administration. Trauma-Informed Care and Alternatives to Seclusion and Restraint. 2015. Available at: http://www. samhsa.gov/nctic/trauma-interventions.

59. Blau G, Caldwell B, Lieberman R. *Residential Interventions for Children, Adolescents, and Families: A Best Practice Guide*. New York: Routledge; 2014.

60. Porter L, Martin K, Anda R. Self-healing communities: a transformational model for improving intergenerational health (executive summary). 2016. Available at: https://rwjf.org/en/library/research/2016/06/self-healing-communities.html.

61. Morgan GB. *Building Community Capacity: A Qualitative Study*. [Unpublished doctoral dissertation.] Seattle, WA: Seattle University; 2015.

62. Scheuler V, Goldstein-Cole K, Longhi D. *Projected Cost Savings Due to Caseloads Avoided: Technical Notes*. Olympia, WA: Washington State Family Policy Council; 2009.

63. American Occupational Therapy Association. Mental health promotion, prevention, and intervention in occupational therapy practice. *Am J Occup Ther*. 2014;64:S30-S43.

64. Champagne T. *Sensory Modulation in Dementia Care: Assessment and Activities for Sensory Enriched Care*. London, UK: Jessica Kingsley; 2018.

65. Bazyk S. Promotion of positive mental health in children and youth with developmental disabilities. *OT Pract*. 2010; 15(7):CE-1-CE-8.

66. Bazyk, S. *Mental Health Promotion, Prevention, and Intervention with Children and Youth: A Guiding Framework for Occupational Therapy.* Bethesda, MD: AOTA; 2011.

67. Champagne T. *Sensory Modulation and Environment: Essential Elements of Occupation.* 3rd ed, rev. Sydney, Australia: Pearson; 2011.

68. Champagne T. *AOTA Societal statement: stress, trauma and posttraumatic stress disorder.* 2017. Available at: https://www.aota.org/~/media/Corporate/Files/AboutAOTA/.OfficialDocs/SocStmtPTSD-fin. pdf.

69. Jerath R, Barnes VA, Crawford MW. Mind-body response and neurophysiological changes during stress and meditation: central role of homeostasis. *J Biol Regul Homeost Agents.* 2014;24:545-554.

70. Rogers C, Mallinson T, Peppers D. High-intensity sports for posttraumatic stress disorder and depression: feasibility study of ocean therapy with veteran of operation enduring freedom and operation Iraqi freedom. *Am Occup Ther Assoc.* 2014;68:395-404.

71. Stoller C, Greuel J, Cimini L, Fowler M, Koomar J. Effects of sensory-enhanced yoga on symptoms of combat stress in deployed military personnel. *Am Occup Ther Assoc.* 2012;66:59-68.

72. Substance Abuse Mental Health Services Administration. *Wellness initiative.* 2017. Available at: https://www.samhsa.gov/wellness-initiative.

73. Substance Abuse and Mental Health Services Administration. (2012). *SAMHSA's working definition of recovery.* Available at https://store.samhsa.gov/system/files/pep12-recdef.pdf

74. Substance Abuse Mental Health Services Administration. *Recovery and Recovery Support.* 2017. Available at: https://www.samhsa.gov/recovery.

75. American Occupational Therapy Association. Occupational therapy practice framework: domain and process. *Am J Occup Ther.* 2014b;68:S1-S51.

76. Massachusetts Department of Mental Health. Resource Guide: Creating Positive Cultures of Care. 2013. Available at: https://www.mass.gov/files/documents/2016/07/vq/restraint-resources.pdf.

77. Herman J. *Trauma and Recovery: The Aftermath of Violence—From Domestic Abuse and Political Terror.* New York: Basic Books; 1992.

78. Cook A, Spinnazzola J, Ford J, et al. Complex trauma in children and adolescents. *Psychiatr Ann.* 2005;35(5):390-398.

79. Melby-Lervag M, Hulme C. Is working memory training effective: A meta-analytic review. *Dev Psychol.* 2013;49:270-291.

80. Perry BD. The neurosequential model of therapeutics: applying principles of neuroscience to clinical work with traumatized and maltreated children. In: Boyd Webb N, ed. *Working with Traumatized Youth in Child Welfare.* New York: Guilford Press; 2006:22-52.

81. Champagne T. Attachment, trauma and occupational therapy practice. *OT Pract.* 2011;16:CE1-CE8.

82. Jaffee SR, Bowes L, Ouellet-Morin I, Fisher HL, Moffitt TE, Merrick MT, et al. Safe, stable, nurturing relationships break the intergenerational cycle of abuse: a prospective nationally representative cohort of children in the United Kingdom. *J Adolesc Health.* 2013;53:S4-S10.

83. Merrick M, Leeb R, Lee R. Examining the role of safe, stable, and nurturing relationships in the intergenerational continuity of child maltreatment. Introduction to the special issue. *J Adolesc Health.* 2013;53:S1-S3.

84. Schofield T, Lee R, Merrick M. Safe, stable, nurturing relationships as a moderator of intergenerational continuity of child maltreatment: a meta-analysis. *J Adolesc Health.* 2013;53:S32-S38.

85. Champagne T. Creating occupational therapy groups for children and youth in community-based mental health practice. *OT Pract.* 2012;13-18.

86. Champagne T. The influence of posttraumatic stress disorder depression and sensory processing patterns on occupational engagement: a case study. *WORK: J Prev Assess Rehabil.* 2011;38(1):67-75.

87. Ayres AJ. *Sensory Integration and the Child.* Los Angeles: Western Psychological Services; 1979.

88. Champagne T, Stromberg N. Sensory approaches in inpatient psychiatric settings: innovative alternatives to seclusion and restraint. *J Psychosoc Nurs.* 2004;42:35-44.

89. Novak T, Scanlan J, McCaul D, MacDonald N, Clarke T. Pilot study of a sensory room in an acute inpatient psychiatric unit. *Aust Psychiatry.* 2012;20:401-440

90. Sutton D, Nicholson E. *Sensory Modulation in Acute Mental Health Wards: A Qualitative Study of Staff and Service user Perspectives.* 2011. Available at: http://aut.researchgateway. ac.nz/bitstream/handle/10292/4312/Sutton%20sensory%20modulation%20in%20acute%20mental%20health%20wards.pdf?sequence=6.

91. Sutton D, Wilson M, Van Kessel K, Vanderpyl J. Optimizing arousal to manage aggression: a pilot study of sensory modulation. *Int J Ment Health Nurs.* 2013;22:500-511.

92. Gronski, MP, Bogan KE, Kloeckner J, Russell-Thomas D, Taff SD, Walker KA, et al. Childhood toxic stress: a community role in health promotion for occupational therapists. *Am J Occup Ther.* 2013;67:148-153.

93. LeBel J, Champagne T, Stromberg N, Coyle R. Integrating sensory and trauma-informed interventions: a Massachusetts state initiative, part 1. *Mental Health Spec Interest Sect Q.* 2010;33(1):1-4.

94. LeBel J, Champagne T. Integrating sensory and trauma-informed interventions: a Massachusetts state initiative, part 2. *Mental Health Spec Interest Sect Q.* 2010;33(2):1-4.

95. Kabat-Zinn, J. *Coming to Our Senses: Healing Ourselves and the World Through Mindfulness.* New York: Hyperion; 2005.

96. Smith-Forbes E, Najera C, Hawkins D. Combat operational stress control in Iraq and Afghanistan: Army occupational therapy. *Mil Med.* 2014;179:279-284.

97. Solomon E, Solomon R, Heide K. EMDR: evidenced-based treatment for victims of trauma. *Vict Offender.* 2009;4:391-397.

98. Cohen JA, Mannarino AP, Iyengar S. Community treatment of posttraumatic stress disorder for children exposed to intimate partner violence: a randomized controlled trial. *Arch Pediatr Adolesc Med.* 2011;165(1):16-21.

99. Blaustein M, Kinniburgh K. *Treating Traumatic Stress in Children and Adolescents: How to Foster Resilience Through Attachment, Regulation and Competency*. New York: Guilford Press; 2010.

100. Linehan M. *Skills Training Manual for Treating Borderline Personality Disorder*. New York: Guilford Press; 1993.

101. Matulis S, Resick PA, Rosner R, Steil R. Developmentally adapted cognitive processing therapy for adolescents suffering from posttraumatic stress disorder after childhood sexual or physical abuse: A pilot study. *Clin Child Fam Psychol Rev*. 2013;17:173-190.

102. Ogden P, Minton K, Pain C. *Trauma and the Body: A Sensorimotor Approach to Psychotherapy*. New York: WW Norton; 2007.

103. Powell B, Cooper G, Hoffman K, Marvin B. *The Circle of Security Intervention: Enhancing Attachment in Early Parent-Child Relationships*. New York: Guilford Press; 2013.

104. Booth P, Jernberg J. *Theraplay: Helping Parents and Children Build Better Relationships Through Play*. San Francisco: Wiley; 2010.

105. Greenspan S, Wieder L. *Engaging Autism: Using the Floortime Approach to Help Children Relate Communicate and Think*. Cambridge, MA: Perseus Books; 2006.

106. Bonanno GA, Mancini AD. The human capacity to thrive in the face of extreme adversity. *Pediatrics*. 2008;121:369-375.

107. Bowlby J. *A Secure Base: Parent-Child Attachment and Healthy Human Development*. New York: Basic Books; 1988.

108. McCrory E, De Brito SA, Viding E. Research review: the neurobiology and genetics of maltreatment and adversity. *J Child Psychol Psychiatry*. 2010;51:1079-1095.

109. Reynolds AJ, Robertson DL. School-based early intervention and later child maltreatment in the Chicago Longitudinal Study. *Child Development,* 2003;74:3-26.

110. Thompson M. *Trauma Resilience Scale for Children: Validation of Protective Factors Associated with Positive Adaptation Following Violence* [dissertation]. Tallahassee, FL: Florida State University; 2010.

111. US Department of Health and Human Services. Developing trauma-informed systems of care. 2003. Available at: https://www.nasmhpd.org/sites/default/files/ TraumaExpertsMtgreport-final.pdf.

18

Wellness, Prevention, and Advocacy

Carol Lambdin-Pattavina

LEARNING OBJECTIVES

1. Understand the concepts of wellness, prevention, and advocacy for mental health.
2. Assess the current state of mental health in the United States and the health disparities of those diagnosed with a mental illness.
3. Describe the frameworks for prevention, wellness, and advocacy as related to mental health and well-being.
4. Discuss examples of complementary approaches for wellness.
5. Articulate occupational therapy's role and opportunities in mental health prevention, wellness, and advocacy.

INTRODUCTION

Dr. Brock Chisholm, the first Director-General of the World Health Organization (WHO), is credited with coining the now familiar truism, "without mental health there can be no true physical health,"[1] which, in popular culture, has been shortened to "there is no health without mental health." In lay terms, there is a direct and inextricable link between our physical and mental health; one affects the other, and the whole person must be addressed and supported at all times in any health care environment if optimal health is to be achieved. Individual journeys of recovery through mental illness have been formally documented for over 200 years[2,3]; the outgrowth of these voices is our current recovery-oriented mental health system, which is the antithesis of the more reductionistic medical approach that reigned in the United States during most of the 20th century. The Recovery Model formally became part of the national landscape when the Substance Abuse and Mental Health Services Administration (SAMHSA) hosted the National Summit on Mental Health Recovery in 2006 and published the subsequent *National Consensus Statement on Mental Health Recovery*.[4] Unlike the previous approach to mental illness, which focused heavily on symptom reduction, the Recovery Model charges the service user with directing their own recovery and becoming more proactive in preventing illness, thus augmenting efforts to improve their wellness and advocating for continued services and supports needed to experience a life well-lived.

Occupational therapy's tradition of client-centeredness, holism, and focus on prevention, wellness, and advocacy can be traced back to its inception in 1917, and is a perfect fit for the current climate of mental health care in this country. Mary Reilly's famous 1961 quote "Man, through the use of his hands, as they are energized by mind and will, can influence the state of his own health,"[5] speaks directly to our ability potentially to alter the course of our health through the choices that we make. Occupational therapists are poised to support individuals, communities, and populations in accessing and developing the relevant information and skills needed to move toward greater health and wellness. In this chapter, we will explore concepts related to prevention, wellness, and advocacy, including definitions, national prevention efforts, wellness and advocacy initiatives, relationship of these constructs to the practice of occupational therapy, and intervention implications for those living with a label of mental illness. Also, we will explore frameworks that can be used in occupational therapy practice to support these interventions. Finally, we will explore complementary and integrative therapies, evidence related to these therapies, and how they can be used by and with service users as interventions to enhance their health and wellness.

Modern definitions of health are slowly coming full circle to the more holistic sensibilities regarding health set forth by the Greeks; modern health has come to mean so much more than simply the absence of disease, as articulated by a series of seminal documents and proclamations. In 1948, WHO provided a definition of health in its constitution, which read, "Health is a state of complete physical, mental and social well-being and not merely the absence of disease or infirmity. The enjoyment of the highest attainable standard of health is one of the fundamental rights of every human being without distinction of race, religion, political belief, economic or social condition."[6]

An earlier version of WHO's global strategy additionally cited literacy, undernutrition, and constant engagement in survival-related activities as contributing factors to poorer health outcomes.[7] In 1986, the first International Conference on Health Promotion was held in Ottawa, Canada, and resulted in the publication of the Ottawa Charter (Box 18.1; Fig. 18.1). The charter introduced the notion that health is

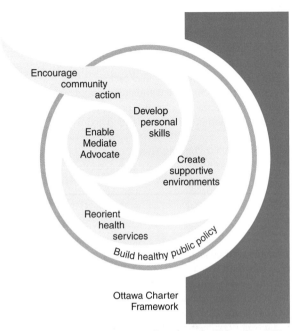

Fig. 18.1 The Ottawa Charter. (Courtesy the Whanganui District Health Board; available at: https://wdhb.org.nz.)

BOX 18.1 Ottawa Charter: Key Actions Necessary for Health Promotion

Building healthy public policy: Provide additional education and training to future and current occupational therapy practitioners in advocacy and political activism to effect policy change at the local, state and national levels.

Creating supportive environments: Work interprofessionally to support environmental changes that will enable individuals, communities, and populations to make choices that support healthier lifestyles.

Strengthening community action: Teach and support communities to self-advocate for their members and teach skills necessary for communities to increase self-sufficiency and sustainability.

Developing personal skills: Address ambivalence related to making healthier life choices through motivational interviewing, provide ongoing education related to health, and teach skills necessary to engage in health-promoting activities and occupations.

Reorienting health care services toward prevention of illness and promotion of health: Increase research efforts to further demonstrate the health benefits of occupational participation, explore interprofessional opportunities to initiate or join community-based prevention efforts, and focus on education related to preventing further complications and illness for those already receiving services.

Adapted from The Ottawa Charter for Health Promotion. Available at: http://www.who.int/healthpromotion/conferences/previous/ottawa/en/index1.html.

a dynamic interaction between the individual and their contexts and environments[8]; humans are not merely passive recipients of states of health or illness, but rather agents who can change modifiable risk factors. As health care workers, we must understand the influence that motivation has on decisions related to personal, community, and population health. Most recently, WHO has been grappling with how best to include spirituality into the dimensions of health.[9] Spirituality speaks to a sense of fulfillment, peace, self-concept, and feelings of wholeness and relatedness to the world at large[10] that comes from being deeply rooted in daily activities (doing) while simultaneously being detached enough (being) to release and replace anger, ego, and jealousy with compassion, love, and equanimity.[9] This process results in "becoming" or transforming into our authentic selves, as Wilcock described in her seminal article, "Reflections on Doing, Being and Becoming."[11] This recent recognition by WHO more closely reflects the holistic or mind-body-spirit nature of occupational therapy practice. Definitions of health have and continue to morph because no one definition perfectly threads together the nuances, internal and external to the individual, community, or population that can create a state of health.

Prevention

Prevention of costly illnesses, injuries, and ultimately disability has gained national prominence and momentum

BOX 18.2   **Primary Prevention Exemplars**

AOTA Backpack Awareness Day: A national campaign to prevent future pain and injury that can result from improperly packing and wearing a backpack.

Let's Move: A national campaign initiated by First Lady Michelle Obama to prevent obesity by encouraging youth engagement in healthy eating and exercise habits and routine.

Campaign for Tobacco-Free Kids: A global campaign targeting youth that seeks to prevent future illness and death caused by smoking.

AOTA, American Occupational Therapy Association

BOX 18.3   **Examples of Primary Mental Wellness Intervention**

Every Moment Counts: A mental health promotion initiative developed by occupational therapist, Susan Bazyk, to support mental wellness in school-based settings.

I'm Thumbody: A program for kindergarten-age children to enhance self-esteem and uniqueness sponsored by an affiliate of Mental Health America.

May is Mental Health Month: A month-long informational endeavor sponsored by Mental Health America to raise awareness of the impact of overall wellness on mental health.

over the past 60 years. Prevention is generally conceptualized based on when intervention occurs to prevent further decline or complications. The most common framework for categorizing levels of intervention stem from the work of Leavell and Clark, who first described prevention tiers in their text, *Textbook of Preventive Medicine*.[12] These tiers included primary, secondary, and tertiary. At the primary level, prevention efforts seek to intervene where no illness, injury, and/or disability previously existed. Primary interventions include development of local, state, and national initiatives and policies, as well as campaigns such as anti-smoking, getting a yearly flu shot, and healthy eating (Box 18.2). Secondary prevention efforts target individuals, communities, and populations that are at greater risk due to social determinants of health and health-related disparities. These efforts may include health screenings related to blood pressure, alcohol use, and diabetes and health-related informational or activity groups related to topics such as effective parenting, exercise, nutrition, and health outcomes of illicit drug use. Finally, tertiary intervention is tailored to health challenges that have already manifested as a result of an illness, injury, or disability. Tertiary level interventions seek to prevent further complications associated with or progression of the condition.[13] In addition to this older three-level classification model of interventions, an additional taxonomy of prevention classification was introduced by the Institute of Medicine in 1994. This included universal, selective, and indicated prevention. Universal prevention efforts target populations at large, selective prevention targets groups or individuals who are at risk, and indicated prevention efforts target those who manifest early symptoms of a condition but who have not yet been diagnosed.[14] Overlap exists in each of these classification systems; the consensus is that efforts be concentrated on preventing costly conditions from occurring—costly in terms of direct costs to the system

and consumers, indirect costs associated with lost wages and consumerism, and costs associated with social injustices arising from inequitable care.

Primary, secondary, and tertiary prevention efforts targeting mental health have gained increasing momentum in the United States as a result of the growing recognition that mental illness is not a "sentence to a bleak and painful life."[15] In fact, greater awareness of the impact of genetics and epigenetics, social determinants of health, trauma, and brain mapping has greatly altered the historic narrative that mental illness could be improved by better parenting, lowering one's stress levels, or simply willing oneself to be better. With nearly one in four people experiencing a mental health challenge over the course of their lifetime, efforts to thwart preventable illnesses and promote overall mental well-being have been garnering significant attention.[16]

Primary intervention to support mental health and wellness has included programs targeting children and youth to promote self-esteem and positive coping skills, national campaigns promoting mental wellness and providing information regarding the positive relationship between physical and mental health, and policies that indirectly support mental well-being, such as mandating that healthy beverages be made available in vending machines in school settings. See Box 18.3.

Secondary interventions targeting those already at risk include screenings performed by primary care physicians and others to assess risk for development of a mental illness, School-based support programs and groups for students who may struggle with self-reported challenges including bullying and extension of health coverage for those in higher-risk categories. Tertiary interventions are those most familiar to occupational therapy practitioners because these are the daily occupation-based interventions provided to support service users to prevent further complications and decline in their mental well-being. See Box 18.4.

> **BOX 18.4 Examples of Secondary Mental Wellness Intervention**
>
> Screening Depository: Free screening tools for mental health conditions such as depression, anxiety, and psychosis provided online at Mental Health America.
>
> Screening, Brief Intervention, and Referral to Treatment (SBIRT): Program developed by the Substance Abuse Mental Health Services Administration to capture those at risk for development of a substance use disorder.
>
> Adverse Childhood Experiences (ACE) screenings: Offered via primary and behavioral health care providers to capture those whose history of adverse childhood events such as domestic violence or divorce puts them at increased risk for physical illness such as heart disease and diabetes.

Wellness

If health is more representative of the product of health-related efforts, such as weight, body mass index, and blood pressure, which fall within person-specific limits, then wellness can be compared to the process of generating those outcomes. Wellness is generally viewed as being a state comprised of multiple dimensions, including physical, emotional, and social wellness. Although variables such as genetics predict or even predetermine health status to some degree, wellness involves active engagement on the part of the individual, community, and/or population by choosing to engage in health promotion and supporting activities and occupations. Efforts to support engagement in wellness practices, such as prevention, can occur at the individual, community, or population level. Unlike prevention, where the onus for prevention-oriented efforts is often shared by health care professionals and service users, wellness typically involves maximum participation on the part of the individual, community, or population to manifest a state of wellness—wellness implies choice and, by deduction, implies action. SAMHSA has sponsored a Wellness Initiative,[17] which provides information, resources, and links to support others in developing or augmenting wellness initiatives (see resource list).

Advocacy

If efforts to prevent mental illness rest largely with the "system," including federal entities, systems of health care, and direct care workers, and wellness rests largely with those who act to enhance their current state, then advocacy rests with all interested parties from the politician to the clinician to the individual affected by a mental illness. The dictionary defines advocacy as "the act or process of supporting a cause or proposal."[18] Hence advocacy efforts are unique and dependent on the cause for which an individual, community, or population are advocating. WHO[19] defines advocacy related to mental health as "a relatively new concept, developed with a view to reducing stigma and discrimination, and promoting the human rights of people with mental disorders. It consists of various actions aimed at changing the major structural and attitudinal barriers to achieving positive mental health outcomes in populations."

WHO has proposed nine principles of advocacy, including awareness raising, information, education, training, mutual help, counseling, mediating, defending, and denouncing. Each principle implies action taking—actions that can be taken at all levels, including service users, providers, allies, and politicians.[19] See Table 18.1.

CURRENT STATE OF MENTAL HEALTH IN THE UNITED STATES

What constitutes a national mental health and subsequent public health crisis has yet to be well defined. If the incidence of diagnosable mental illness is trending upward, there is decreased access to and coverage for mental health services,[20] or there is a disease burden for mental and substance use disorders that is higher than any other illness,[21] then the United States is experiencing a crisis of epic proportions. According to the 2018 State of Mental Health in America report, 43 million US citizens have a diagnosed mental health condition. Of those, approximately half have a co-occurring substance use disorder. Every day, 115 people overdose from opiates in the United States,[13] and 30% of those who have been prescribed opioids for chronic pain have misused these drugs.[22] Nearly 10 million Americans have experienced suicidal ideation, and yet the mental health workforce has sharply declined, and access to care becomes an increasing challenge for those who struggle.[20] Currently, 56% of those living with a mental health condition are unable to access needed services. With proposed changes to Medicaid, a primary provider for community-based mental health services, this percentage is expected to increase.[23]

Shortages of mental health professionals has been reaching epic proportions, with a current 6.4% shortage in the psychiatry workforce. By 2025, that percentage is expected to rise to 12%, which translates to a deficit of nearly 7000 psychiatrists needed to treat those who have been diagnosed with a mental health condition.[24] The picture of mental health for children and youth is even more alarming. Within the past 5 years, the prevalence of teen depression has increased from 5.9% to 8.2%, 1.7 million teens with depressive episodes did not receive treatment,[18] and

TABLE 18.1   WHO Principles of Mental Health Advocacy: Suggestions for Action Taking by Occupational Therapy Practitioners

Principle	Individual	Community	Population
Awareness raising	Screen for mental health challenges	Participate in a yearly NAMI walk in your area.	Attend national conferences sponsored by professional organizations other than those targeting occupational therapy practitioners.
Information	Provide literature about mental health and wellness in your practice setting	Ensure that local schools and public gathering sites have access to evidence-based information from reputable sources such as MHA and SAMHSA.	Add to the body of knowledge by conducting research and disseminating findings.
Education	Provide education to all clients regarding ways to maintain and support positive mental health and wellness	Support and provide informational sessions at community gatherings.	Develop and provide programs such as national podcasts, blogs, and webinars, educating practitioners about the role of occupational therapy in mental health and wellness.
Training	Encourage peers to become intentional peer specialist if desired	Provide onsite trainings for staff and peers regarding the importance of mental health to overall wellness.	Train other professionals about the importance of occupation engagement to overall health and well-being.
Denouncing	Encourage and enforce zero tolerance for stigmatizing language in the workplace	Take opportunities to speak about the power of language and the importance of using person-first language.	Participate in national campaigns such as StigmaFree sponsored by NAMI.
Mutual Help	Encourage a positive work atmosphere to support mental health in the workplace	Start a peer to peer mentor program in the community.	Join a community of practice (CoP) around the issue of mental health and OTs role is supporting those who struggle.
Counseling	Encourage clients to seek additional support if their concerns are beyond the scope of your practice	Become part of a network of mental health professionals to enable referrals as needed.	Engage in national efforts that destigmatize those seeking help to maintain mental wellness.
Mediating	Serve as a health advocate for those struggling with a mental health challenge	Support expansion of mental health services in your community.	Serve on national boards such as AOTA to advocate for occupational therapy's role in mental health and wellness.
Defending	When anyone uses stigmatizing language, be the first to correct their phrasing (kindly)	Walk the talk, and be willing to disclose personal struggles to benefit the community.	Vote for those in favor of supporting mental health initiatives and funding.

AOTA, American Occupational Therapy Association; *MHA,* Mental Health America; *NAMI,* National Alliance on Mental Illness; *SAMHSA,* Substance Abuse and Mental Health Services Administration.

suicide is the third leading cause of death in those ages 10 to 24 years.[25] Whether the apparent "crisis" is due to an increase in the US population[26] or a greater willingness to disclose a mental health condition in the wake of major antistigma campaigns,[27] the implications are the same. Prevention efforts must be augmented at all levels of intervention, a wellness-oriented lifestyle must become the norm rather than the exception, and service providers and users must unite to advocate for evidence-based, person-centered supports to enable access to a full spectrum of occupational choices and participation.

HEALTH DISPARITIES OF THOSE DIAGNOSED WITH A MENTAL ILLNESS

The numbers do not lie; mental health challenges are on the rise and, as much as they may represent a personal crisis, they represent a public health crisis as well. Members of our community who experience a mental health condition are likely experiencing health disparities. According to *Healthy People 2020*, a health disparity is defined as[28]:

> a particular type of health difference that is closely linked with social, economic, and/or environmental disadvantage. Health disparities adversely affect groups of people who have systematically experienced greater obstacles to health based on their racial or ethnic group; religion; socioeconomic status; gender; age; mental health; cognitive, sensory, or physical disability; sexual orientation or gender identity; geographic location; or other characteristics historically linked to discrimination or exclusion.

Mental illness is no respecter of persons; people of all races, ethnicities and genders can and do develop mental health conditions. Health disparities arise due to access and quality of care afforded to those who struggle. These disparities often result from social and economic inequities that translate to poorer health outcomes. It has been well established that those with a severe and chronic mental illness die 10 to 25 years earlier than their counterparts who have not experienced a severe and chronic mental illness.[29] What accounts for this significant differential? Those diagnosed with a mental health condition, particularly those with a severe and chronic condition, are at greater risk for a number of health conditions related to the following[30-32]:

- Low socioeconomic status, which limits coverage and hence access to needed services, including medications and follow-up care
- Sedentary lifestyle due to side effects of many psychotropic medications that can promote obesity and lethargy
- Limited access to wellness-rich practices and environments

- Stigma that limits or prevents participation in the community that could nurture psychoemotional and physical health
- Health practices that reflect lack of resources

Poor health–promoting routines, including smoking, poor eating habits, and poor sleep hygiene, suicide, cardiovascular disease, and cancer are largely responsible for the decrease in life expectancy in this population.[33] Suicide is the tenth leading cause of death in the United States, and nearly 50,000 lives are claimed each year by suicide, a rate twice that of those lost to homicide.[34] The rate of cardiovascular disease (CVD) is two or three times higher in those diagnosed with a mental health condition than in the general population.[35] Contributors to CVD include obesity, diabetes, high cholesterol levels, and hypertension. Results from the Clinical Antipsychotic Trials of Intervention Effectiveness (CATIE) have indicated that individuals with severe and persistent mental illness experience diabetes at rates four times higher than the matched control population and hypertension rates twice those of the control group.[36] Many of the contributing factors to the high incidence of CVD are modifiable, including poor diet and smoking. Some are related to medications used to treat the symptoms of the mental illness, which can result in the metabolic syndrome (a cluster of symptoms that increases the risk of CVD). Other factors include poor access to and inadequate mental health care, as well as the stigma associated with mental illness, which often prevents individuals from wanting to interact with health care in all realms.[35] Those with a mental illness experience cancer at rates similar to those in the general population. Interestingly, cancer proves more fatal (30% higher mortality rate) for those with a mental illness than for those without.[33] Hypotheses regarding this health disparity relate to poorer access to advanced screenings, limited access to specialists and advanced care, and insurance-related limitations on access to needed medications.[33]

In addition to poorer physical health status resulting from issues directly related to a mental illness, those who struggle with a mental health condition are often diagnosed with a co-occurring substance use disorder. Nearly 8 million people are diagnosed with a co-occurring substance use disorder, and those with a mental illness are more likely to be diagnosed with a substance use disorder than the general population.[37] It can be difficult to determine which diagnosis manifested first but, in either case, the resulting challenges of managing two significant diagnoses can become a "merry go round" that seemingly will not come to a complete stop. Symptoms related to the mental illness may result in increased use of substances to cope with the exacerbation. As a result of increased substance use, symptoms related to the mental illness, such as depression and feelings of hopelessness or anxiety and uncontrolled fears, may accelerate. In many cases, one diagnosis may be addressed to the exclusion of the other. This is an approach that is outdated, and all presenting diagnoses and concerns must be addressed simultaneously to achieve the best outcomes.[38]

Occupational implications of these health disparities, specifically the disparity of having a mental illness and associated implications and complications, are numerous and cannot be underestimated. As a result of the waiting process—waiting to gain access to services, waiting for medications to take effect, waiting to be more recovered to engage with an occupational life—activity patterns in those with a mental health condition are frequently disrupted.[39]

FRAMEWORKS FOR PREVENTION, WELLNESS, AND ADVOCACY TO GUIDE OCCUPATIONAL THERAPY INTERVENTION

From its inception, the profession of occupational therapy has been guided by principles of wellness and a desire to support individuals, communities, and populations in reaching their full and desired potential as occupational beings. Individuals who have been labeled with a mental illness are at greater risk for poorer health,[40-42] and wellness practices by and with this population have been largely overlooked due to health disparities.[43,44]

As is the case in all practice settings and with all consumers of occupational therapy services, occupational therapists are compelled to base their approach in theory that explains the phenomenon in question and provides a path to creating a framework for subsequent intervention. Engaging in the processes of prevention, wellness, and advocacy are no different, and all relate back to the foundational roots of the profession—most specifically, humanism. Humanism arguably dates to ancient Greece and Rome and, since then, has been subdivided into other categories. Definitions will vary, depending on the type of humanism to which one is referring. Used in this context, humanism will refer to the principles on which occupational therapy was founded; these include principles of holism, the belief that all humans are inherently good and possess potential to do good, and that therapy can and should highlight strengths rather than weaknesses. In keeping with humanism, therapists can look to Moral Treatment, the Recovery Model, Swarbrick's Eight Dimensions of Wellness, and the Occupational Therapy Practice Framework III to drive the clinical reasoning process with regard to prevention, wellness, and advocacy.

"Moral Treatment" was coined by Philippe Pinel in the 17th century. Pinel, 1745–1826, was a French physician who worked at the Hospice de Bicètre. Under his direction,

and much to the consternation of the other physicians, he ordered that the asylum inmates be released from the shackles that bound them. Contrary to popular thought, these men did not capture guards and seize the asylum; rather, they flourished in their new environment that was now predicated on approaching the inmates as humans, full of potential, who could lead productive lives. His belief that those suffering from mental illness were not evil but warranted care and compassion was radical and initially not well received. His work, however, was a precursor to the profession of occupational therapy and set a precedent of enabling those with whom we collaborate to design and lead an occupational fulfilling life.

Now, occupational therapists can look to the Recovery Model to frame prevention, wellness, and advocacy efforts. Although the Recovery Model was officially introduced to the world in 2006 at the National Summit on Mental Health Recovery, the consumer, survivor, and ex-patient movement had developed long before then. Clifford Beers, in his groundbreaking autobiography, *A Mind That Found Itself*, spearheaded a revolution that gave voice to the silence of those struggling with mental illness in a system that completely demoralized and dehumanized their very existence. This same movement sparked a desire for self-directed care, which resulted in the development of the Clubhouse Model in the late 1940s and the use of peer support in the 1970s. More recently, Dr. Pat Deegan, an ex-patient and survivor herself, has, among others, led the movement to embrace voice and choice when describing personal journeys of recovery and to advocate for consumers' rights to have equal rights in directing systems of care.

A modern outgrowth of these pivotal figures and movements is the Recovery Model. This model (described in detail in Chapter 1) is founded on four pillars deemed necessary for recovery and includes 10 principles. Home, health, community, and purpose constitute the four pillars (or foundation) necessary for recovery. The principles of recovery include recovery that is person-driven, may take many pathways, addresses trauma, is holistic, includes peer support, is relational, is culturally influenced and guided, is hope-based, focuses on strengths and responsibility, and is based on respect.[45] The pillars of health and purpose and the principles of person-driven and holistic care can serve as a framework for understanding and developing interventions around the issues of prevention, wellness, and advocacy.[a]

---

[a]In concert with efforts to advocate, it must be noted that some service users do not embrace the idea of recovery because it implies that there is something from which someone needs to recover, and that there is an endpoint of wellness that will be reached. An alternative for framing future discussion includes the "journey of discovery."

The pillar of health represents the outgrowth of wellness efforts, as well as those related to prevention at all levels—primary, secondary, and tertiary. Purpose is a well-researched concept related to those who struggle with mental health challenges and is often affected by systemic marginalization and injustice.[46-50] The recovery principle of being person-driven is aligned with the notion of advocacy and its associated actions. Additionally, in this model, service users are tasked with crafting their own vision of health and development of wellness practices that will support that vision. Prevention of further conditions or complications associated with the mental illness also rests largely with the service user.

Recovery is holistic and therefore requires that all facets of the individual embedded in context and environment be addressed in the journey. Honoring the mind-body-spirit connection is evidence-based and sanctioned by practices such as integrative primary care and wrap-around services. Integrative primary care addresses the whole person, focuses on the importance of the therapeutic relationship, and encourages use of traditional and alternative methods of healing within the context of primary care.[51] Wrap-around services reflect the concept of "it takes a village." These services wrap around the individual to support that person in all ways to move toward greater health and wellness. This approach is strength-driven and family-oriented; it may include formal services such as case management or

psychiatry and informal supports such as friends providing social support or caregivers providing financial support. This model promotes inclusion and continuity of care and helps maintain the service user at the center of care.[52]

Margaret Swarbrick's Eight Dimensions of Wellness[53] was adopted by SAMHSA as a model for service providers and users to view the construct of wellness in crafting individual recovery. Swarbrick is an occupational therapist, and her work around wellness brought national attention to the power and scope of occupational therapy in mental health settings. The Eight Dimensions of Wellness include social, emotional, environmental, financial, intellectual, physical, spiritual, and occupational (Fig. 18.2).

The social dimension encompasses the sense of belonging that one has and the degree that one establishes and uses a support system. Occupational therapy practitioners can support this dimension by helping the individual do the following: (1) develop effective communication skills; (2) establish formal and informal supports such as face to face or virtual support groups and programs; and (3) identify ways in which they can give back to their mental health community, such as becoming a peer supporter. The emotional dimension speaks to one's ability to experience and regulate emotions in a satisfying way. Occupational therapy practitioners can support this dimension by enabling knowledge and skill development, including acquisition of coping skills and sensory strategies, such as grounding and

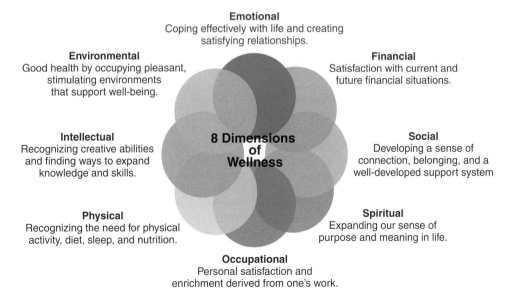

Fig. 18.2 The dimensions of wellness. (Adapted from Swarbrick M. A wellness approach. Available at: http://search.ebscohost.com.une.idm.oclc.org/login.aspx?direct=true&db=ccm&AN=106170829&site=ehost-live&scope=site.)

self-calming. The environmental dimension supports mental well-being by surrounding an individual with a physical environment that is safe and meets their cognitive, psychological, and sensory needs. Occupational therapy practitioners are well suited to assess the environment and alter it accordingly based on these needs. One service user may need to declutter the environment to lessen feelings associated with anxiety, whereas another may need visual cues to assist in sequencing through daily routines.

The next dimension, financial, reflects one's satisfaction with their current and prospective financial state. Occupational therapy practitioners may be able to support this dimension by engaging the client in supported employment efforts, helping them acquire the skills to manage their funds independently, and support acquisition of compensatory financial strategies.

The intellectual dimension refers to expanding one's creative abilities by actively seeking opportunities to acquire information and expand the base of knowledge. Occupational therapy practitioners readily use learning theories on a daily basis in the form of constructivism and social and behavioral learning, among others. These teaching and learning approaches enable service users to expand their knowledge and hence expand their capacity for self-advocacy.

The next dimension, physical, directly affects the state of one's mental health. Due to the holistic nature of occupational therapy, practitioners are trained to observe and intervene with physical concerns and recognize acutely the potential impact of overall health and well-being.

The spiritual dimension addresses age-old questions such as "why am I here? and "what is my purpose in life?" These are difficult questions and, historically, not those that occupational therapy practitioners have eagerly addressed. Spiritual occupations are, however, a part of our guiding practice document, the occupational therapy practice framework. Meaning and purpose often come not just from being but from doing, which is the cornerstone of occupational therapy intervention.

The final dimension as described by Swarbrick is the occupational dimension. In this context, occupation refers to one's work. Unemployment rates for those labeled with a mental illness have been reported as high as 80%.[54] Occupational therapy practitioners can support this dimension by working with and for supported employment programs, educating community businesses about this untapped pool of reliable employees, and advocating for continued and needed mental health supports for those who are working. These dimensions can be used to guide occupational therapy practitioners in developing intervention plans to support recovery by providing a framework to support wellness practices (Case Study 18.1).

CASE STUDY 18.1

Dave is 67 years old. He retired 6 months ago from a large company, where he was employed as an engineer for 40 years. Dave loved his job and often worked 60 to 70 hours a week. He is proud of the years of service he gave to his company. He has a Master's degree in electrical engineering.

Prior to his retirement, Dave experienced mixed feelings regarding this life change. Although not spoken, he was under the impression that the company wanted him to retire to hire new graduates to do the same job for less money. At the same time, he was feeling a bit weary and looked forward to doing things that he had not been able to do as a full-time employee.

During the first several weeks following his retirement, Dave simply rested. He believed he was entitled to sleep late and take frequent naps during the day. He thought to himself that once he had fully "rested up," he would be ready to undertake new projects.

Weeks turned into months. Dave's wife of 43 years, Marianne, believed at first that this was a passing phase. Marianne has taken care of the house for the duration of their marriage. She looked forward to doing more things with Dave on his retirement. However, Dave's constant sleeping began to put a strain on their marriage, and Marianne thought she had more responsibilities now than she had when Dave was working.

Dave has three children, Alex age 42, Brenda age 40, and Brian age 37. Dave also has six grandchildren, ranging in age from 2 to 15 years. Alex and Brenda both live out of state, and Dave has only seen his grandchildren three times over the past 6 years. Brian, the youngest, lives in the next town over, but their relationship has always been strained because Brian has a history of substance use and, according to Dave, lacks direction.

Over the past several weeks, Marianne has become increasingly more concerned and frustrated with the situation. Dave rarely gets out of bed. He has not bathed in over a week and his appetite has decreased considerably. Dave has made statements to the effect that he has nothing to live for.

Two days ago, Marianne told Dave that Brian was very ill and that Dave had to go see him. Instead, Marianne

CASE STUDY 18.1—cont'd

drove Dave to the local emergency room to have him admitted. Dave attempted to walk out but after he expressed a desire to commit suicide, the staff was mandated to commit him to the facility involuntarily. Although not convinced that anyone could help him, Dave has agreed to remain in the hospital because Marianne told him that he was not permitted to return home until the doctor released him.

Dave has never before experienced an episode like this. Although deeply distraught by the death of his mother when he was 48 years old, Dave threw himself even deeper into his work and seemed to recover without further incident.

Guided Thinking
- Discuss Dave's status with regard to the Eight Dimensions of Wellness.
- Select three dimensions, and discuss how occupational therapy could support Dave in his recovery by developing a plan targeting these areas of wellness:
  - While in the inpatient psychiatric unit
  - At home in the community

In addition to using concepts derived from the era of Moral Treatment, the Recovery Model, and/or the Eight Dimensions of Wellness to drive thinking about prevention, wellness, and advocacy interventions, occupational therapists need look no further than the professional document designed to guide the occupational therapy process, the *Occupational Therapy Practice Framework* (OTPF), now in its third edition. In this document, prevention is an approach and outcome of occupational therapy services. Approaches are "specific strategies selected to direct the process of evaluation and intervention planning, selection, and implementation on the basis of the client's desired outcomes, evaluation data, and evidence"; outcomes "are the end result of the occupational therapy process."[55] Occupational therapy's role in using prevention as an approach and/or an outcome is clearly outlined in the OTPF and reflects a strong professional emphasis on taking a proactive stance with all service users. Wellness is also an outcome; it occurs as a result of actions taken by an individual, community, or population to affect the state of their own health. Advocacy is an OTPF intervention directed at both the client (self-advocacy) and the occupational therapist (advocacy).[55] Advocacy involves developing skills related to voice and choice. Voice represents the skill to communicate needs and desires, and choice effectively is derived from an environment that is occupationally just.

OPPORTUNITIES FOR PREVENTION IN OCCUPATIONAL THERAPY

Although genetics certainly contribute to the manifestation of a mental illness, occupational therapists have the opportunity to effect change by assuming a proactive stance on the prevention of mental illness. Whether engaged in primary, secondary, or tertiary levels of prevention, occupational therapists are uniquely poised to contribute to national, state, and local dialogues regarding modifiable risk factors associated with the development or exacerbation of mental illness. These factors broadly include the stigma associated with mental illness, quality of attachments to primary caregivers, poverty, social disadvantage, food insecurity, coping with 21st century stressors, including exposure to extreme violence, and access to prevention-oriented services.[31,32] Primary- or population-level prevention efforts often come in the form of education. Stigma can prevent individuals from proactively seeking support where no mental illness exists. Meeting one's psychoemotional needs on a regular basis, whether through formal channels such as a psychologist or counselor or via informal channels such as journaling or chatting with supportive friends, is no different than meeting one's physical needs by working out at the gym on a weekly basis.

Occupational therapists possess the skills necessary to articulate the holistic nature of well-being that includes mental wellness. Prevention at the population level includes population-oriented research, antistigma campaigns, and early intervention with youth to discuss mental health and wellness as part of the culture. Quality attachments to primary caregivers are foundational for the development of current and future healthy relationships. Occupational therapists receive training on attachment theory and know firsthand the impact of avoidant, ambivalent, or disorganized attachments on the psychological, social, and emotional development of a child. Family structure, as well as the activity patterns surrounding primary caregivers, has drastically changed over the last century, leading to fewer children and fewer opportunities to role-model healthy parenting. This is a prime opportunity to join or initiate national campaigns to support nurturing parenting practices and encourage new parents to reach out for the support and skill building they need to raise healthy children psychologically, socially, and emotionally.

For those who are at greater risk of developing a mental illness due to factors such as poverty, social disadvantage, and food insecurity, occupational therapists can join forces with local communities to develop, support, and engage in health and wellness practices that are sustainable and promote self-reliance. Sustainable practices might take the form of community gardens or programming, such as pairing older adults as mentors for local youth, which serves to prevent isolation in the older adults and promote healthy development in the younger individuals. There are many 21st century stressors, not the least of which are exposure to extreme violence due to increased prevalence and repetitive exposure through various media outlets. According to the Centers for Disease Control and Prevention (CDC), nearly 62,000 people died as a result of violence in 2015. Of these, 65% were suicides and nearly 25% were homicides. Homicides typically included a firearm and often followed an interpersonal conflict.[56] Helping individuals develop a sense of meaning or purpose and addressing the many underlying factors and environmental forces that inhibit the development of healthy interpersonal relations is the cornerstone of occupations related to social interaction. Additionally, coping skills involving cognitive restructuring, sensory modulation, and habit training, to name a few, have been in the repertoire of occupational therapy intervention since its inception.

Finally, efforts to reach individuals to provide prevention-oriented initiatives can be a logistic challenge. Many of the neediest communities are remotely located as a result of being economically disadvantaged. Approximately 20% of Americans live in what is considered a rural area, defined by the US Census Bureau as areas that are sparsely populated, have low housing density, and are far from urban areas.[57] To reach these rural communities, telehealth is a promising way to link current prevention efforts with those who need it most. Telehealth dates back to the 1920s, when radios were used to transmit medical information to ships at sea. Occupational therapists have a history of creativity in developing approaches and interventions that meet the needs of those served. Using a virtual platform is merely an extension of that creativity. Never more has the profession needed to address these critical public health challenges that face the world today. Public health trickles down to personal well-being. Although individual treatment remains a relevant and critical piece of daily practice, it is apparent that to affect long-standing change that will result in global improvements in health and wellness, occupational therapy will need to continue to develop significant and sustainable prevention efforts at all levels of intervention.

OPPORTUNITIES FOR WELLNESS IN OCCUPATIONAL THERAPY

US citizens have increasingly become more proactive in the development of and participation in personal wellness practices.[58] Use of complementary and alternative medicines (CAMs) has seen a significant increase in the 1990s, and their use has remained consistent in the new millennium.[59] Complementary medicine and approaches are considered adjunctive to conventional medicine, whereas alternative medicine and approaches would be those used in place of conventional medicine. Integrative health care combines the best of both worlds, conventional and complementary medicine, into holistic care that is coordinated and person-centered.[60] According to the most recent National Health Statistics report, the top five complementary approaches to personal wellness include nonvitamin nonmineral dietary supplements, deep breathing, yoga, tai chi, qi gong, chiropractic manipulation, and meditation.[59] Occupational therapy is well suited to use many of these approaches to enhance occupational engagement and participation. Most recently, the American Occupational Therapy Association (AOTA) published a position paper, *Occupational Therapy and Complementary Health Approaches and Integrative Health*, which outlines the scope of practice regarding the use of complementary approaches and delineates how these approaches can be used as interventions in all applicable practice settings.[61] According to this document, these approaches can be used in the following ways: (1) as methods or tasks to prepare the individual for engagement in activities and occupations such as deep breathing; (2) as activities to promote skill building, such as yoga poses to enhance balance; and (3) as occupations if the person wishes to return to or develop occupations related to complementary practices, such as role participation as a student in a tai chi class. Evidence for use of these approaches has been growing and includes positive outcomes for the use of guided imagery to improve socialization in withdrawn youth,[62] aromatherapy to reduce agitation in older adults with dementia,[63] and tai chi to help prevent falls and improve motor skills.[64,65] It is beyond the scope of this chapter to review the evidence related to all complementary approaches fully; however, three of those used most often used—breathing, mindfulness, and yoga—will be reviewed here. Evidence related to emerging complementary methods, including Reiki, Emotional Freedom Technique (EFT), and drumming are also provided. See Table 18.2.

Mindfulness

A commonly used and well-researched complementary self-healing interventions is mindfulness. The Western

TABLE 18.2 Promising Complementary Approaches to Support Mental Health and Wellness

Complementary Approach	Definition	Evidence Bytes
Reiki	Reiki originates from Japan and means universal life force. It is a form of energy healing that typically involves channeling universal energy (biofield energy) through the practitioner's hands. Energy can also be remotely channeled by setting the intention on the person in need of the healing energy.	Reiki's effectiveness is inconclusive due to the paucity of robust, randomized controlled trials (RCTs). Favorable results. However, have been found with Reiki to decrease emotional exhaustion, depersonalization, and parasympathetic nervous system responses such as decreased cortisol levels, lower diastolic blood pressure, and salivary response related to improved immune functioning Biofield therapies including Reiki hold promise for decreasing signs and symptoms associated with anxiety and improving mood and general mental health and wellness.
Drumming	Therapeutic drumming is the intentional use of sounds and rhythms made with a variety of drumlike instruments to improve a variety of conditions related not only to mental health but to spiritual, socioemotional, and physical health as well.	Improved anxiety, depression, social resilience, and antiinflammatory response in mental health service users Individuals with high levels of self-reported anxiety and depression significantly benefited on six dimensions of Stellenbosch Mood Scale Drumming shown to support feelings of belongingness, acceptance, and safety among peers
Emotional freedom technique (EFT)	A method developed by Gary Craig in the mid-1990s designed to heal psychoemotional "wounds" by tapping on the body's meridians. First identified and used in the Chinese culture.	Meta-analysis reveals that EFT significantly improves symptoms associated with PTSD. EFT significantly decreased levels of anxiety in an RCT with high-ability adolescents.

EFT, Emotional freedom technique; *PTSD*, posttraumatic stress disorder.
Adapted from references 6 and 66 to 75.

understanding and practice of mindfulness originated in eastern Buddhist practices and refers to "the awareness that emerges through paying attention on purpose: in the present moment and non-judgmentally."[76] Mindfulness creates space to be present for what is happening in the moment. Given that effective therapeutic use of self relies heavily on interactive or moment to moment reasoning, we can directly link mindfulness to improved client-practitioner rapport, as well as the rapport that clients may be seeking with themselves. Remaining present or mindful, which encourages awareness and merging of somatic, psychological, and emotional experiences, can help mitigate depersonalization, which is a hallmark of many mental health diagnoses (e.g., borderline personality disorder, dissociative identity disorder, and trauma-related disorders such as posttraumatic stress disorder (PTSD).[77,78] Recent research

in mindfulness practices has been focused on dosing, frequency, and duration to inform mindfulness practices and programs. The gold standard to date has been the mindfulness-based stress reduction (MBSR) program. The evidence-based protocol for MBSR typically includes 2- to 3-hour sessions once a week for 8 weeks. The program consists of meditation, yoga, and psychoeducation.[79] However, current health care constraints, directly related to productivity standards and outcome thresholds, necessitate that mindfulness interventions have the most effect for the smallest investment of resources, including practitioner time and organizational funds. Several studies have yielded positive results by delivering mindfulness education, training, and practice either online or in smaller doses, which may prove as effective as face to face delivery and more conducive to the current health care climate.

TABLE 18.3   Studies Supporting Use of Mindfulness-Based Stress Reduction (MSBR) in Mental Health Care

Study	Comments
Janssen et al[82]	In this systematic review, 1790 articles were gathered in 2015. Of those, 24 met inclusion criteria and were evaluated for the purposes of this review. Findings indicated that MBSR may be useful for reducing exhaustion, stress, psychological distress, depression, and anxiety. MBSR may also yield improvements in one's ability to be mindful, quality of sleep, and sense of accomplishment.
Polusny et al[78]	Controlled trial in which participants were randomly assigned to the experimental group that received MBSR ($n = 58$) or a present-centered group ($n = 58$) in which participants focused on current life concerns for a total of eight weekly sessions. Results indicated that the MBSR group reported greater improvement on symptoms related to the PTSD than the control group at both discharge and 2-month follow-up.
Zainal et al[83]	In this meta-analysis, nine studies up through 2011 met inclusion criteria. Markers of mental health concern for this population included stress, depression, and anxiety. Effect size for MSBR for each of these respectively was 0.710, 0.575 and 0.733, which indicates that MBSR may prove effective in mitigating these concerns (stress, depression, anxiety) in other populations.
Goldin & Gross[84]	Using MRI to assess pre- and postintervention brain behavior changes, 14 participants diagnosed with social anxiety disorder demonstrated decreased anxiety and depression and improved self-esteem when using MBSR to combat negative self-beliefs and emotions.

PTSD, posttraumatic stress disorder.

Remote interventions delivered via telehealth also hold promise to reach those who are marginalized due to factors such as low socioeconomic status or living in rural areas devoid of access to regular health care.[79-81] See Table 18.3 for a synopsis of recent studies supporting the use of MBSR.

There is a myriad of resources related to mindfulness training and practices (see below, "Mindfulness-Based Stress Reduction Resources"), but they generally share the same principles that being present or mindful, not just with our minds but with our whole body, can reduce anxiety, depression, and symptoms related to trauma, as well as improve quality of life and functioning. [77,79,81] How does mindfulness work, and how can occupational therapists use this approach in the context of everyday interventions? Mindfulness simultaneously requires and enhances attention regulation, body awareness, emotional regulation, interoception or experience of self, and cognitive flexibility.[85,86] Mechanisms of action appear to be seated in the anterior cingulate cortex, insula, temporoparietal junction, frontolimbic network, and default mode network structures, which work in tandem to support self-regulation.[85] Mindfulness at its core is a spiritual practice, however, and that should not go unnoticed or unappreciated. Being in tune with the self and connecting in a meaningful and deeply spiritual way to the universe to discover one's truth and existential purpose is a personal experience and journey, which cannot be relegated to objective markers of competency. Some would argue that mindfulness is not a practice at all, but a natural state that becomes clouded by thoughts.[87] Mindfulness is an everyday, all-day practice that results in a way of being that alters every physical manifestation of self in the world. In fact, the stillness of being mindful would seemingly put it at odds with "doing," which serves as the symbolic core of the occupational therapy profession. One could argue, however, that the changes in the physical manifestations of self through mindfulness practices are reflected in what and how and why individuals do what they do—from socializing with friends and loved ones to habits and ways of being while driving to the choices made about engagement in practices of self-care. Although mindfulness is not, like therapeutic use of self, a tool to be picked up at will, it is a practice that clinicians and service users alike can strive to consistently engage in and improve daily.

Implications for use of mindfulness in occupational therapy include practice by the clinician to enhance therapeutic use of self, listening, and acceptance to enhance general outcomes for service users.[88-91] Additionally, practitioners can use this understanding of mindfulness to

TABLE 18.4 Encouraging Mindfulness

Action	Comments
Engage in diaphragmatic breathing; take several breaths where you expand your belly.	Intentionally notice your bodily sensations; the chair on which you are sitting, the rumble in your stomach, and the cold pen you are holding.
Intentionally notice the sights, sounds, and smells around you.	Take 5 to 10 minutes to do nothing and simply notice your surroundings.
Accept your thoughts without judgment or attempts to deny them.	Ask yourself whether you are truly listening if engaged in social interaction.

create client-centered interventions that support wellness and enable the service user to take greater control over thoughts and feeling states. which can and often lead to occupational challenges such as poor quality of social and work-related interactions and decreased ability to cope with daily stressors and disrupted habits, roles, and routines.[92] See Table 18.4.

Yoga

Another person-centered, evidence-based intervention used to support those with a variety of mental health challenges is yoga. Yoga is an ancient practice, probably dating back 5000 years or more. The word yoga means "union," union of one's consciousness with universal consciousness, as well as the union between the mind, body, and spirit. Pantanjali, a philosopher who is often cited as the "father of modern yoga," described a yoga practice consisting of eight paths[93]:

1. *Yama*—practice of morality, such as truthfulness, kindness, and selflessness
2. *Niyama*—practice of self-care, such as contentment and exercise
3. *Asana*—practice of yogic poses through which one connects their earthly energy with that of their higher or spiritual selves
4. *Pranayama*—practice of breathing that enables one to channel the life force
5. *Pratyahara*—practice of calming and becoming less responsive to outside stimuli
6. *Dharana*—practice of concentration
7. *Dhyana*—practice of meditation
8. *Samahdi*—practice of spiritual connection or achieving a state of "flow"

Yoga has routinely been used to combat mental health challenges, including depression, attentional issues, substance use disorder, trauma, and stressor-related disorders and anxiety.[94-97] Tools and equipment often associated with yoga include special clothing, mats, blocks and bolsters, and enough space to execute the poses adequately. Many poses, however, can be executed while sitting or standing, which provides additional flexibility for clients who have balance concerns or are experiencing anergia or, conversely, akathisia and for therapists who may be limited by their physical environment.

Somewhat new to the practice of yoga is trauma-sensitive yoga (TSY). TSY began at the Trauma Center at the Justice Resource Institute in Brookline, Massachusetts, in 2003 and was designed specifically for those who have experienced complex trauma and PTSD. Complex trauma (see Chapter 17 for a more in-depth review of trauma) may be present in survivors of war, sexual assault, and childhood abuse and neglect or in those who are at risk as a result of contextual and environmental circumstances.[98] TSY differs significantly from other forms of yoga; these differences revolve around creating a safe environment for the participants to enable exploration and control of their own bodies and associated psychological and emotional states. A hallmark of TSY is inviting participation versus providing directives to the next asana. Another distinct difference is that the facilitator remains in clear view of all participants and there is no laying on of hands; this creates a sense of safety in that participants are in full control of their participation throughout the session and are able to choose when and how they might participate. This choice is in stark contrast to the lack of control experienced by trauma survivors during the circumstances surrounding their trauma history.

Yoga and now TSY have been used with a variety of populations, with relative success. Although the choice may be engaging in traditional yoga practices or one that involves the newer TSY, yoga can serve as a lifelong practice to promote wellness. See Tables 18.5 and 18.6.

OPPORTUNITIES FOR ADVOCACY IN OCCUPATIONAL THERAPY

Shifting focus to prevention and wellness efforts leads to improved population health, decreased costs associated with health care, including lost wages, and a shift in mind set from being reactive to being proactive.[103] Shifting mind set is challenging and necessary for the profession to take a leadership role in moving all individuals, communities, and populations toward greater health and wellness. To that end, occupational therapy practitioners must cultivate their

TABLE 18.5	**Studies Supporting Use of Yoga in Mental Health Care**
Study	**Comments**
Pascoe et al[99]	This meta-analysis included 42 studies. Findings indicated that interventions that included yoga asanas or poses improved sympathetic nervous system regulation and improved aspects of the hypothalamic-pituitary-adrenal system, such as decreasing cortisol levels during rest and wakeful states and lowering heart rate.
Macy et al[100]	This study reviewed 13 previously conducted literature reviews, including one meta-analysis; the total included 185 studies. Results indicated that yoga is promising in terms of providing ancillary support in cases of depression, anxiety, and PTSD.
van der Kolk et al[101]	This controlled trial randomly assigned 64 women (60 completed the study) diagnosed with treatment-resistant PTSD to a trauma-sensitive yoga group or a group that provided supportive women's health education. At the conclusion of the study, 16 of the 31 participants assigned to the yoga group no longer met criteria for PTSD, as compared with 6 of the 29 participants in the education group. The effect sizes were similar to those found with comparable psychopharmacologic and psychotherapeutic approaches.
Vollbehr et al[102]	This meta-analysis included 18 studies. Most studies were heterogeneous and of lower quality, which indicated the need to use greater rigor when executing research to determine yoga's effectiveness with various populations and conditions. Results did indicate that yoga was more effective than psychoeducation for improving depression.

PTSD, posttraumatic stress disorder.

TABLE 18.6	**Yoga Versus Trauma-Sensitive Yoga**
Yoga	**Trauma-Sensitive Yoga (TSY)**
Focus may vary but is often on enhancing core strength and flexibility.	Focus is on reclamation of the body and inner experience
Instructor often provides physical touch to support engagement in the asanas.	Few or no physical assistance provided, given the potential triggering effect of touch.
Environment often has colored lighting and may have symbolic wall decorations such as mandalas or artwork.	Environment is generally plain with clear but warm lighting. Mirrors should be covered if present. Participants are invited to occupy a space of their choosing, and the exit is in line of sight and easily accessed. The instructor remains in the line of sight at all times.
Verbal directives are provided to enter into the next asana.	Participants are verbally invited to engage (or not) in each of the poses. For example, "You may want to lay down on your back for our final resting pose or you may want to simply remain where you are now in a sitting position."
The type of yoga may vary, from restorative yoga with its focus on centering and relaxation to "hot" yoga, which is generally rigorous in nature.	TSY is generally less rigorous, with emphasis on posing that evoke a sense of safety such as the child's pose or ones that evoke a sense of strength such as the warrior pose.

Adapted from Emerson D, Sharma R, Chaudhry S, Turner J. (2009). Trauma-sensitive yoga: principles, practice, and research. *Int J Yoga Therapy.* 2009;19(1):123-128.

ability to advocate for their clients, for their profession, and for the public at large. Advocacy on an individual level may take many forms. Practitioners may advocate for expanded mental health supports for peers, such as additional programming or funding. Using a recovery and trauma-informed approach that includes person-centered language is, on a daily basis, perhaps the most meaningful advocacy of all. Practitioners may also support skill development so that peers engage in self-advocacy to enable them to seek needed services or platforms from which they can teach and empower. On a community level, advocacy may take the form of attending local events such as National Alliance on Mental Illness (NAMI) walks, which are held around the country and enable all stakeholders to join with one voice to eradicate stigma and support mental health prevention and wellness. Opportunities abound to speak to local agencies, programs, and entities such as local schools about the

importance of holistic self-care, which includes a rigorous mental wellness regimen. Local universities that have occupational therapy programs are rich with resources to support community advocacy, and forging these partnerships is mutually beneficial. At the population level, advocacy efforts often include becoming politically aware and active with groups that share similar views on the importance of mental wellness and getting those who have been diagnosed the services and benefits that they need to engage in daily occupations meaningfully. Voting to support mental wellness initiatives and those labeled with a mental illness is a common advocacy effort, which may or may not be in concert with personal party affiliations. National organizations, including AOTA, NAMI, and Mental Health America (MHA) are a few of the national organizations with opportunities related to advocacy (see Table 18.7 for additional information regarding these and other organizations).

TABLE 18.7 National Mental Health Advocacy Organizations

Organization	Mission	Advocacy Efforts Useful for Occupational Therapy Practice
American Occupational Therapy Association (AOTA)	This organization seeks to advance the occupational therapy profession and serve the public interest by setting standards.	Membership in AOTA affords the practitioner access to a variety of mental health occupational therapy–related resources, including practice guidelines and evidence-based resources. It also affords the practitioner a voice when voting for leadership positions and positions of the association at large.
BringChange2Mind	BringChange2Mind is a nonprofit organization dedicated to increasing awareness about mental illness and demystify those who live with these challenges.	BringChange2Mind offers opportunities for involvement through advocacy and provides information for peers and professionals as how best to communicate in an empathetic, nonthreatening manner using the "Talk Tool."
Healing Voices	Healing Voices is a social change video that has sparked dialogue around the globe and goes far beyond the screen.	The video can be used with peers and staff to spark dialogue about how society views mental illness and the endless possibilities for co-creating new and innovative views.
Mental Health America (MHA)	With affiliates around the nation, MHA was begun by an ex-patient, Clifford Beers, and is the oldest and most well-established nonprofit organization to promote awareness of mental illness.	MHA offers a wide array of online services (e.g., screenings for major mental illnesses such as depression and anxiety). Also, the organization offers up to date statistics, legislative updates, and printable pamphlets and posters. Many local affiliates exist and may offer additional brick and mortar programs for members of the community.

Continued

TABLE 18.7 National Mental Health Advocacy Organizations—cont'd

Organization	Mission	Advocacy Efforts Useful for Occupational Therapy Practice
Substance Abuse and Mental Health Services Administration (SAMHSA)	SAMHSA is a federally funded organization that seeks to improve the mental health of all Americans through awareness and education.	SAMHSA is a repository of evidence-based programs and protocols, up to date statistics, and illness-related information and provides this information in a variety of formats and targets a number of audiences, including peers, professionals, and care providers.

CONCLUSION

The more globally connected and technologically savvy the world becomes, the less we can ignore the impact of mental wellness and, conversely, illness on overall individual, community, and population health. No one person, profession, or policy can prevent all illnesses, injuries, and disabilities nor would that be the goal; striving for the eradication of such conditions can be compared to the practice of eugenics. However, striving for greater health and wellness, regardless of illness, injury, and/or disability, is a goal that occupational therapy practitioners can rally around and support. Mental health, as inextricably linked to overall health and well-being, is no longer a notion but rather an accepted and evidence-based fact. Similarly, a holistic approach to health care is no longer an option but rather a necessity, a necessity that requires occupational therapy professionals to embed their practice with principles of and efforts toward prevention, wellness, and advocacy.

WELLNESS RESOURCES

Holistic OT: An online community of occupational therapy practitioners who are dedicated to promoting health and well for themselves and persons served. Available at: http://holisticot.org.

National Wellness Institute: Organization dedicated to providing health and wellness resources for professionals who work with a variety of client populations. Available at: https://www.nationalwellness.org.

Substance Abuse and Mental Health Services Administration (SAMHSA) Wellness Initiative: National effort to raise awareness of the health disparities that exist early death. Available at: https://www.samhsa.gov/wellness-initiative.

SAMHSA Program to Achieve Wellness (PAW): National program that supports organizational and service user efforts to promote and implement best practices related to wellness for those living with mental illness and substance use. Available at: https://www.samhsa.gov/wellness-initiative/program-achieve-wellness.

Wellness Recovery Action Plan (WRAP): Provides resources for providers and service users regarding use of WRAP to promote mental health and wellness. Available at: http://mentalhealthrecovery.com/wrap-is.

ULifeline: Online community dedicated to supporting the mental health and wellness of college students. Available at: http://www.ulifeline.org/stay_well.

US Department of Veterans Affairs Mental Health: Federal department that supports and provides care for US citizens who have served the country in a military capacity. Available at: https://www.mentalhealth.va.gov.

MINDFULNESS-BASED STRESS REDUCTION RESOURCES

Guided Mindfulness Meditation Practices with Jon Kabat-Zinn: Website provides links to purchase of guided meditations created by the founder of Mindfulness-Based Stress Reduction (MSBR), Jon Kabat-Zinn. Available at: https://palousemindfulness.com.

HolisticOT.com: Online community of occupational therapy practitioners dedicated to the promotion and inclusion of complimentary therapies in practice.

PESI: Website that provides cost-effective continuing education opportunities specific to mental and behavioral health, including MBSR. Available at: https://www.pesi.com.

Mindfulness Attention Awareness Scale: Available at: https://ppc.sas.upenn.edu/resources/ questionnaires-researchers/mindful-attention-awareness-scale-15-item self-report measure of mindfulness (no charge).

National Center for Complementary and Integrative Health: This is part of the larger National Institute of Health. The website provides links to up to date information and research related to MBSR. Available at: https://nccih.nih.gov.

Occupational Therapy Complementary Health Approaches and Integrative Health: AOTA's position paper on the use of complementary therapies in the occupational therapy process. Available at: https://www.aota.org/~/media/

Corporate/Files/Secure/AboutAOTA/ OfficialDocs/AJOT/ Complementary-Health-Approaches-Integrative-Health.pdf.
University of Massachusetts, History of MSBR: Website provides a history of the development of MSBR by Jon Kabat-Zinn while serving as the Founding Executive Director of the Center for Mindfulness at the University of Massachusetts. Available at: https://www.umassmed .edu/cfm/

University of Massachusetts, Mindfulness-Based Programs: Website provides links to several MBSR programs offered by the University of Massachusetts, the originating institution of MBSR.

REFERENCES

1. World Health Organization. Outline for a Study Group on World Health and the Survival of the Human Race. Geneva: World Health Organization; 1954.

2. Rissmiller DJ, Rissmiller JH. Evolution of the antipsychiatry movement into mental health consumerism. 2006. Available at: http://search.ebscohost.com.une.idm.oclc.org/login. aspx?direct=true&db=ccm&AN=106350328&site=ehost-live&scope=site.

3. Brandon D. A friend to alleged lunatics John Perceval. 2007. Available at: http://search.ebscohost.com.une.idm.oclc.org/ login.aspx?direct=true&db=ccm&AN=106000035&site= ehost-live&scope=site.

4. Substance Abuse and Mental Health Services Administration. National Consensus Statement on Mental Health Recovery. Rockville, MD: Center of Mental Health Services, Substance Abuse and Mental Health Services Administration; 2006.

5. Reilly M. Occupational therapy can be one of the greatest ideas of 20th century medicine. 1961 Eleanor Clarke Slagle Lecture. *Am J Occup Ther.* 1962;16:1-9.

6. World Health Organization. Constitution of the World Health Organization. 1948. Available at: https://www.loc .gov/law/help/us-treaties/bevans/m-ust000004-0119.pdf.

7. World Health Organization. Global strategy for health for all by the year 2000. 1981. Available at: http://iris.wpro.who.int/ bitstream/handle/10665.1/6967/WPR_RC032_Global Strategy_1981_en.pdf

8. World Health Organization. Ottawa Charter for Health Promotion: First International Conference on Health Promotion Ottawa 21 November 1986. 1986. Available at: https://www.healthpromotion.org.au/images/ottawa_ charter_hp.pdf.

9. Dhar N, Chaturvedi SK, Nandan D. Spiritual health, the fourth dimension: a public health perspective. *WHO South-East Asia J Public Health.* 2013;2(1):3-5.

10. Svalastog AL, Donev D, Jahren Kristoffersen N, Gajović S. Concepts and definitions of health and health-related values in the knowledge landscapes of the digital society. *Croat Med J.* 2017;58(6):431-435.

11. Wilcock A. Reflections on doing, being and becoming. 1998. Available at: http://search.ebscohost.com.une.idm.oclc.org/ login.aspx?direct=true&db=amed&AN=9172110&site= ehost-live&scope=site.

12. Leavell H, Clark E. *Textbook of Preventive Medicine.* New York: McGraw-Hill; 1953.

13. CDC/NCHS, National Vital Statistics System. Mortality. Atlanta: US Department of Health and Human Services; 2017.

14. Institute of Medicine (US) Committee on Prevention of Mental Disorders; Mrazek PJ, Haggerty RJ, editors. *Reducing Risks for Mental Disorders: Frontiers for Preventive Intervention Research.* Washington, DC: National Academies Press; 1994. Available from: https://www.ncbi.nlm.nih.gov/books/ NBK236319/ doi: 10.17226/2139

15. Saks E. Stories of hope and recovery. 2013. Available at: https://www.youtube.com/ watch?v= U_4O3U5CWis.

16. World Health Organization. Prevention of mental disorders: effective interventions and policy options. 2004. Available at: http://www.who.int/mental_health/evidence/en/prevention_ of_mental_disorders_sr.pdf.

17. Substance Abuse Mental Health Services Administration. Wellness initiative. 2018. Available at: https://www.samhsa .gov/wellness-initiative.

18. Merriam-Webster. Definition of advocacy. 2018. Available at: https://www.merriam-webster.com/dictionary/advocacy.

19. World Health Organization. *Advocacy for Mental Health.* Geneva: World Health Organization; 2003.

20. Mental Health America. The state of mental health in america. 2018. Available at: https://www.mentalhealthamer-ica.net/sites/default/files/2018%20The%20State%20of %20MH%20in%20America%20-%20FINAL.pdf.

21. Kamal R, Cox C, Rousseau D. Costs and outcomes of mental health and substance use disorders in the US. *JAMA.* 2017;318(5):415.

22. Vivolo-Kantor AM, Seth P, Gladden RM, et al. Vital signs: Trends in emergency department visits for suspected opioid overdoses—United States, July 2016-September 2017. *Morb Mortal Wkly Rep.* 2018;67(9):279-285.

23. National Alliance on Mental Illness. New bill puts mental health coverage at risk. 2017. Available at: https://www.nami .org/About-NAMI/NAMI-News/New-Bill-Puts-Mental-Health-Coverage-At-Risk.

24. National Council for Behavioral Health. Psychiatric shortage: causes and solutions. 2017. Available at: https:// www.thenationalcouncil.org/wp-content/uploads/2017/03/ Psychiatric-Shortage_National-Council-.pdf.

25. National Institute of Mental Health. Any mental illness (AMI) among adults. Available at: http://www.nimh.nih.gov/health/ statistics/prevalence/any-mental-illness-ami-among-adults .shtml.

26. US Census Bureau. US and World Population Clock. Available at: https://www.census.gov/popclock.

27. Itkowitz C. Unwell and unashamed. 2016. Available at: https://www. washingtonpost.com/sf/lo-cal/2016/06/01/unwell-and-unashamed/?utm_ term=.8e01f714f1fc.

28. US Department of Health and Human Services. The Secretary's Advisory Committee on National Health Promotion and Disease Prevention Objectives for 2020. Phase I report: recommendations for the framework and format of Healthy People 2020. Section IV: Advisory Committee findings and recommendations. Available at: http://www.healthypeople.gov/sites/default/files/PhaseI_0.pdf.

29. National Association of State Mental Health Program Directors Council. *Morbidity and Mortality in People with Serious Mental Illness.* Alexandria, VA: National Association of State Mental Health Program Directors Council; 2006.

30. Goldman ML, Spaeth-Rublee B, Pincus HA. The case for severe mental illness as a disparities category. *Psychiatr Serv.* 2018;69(6):726-728.

31. Walker E, McGee R, Druss B. Mortality in mental disorders and global disease burden implications: a systematic review and meta-analysis. *JAMA Psychiatry.* 2015;72(4):334-341.

32. Safran MA, Mays RA, Huang LN, et al. Mental health disparities. *Am J Publ Health.* 2009;99(11):1962-1966.

33. Kisely S, Crowe E, Lawrence D. Cancer-related mortality in people with mental illness. *JAMA Psychiatry.* 2013;70(2):209-217.

34. National Institute of Mental Health. Suicide. Available at: https://www.nimh.nih.gov/health/ statistics/suicide.shtml.

35. Morden NE, Mistler LA, Weeks WB, Bartels SJ. Health care for patients with serious mental illness: family medicine's role. *J Am Board Fam Med.* 2009;22(2):187-195.

36. Daumit GL, Goff DC, Meyer JM, et al. A comparison of ten-year cardiac risk estimates in schizophrenia patients from the CATIE study and matched controls. Available at: http://search.ebscohost.com.une.idm.oclc.org/login.aspx?direct=true&db=cmedm&AN=16198088&site=ehost-live&scope=site.

37. Substance Abuse and Mental Health Services Administration. Behavioral health trends in the United States: results from the 2014 National Survey on Drug Use and Health. 2015. Available at: https://www.samhsa.gov/data/sites/default/files/NSDUH-FRR1-2014/NSDUH-FRR1-2014.pdf.

38. National Alliance on Mental Illness. Dual diagnosis. 2018 Available at: https://www.nami.org/Learn-More/Mental-Health-Conditions/Related-Conditions/Dual-Diagnosis.

39. Davidson L. Habits and other anchors of everyday life that people with psychiatric disabilities may not take for granted. Available at: http://search.ebscohost.com.une.idm.oclc. org/login.aspx?direct=true&db=ccm&AN=105889313&site=ehost-live&scope=site.

40. Colton CW, Manderscheid RW. Congruencies in increased mortality rates, years of potential life lost, and causes of death among public mental health clients in eight states. Available at: http://search.ebscohost.com.une.idm.oclc.org/login.aspx?direct-true&db-cmedm&AN-16539783&site-ehost-live&scope-site.

41. DE Hert M, Correll CU, Bobes J, et al. Physical illness in patients with severe mental disorders. I. Prevalence, impact of medications and disparities in health care. *World Psychiatry.* 2011;10(1):52-77.

42. Suryavanshi MS, Yang Y. Clinical and economic burden of mental disorders among children with chronic physical conditions, United States, 2008-2013. *Prev Chronic Dis.* 2016;13:E71.

43. Lawrence D, Kisely S. Inequalities in health care provision for people with severe mental illness. *J Psychopharmacol.* 2010;24(suppl 4):61-68.

44. Scott D, Happell B. The high prevalence of poor physical health and unhealthy lifestyle behaviours in individuals with severe mental illness. *Issues Ment Health Nurs.* 2011;32(9):589-597.

45. Substance Abuse and Mental Health Services Administration. SAMHSA's working definition of recovery: 10 guiding principles of recovery. publication id: PEP12-RECDEF. 2012. Available at: https://store.samhsa.gov/product/SAMHSA-s-Working-Definition-of-Recovery/PEP12-RECDEF.

46. Hamer HP, Kidd J, Clarke S, Butler R, Lampshire D. Citizens un-interrupted: practices of inclusion by mental health service users. *J Occup Sci.* 2017;24(1):76-87.

47. Cleary M, Horsfall J, Escott P. Marginalization and associated concepts and processes in relation to mental health/illness. *Issues Ment Health Nurs.* 2014;35(3):224-226.

48. Ehrlich-Ben Or S, Hasson-Ohayon I, Feingold D, Vahab K, Amiaz R, Weiser M, et al. Meaning in life, insight and self-stigma among people with severe mental illness. Compr Psychiatry. 2013;54(2):195-200.

49. Sutton DJ, Hocking CS, Smythe LA. A phenomenological study of occupational engagement in recovery from mental illness. *Can J Occup Ther.* 2012;79(3):142-150.

50. Walsh J. Spiritual interventions with consumers in recovery from mental illness. *J Spiritual Ment Health.* 2012;14(4), 229-241.

51. Fortney L, Rakel D, Rindfleisch JA, Mallory J. Introduction to integrative primary care: the health-oriented clinic. *Prim Care.* 2010;37(1):1-12.

52. Winters NC, Metz WP. The wraparound approach in systems of care. *Psychiatr Clin North Am.* 2009;32(1):135-151.

53. Swarbrick M. A wellness approach. 2006. Available at: Mindfulness-Based Stress Reduction posttraumatic stress disorder American Occupational Therapy Association National Alliance on Mental Illness (.

54. National Alliance on Mental Illness. Road to recovery: employment and mental illness. 2014. Available at: http://www.nami.org/work.

55. American Occupational Therapy Association. Occupational therapy practice framework: domain and process (3rd edition). *Am J Occup Ther.* 2014;68(suppl 1):S1-S48.

56. Jack S, Petrosky E, Lyons B, Blair JM, Ertl AM, Sheats KJ, et al. Surveillance for violent deaths—national violent death reporting system, 27 states, 2015. *MMWR Surveill Summ.* 2018;67(suppl 11):1-32. doi:10.15585/mmwr.ss6711a1.

57. Ratcliffe M, Burd C, Holder K, Fields A. Defining Rural at the U.S. Census Bureau. Washington, DC: U.S. Census Bureau; 2016.

58. Zhang Y, Peck K, Spalding M, Jones BG, Cook RL. Discrepancy between patients' use of and health providers' familiarity with CAM. *Patient Educ Couns.* 2012;89(3):399-404.

59. Clarke T, Black L, Stussman B, Barnes P, Nahin R. *Trends in the Use of Complementary Health Approaches Among Adults: United States, 2002-2012.* Hyattsville, MD: National Center for Health Statistics; 2015.

60. National Center for Complimentary and Integrative Health Care. Complementary, alternative, or integrative health: what's in a name? 2018. Available at: https://nccih.nih.gov/health/integrative-health.

61. American Occupational Therapy Association. Occupational therapy and complementary health approaches and integrative health. *Am J Occup Ther.* 2017;71(suppl 2):7112410020.

62. Arbesman M, Bazyk S, Nochajski SM. Systematic review of occupational therapy and mental health promotion, prevention, and intervention for children and youth. *Am J Occup Ther.* 2013;67:e120-e130.

63. Padilla R. Effectiveness of environment-based interventions for people with Alzheimer's disease and related dementias. *Am J Occup Ther.* 2011;65:514-522.

64. Chase CA, Mann K, Wasek S, Arbesman M. Systematic review of the effect of home modification and fall prevention programs on falls and the performance of community-dwelling older adults. *Am J Occup Ther.* 2012;66:284-291.

65. Foster ER, Bedekar M, Tickle-Degnen L. Systematic review of the effectiveness of occupational therapy–related interventions for people with Parkinson's disease. *Am J Occup Ther.* 2014;68:39-49.

66. Stein D. *Essential Reiki: A Complete Guide to an Ancient Healing Art.* New York: Crossing Press; 1995.

67. Díaz-Rodríguez L, Arroyo-Morales M, Cantarero-Villanueva I, Férnandez-Lao C, Polley M, Fernández-de-las-Peñas C. The application of Reiki in nurses diagnosed with burnout syndrome has beneficial effects on concentration of salivary IgA and blood pressure. *Rev Lat Am Enfermagem.* 2011;19(5):1132-1138.

68. Rosada R, Rubik B, Mainguy B, Plummer J, Mehl-Madrona L. Reiki reduces burnout among community mental health clinicians. *J Altern Complement Med.* 2015;21(8):489-495.

69. Mangione L, Swengros D, Anderson JG. Mental health wellness and biofield therapies: an integrative review. *Issues Ment Health Nurs.* 2017;38(11):930-944.

70. Wood L, Ivery P, Donovan R, Lambin E. To the beat of a different drum: improving the social and mental wellbeing of at-risk young people through drumming . . . discovering relationships using music—beliefs, emotions, attitudes, & thoughts. J Public Ment Health. 2013;12(2):70-79.

71. Fancourt D, Perkins R, Ascenso S, Carvalho LA, Steptoe A, Williamon A. Effects of group drumming interventions on anxiety, depression, social resilience and inflammatory immune response among mental health service users. *PLoS One.* 2016;11(3):e0151136.

72. Plastow NA, Joubert L, Chotoo Y, Nowers A, Greeff M, Strydom T, et al. The immediate effect of African drumming on the mental well-being of adults with mood disorders: an uncontrolled pretest-posttest pilot study. *Am J Occup Ther.* 2018;72(5):1-6.

73. Perkins R, Ascenso S, Atkins L, Fancourt D, Williamon A. Making music for mental health: How group drumming mediates recovery. *Psychol Well-Being.* 2016;6(1):11.

74. Church D, Yount G, Rachlin K, Fox L, Nelms J. Epigenetic effects of PTSD remediation in veterans using clinical emotional freedom techniques: a randomized controlled pilot study. *Am J Health Promot.* 2018;32(1):112-122.

75. Gaesser AH, Karan OC. A randomized controlled comparison of Emotional Freedom Technique and cognitive-behavioral therapy to reduce adolescent anxiety: a pilot study. *J Altern Complement Med.* 2017;23(2):102-108.

76. Kabat-Zinn J. Mindfulness-based interventions in context: past, present, and future. *Clin Psychol: Sci Pract.* 2003;10(2):144-156.

77. Gilmartin H, Goyal A, Hamati MC, et al. Brief mindfulness practices for health care providers—a systematic literature review. *Am J Med.* 2017;130(10):1219.e1-1219.e17.

78. Polusny MA, Erbes CR, Thuras P, Moran A, Lamberty GJ, Collins RC, et al. Mindfulness-based stress reduction for posttraumatic stress disorder among veterans a randomized clinical trial. *JAMA.* 2015;314(5):456-465.

79. Heeter C, Lehto RH, Allbritton M, Day T, Wiseman M. Effects of a technology-assisted meditation program on health care providers' interoceptive awareness, compassion fatigue, and burnout. *J Hosp Palliat Nurs.* 2017;19(4):314-322.

80. Horner JK, Piercy BS, Eure L, Woodard EK. A pilot study to evaluate mindfulness as a strategy to improve inpatient nurse and patient experiences. *Appl Nurs Res.* 2014;27(3):198-201.

81. Sevilla-Llewellyn-Jones J, Santesteban-Echarri O, Pryor I, McGorry P, Alvarez-Jimenez M. Web-based mindfulness interventions for mental health treatment: systematic review and meta-analysis. *J Med Internet Res.* 2018;20(9):60.

82. Janssen M, Heerkens Y, Kuijer W, van der Heijden B, Engels J. Effects of mindfulness based stress reduction on employees' mental health: a systematic review. *PLoS ONE.* 2018;13(1):e0191332.

83. Zainal NZ, Booth S, Huppert FA. The efficacy of mindfulness-based stress reduction on mental health of breast cancer patients: a meta-analysis. *Psychooncology.* 2013;22(7):1457-1465.

84. Goldin PR, Gross JJ. Effects of mindfulness-based stress reduction (MBSR) on emotion regulation in social anxiety disorder. *Emotion.* 2010;10(1):83-91.

85. Hölzel BK, Lazar SW, Gard T, Schuman-Olivier Z, Vago DR, Ott U. How does mindfulness meditation work? Proposing mechanisms of action from a conceptual and neural perspective. *Perspect Psychol Sci.* 2011;6(6):537-559.

86. Sagui-Henson SJ, Blevins CL, Levens SM. Examining the psychological and emotional mechanisms of mindfulness that reduce stress to enhance healthy behaviours. *Stress Health.* 2018;34(3):379-390.

87. Kelley TM, Lambert EG, Pransky J. Inside-out or outside-in: understanding spiritual principles versus depending on techniques to realize improved mindfulness/mental health. *J Spiritual Ment Health.* 2015;17(3):153-171.

88. Howgego IM, Yellowlees P, Owen C, Meldrum L, Dark F. The therapeutic alliance: the key to effective patient outcome? A descriptive review of the evidence in community mental health case management. Available at: http://search.ebscohost.com.une.idm.oclc.org/login.aspx?direct=true&db=ccm&AN=106887.491&site=ehost-live&scope=site.

89. McCabe R, Priebe S. The therapeutic relationship in the treatment of severe mental illness: a review of methods and findings. Available at: http://search.ebscohost.com.une.idm.oclc.org/ login.aspx?direct=true&db=ccm&AN=106575812&site=ehost-live&scope=site.

90. Zugai JS, Stein-Parbury J, Roche M. Therapeutic alliance in mental health nursing: an evolutionary concept analysis. *Issues Ment Health Nurs.* 2015;36(4):249-257.

91. Mander J, Neubauer AB, Schlarb A, et al. The therapeutic alliance in different mental disorders: a comparison of patients with depression, somatoform, and eating disorders. *Psychol Psychother.* 2017;90(4):649-667.

92. Read H, Roush S, Downing D. Early intervention in mental health for adolescents and young adults: a systematic review. *Am J Occup Ther.* 2018;72(5):7205190040p1-7205190040p8.

93. Taylor M. Yoga therapeutics: An ancient practice in a twenty-first century setting. In C. Davis (ed.). *Integrative Therapies in Rehabilitation: Evidence for Efficacy in Therapy, Prevention, and Wellness.* 4th ed. Thorofare, NJ: Slack; 2017:181-202.

94. Khanna S, Greeson JM. A narrative review of yoga and mindfulness as complementary therapies for addiction. *Complement Ther Med.* 2013;21(2):244-252.

95. Louie L. The effectiveness of yoga for depression: a critical literature review. *Issues Ment Health Nurs.* 2014;35(4):265-276.

96. Chimiklis AL, Dahl V, Spears AP, Goss K, Fogarty K, Chacko A. Yoga, mindfulness, and meditation interventions for youth with ADHD: systematic review and meta-analysis. *J Child Fam Stud.* 2018;27(10):3155-3168.

97. Wynn GH. Complementary and alternative medicine approaches in the treatment of PTSD. *Curr Psychiatry Rep.* 2015;17(8):600.

98. Emerson D, Sharma R, Chaudhry S, Turner J. Trauma-sensitive yoga: principles, practice, and research. *Int J Yoga Therapy.* 2009;19(1):123-128.

99. Pascoe MC, Thompson DR, Ski CF. Yoga, mindfulness-based stress reduction and stress-related physiological measures: a meta-analysis. *Psychoneuroendocrinology.* 2017;86:152-168.

100. Macy RJ, Jones E, Graham LM, Roach L. Yoga for trauma and related mental health problems: a meta-review with clinical and service recommendations. *Trauma Violence Abuse.* 2018;19(1):35-57.

101. van der Kolk BA, Stone L, West J, et al. Yoga as an adjunctive treatment for posttraumatic stress disorder: a randomized controlled trial. *Journal of Clinical Psychiatry.* 2014;75(6):e559-e565. doi:10.4088/JCP.13m08561.

102. Vollbehr NK, Bartels-Velthuis AA, Nauta MH, et al. Hatha yoga for acute, chronic and/or treatment-resistant mood and anxiety disorders: A systematic review and meta-analysis. *PLoS ONE.* 2018;13(10):0204925.

103. Yong P, Saunders R, Olsen L. (Eds.). The health care imperative: lowering costs and improving outcomes: workshop series summary. 2002. Available at: https://www.ncbi.nlm.nih.gov/books/NBK53920/pdf/Bookshelf_NBK53920.pdf.

Page numbers followed by *f* indicate figures, *t* indicate tables, and *b* indicate boxes.